A Companion to Specialist Surgical Practice
Third Edition

Series Editors
O. James Garden
Simon Paterson-Brown

Breast Surgery
Third Edition

Edited by

J. Michael Dixon
Honorary Senior Lecturer
Clinical and Surgical Sciences (Surgery)
University of Edinburgh
and
Consultant Surgeon
Edinburgh Breast Unit
Western General Hospital

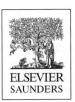

ELSEVIER
SAUNDERS

ELSEVIER
SAUNDERS

An imprint of Elsevier Limited

First edition 1997
Second edition 2001
Third edition 2006
Reprinted 2006, 2007

The right of J.M. Dixon to be identified as editor of this work has been asserted by him in accordance with the Copyright, Designs and Patents Act 1988.

EAN 9780702027383

ISBN 0 7020 2738 3

British Library Cataloguing in Publication Data
A catalogue record for this book is available from the British Library

Library of Congress Cataloging in Publication Data
A catalog record for this book is available from the Library of Congress

Notice
Medical knowledge is constantly changing. Standard safety precautions must be followed, but as new research and clinical experience broaden our knowledge, changes in treatment and drug therapy may become necessary or appropriate. Readers are advised to check the most current product information provided by the manufacturer of each drug to be administered to verify the recommended dose, the method and duration of administration, and contraindications. It is the responsibility of the practitioner, relying on experience and knowledge of the patient, to determine dosages and the best treatment for each individual patient. Neither the Publisher nor the editor assumes any liability for any injury and/or damage to persons or property arising from this publication.
The Publisher

Printed in The Netherlands
Last digit is the print number: 9 8 7 6 5 4 3

Commissioning Editor: Laurence Hunter
Project Development Manager: Sheila Black
Editorial Assistants: Kathryn Mason, Liz Brown
Project Manager: Cheryl Brant
Design Manager: Jayne Jones
Illustration Manager: Mick Ruddy
Illustrator: Martin Woodward
Marketing Managers: Gaynor Jones (UK), Ethel Cathers (USA)

Contents

Contents

Colour plate section follows p. 116

Contributors

Andrew D. Baildam BSc MB ChB MD FRCS
Consultant Oncoplastic Breast Surgeon
Withington Hospital;
Honorary Senior Lecturer in Surgical Oncology
University of Manchester
Manchester, UK

Nicola L.P. Barnes MB ChB MRCS
Surgical Research Fellow
Academic Department of Surgery
University of Manchester
Manchester, UK

Tom Bates MB BS FRCS
Consultant Surgeon
Breast Unit
William Harvey Hospital
Ashford, UK

Melissa A. Bochner MB BS MS FRACS
Consultant Surgeon
Breast, Endocrine and Surgical Oncology Unit
Royal Adelaide Hospital
Adelaide, SA, Australia

Nigel J. Bundred MD FRCS
Professor of Surgical Oncology
Education and Research Centre
University of Manchester;
Consultant Surgeon
South Manchester University Hospital
Manchester, UK

Susan Chua MB BS FRACP
Senior Clinical Research Fellow
Royal Marsden Hospital
London, UK

Krishna Clough MD
Chief of Surgery
Paris Breast Center
Paris, France

Tim Davidson ChM MRCP FRCS
Consultant General and Breast Surgeon
Royal Free Hospital
London, UK

J. Michael Dixon BSc MB ChB MD FRCS FRCS(Ed) FRCP
Honorary Senior Lecturer
Clinical and Surgical Sciences (Surgery)
University of Edinburgh;
Consultant Surgeon
Edinburgh Breast Unit
Western General Hospital
Edinburgh, UK

William C. Dooley MD
G. Rainey Williams Professor of Surgical Oncology and Chair
University of Oklahoma Breast Institute;
Director, Division of Surgical Oncology
University of Oklahoma Health Sciences Center
Oklahoma City, OK, USA

Ian O. Ellis BM BS BMedSc MRCPath FRCPath
Professor of Cancer Pathology
University of Nottingham School of Medicine;
Honorary Consultant Pathologist
City Hospital
Nottingham, UK

D. Gareth Evans MB ChB FRCS
Professor of Medical Genetics
Academic Unit of Medical Genetics
St Mary's Hospital
Manchester, UK

Lesley Fallowfield BSc DPhil
Professor in Psycho-oncology
Cancer Research UK Psychosocial Oncology Group
Brighton and Sussex Medical School
University of Sussex
Brighton, UK

Janet Hardy MD BSc FRACP
Professor of Palliative Care
University of Queensland;
Director of Palliative Care
Mater Health Services
Brisbane, Queensland, Australia

Valerie A. Jenkins BSc DPhil
Senior Research Psychologist
Cancer Research UK Psychosocial Oncology Group
Brighton and Sussex Medical School
University of Sussex
Brighton, UK

James Kollias MB BS MD FRCSA
Senior Consultant Surgeon
Breast, Endocrine and Surgical Oncology Unit
Royal Adelaide Hospital
Adelaide, SA, Australia

Swati Kulkarni MD FACS
Breast Fellow
Division of Surgical Oncology
Northwestern Memorial Hospital
Chicago, IL, USA

R. Douglas Macmillan MD FRCS
Consultant Surgeon and Associate Clinical Director
Nottingham Breast Institute
Nottingham City Hospital
Nottingham, UK

Monica Morrow MD FACS
Professor of Surgery
Northwestern University Feinberg School of Medicine
Director, Lynn Sage Comprehensive Breast Program
Northwestern Memorial Hospital
Chicago, IL, USA

Sarah E. Pinder MB ChB FRCPath
Consultant Breast Pathologist
Addenbrooke's Hospital
Cambridge, UK

Richard M. Rainsbury BSc MS FRCS
Consultant Oncoplastic Breast Surgeon
Royal Hampshire County Hospital
Winchester, UK

Rajendra S. Rampaul MB ChB MD FRCS
Specialist Registrar in Surgery
City Hospital
Nottingham, UK

John F.R. Robertson MB ChB FRCS
Professor of Surgery
University of Nottingham;
Consultant Surgeon
City Hospital
Nottingham, UK

Gillian Ross MB ChB FRCP
Senior Lecturer and Honorary
Consultant Clinical Oncologist
Royal Marsden Hospital
London, UK

J. Richard C. Sainsbury MD FRCS
Senior Lecturer and Consultant Surgeon
University College London
London

Ian E. Smith MD FRCP
Professor of Cancer Medicine and
Consultant Clinical Oncologist
Royal Marsden Hospital and
Institute of Cancer Research
London, UK

Steven Thrush MB BS FRCS(Gen Surg)
Consultant Surgeon
Breast Unit
Worcester Royal Hospital
Worcester, UK

Ander Urruticoechea MD
Clinical Research Fellow
Royal Marsden Hospital
London, UK

Eva M. Weiler-Mithoff MD FRCS(Ed) FRCS(Glasg) FRCS(Plast)
Consultant Plastic Surgeon
Canniesburn Plastic Surgery Unit
Glasgow Royal Infirmary
Glasgow, UK

A. Robin M. Wilson MB ChB FRCR FRCP
Consultant Radiologist
Nottingham Breast Institute
Nottingham City Hospital
Nottingham, UK

Preface

The *Companion to Specialist Surgical Practice* series was designed to meet the needs of surgeons in higher training and practising consultants who wish up-to-date and evidence-based information on the subspecialist areas relevant to their surgical practice. In trying to meet this aim, we have recognised that the series will never be as all-encompassing as many of the larger reference surgical textbooks. However, by their very size, it is rare that the latter are completely up to date at the time of publication. The first edition of this series was published in 1997, with the second following in 2001. In this third edition, we have been able to bring up to date the relevant specialist information that we and the individual volume editors consider important for the practising subspecialist surgeon. Where possible, all contributors have attempted to identify evidence-based references to support key recommendations within each chapter. These should all be interpreted with the help of the guidance summary 'Evidence-based practice in surgery', which follows this preface.

We are extremely grateful to all volume editors and to their contributors to this third edition. It is thanks to their enthusiasm and hard work that the relatively short time frame between each of the editions has been maintained, thereby providing to the reader the most accurate and up-to-date information possible. We were all immensely saddened by the sudden and tragic death of Professor John Farndon, who edited the first and second editions of the volumes *Breast Surgery* and *Endocrine Surgery*. While recognising that he was a unique and talented individual, we are pleased to welcome the additional editorial skills of Mike Dixon and Tom Lennard for this third edition.

We are also grateful for the support and encouragement of Elsevier Ltd and hope that our aim – of providing up-to-date and affordable surgical texts – has been met and that all readers, whether in training or in consultant practice, will find this third edition a valuable resource.

O. James Garden BSc, MB, ChB, MD, FRCS(Glasg), FRCS(Ed), FRCP(Ed)
Regius Professor of Clinical Surgery, Clinical and Surgical Sciences (Surgery), University of Edinburgh, and Honorary Consultant Surgeon, Royal Infirmary of Edinburgh

Simon Paterson-Brown MB, BS, MPhil, MS, FRCS(Ed), FRCS
Honorary Senior Lecturer, Clinical and Surgical Sciences (Surgery), University of Edinburgh, and Consultant General and Upper Gastrointestinal Surgeon, Royal Infirmary of Edinburgh

EVIDENCE-BASED PRACTICE IN SURGERY

The third edition of the *Companion to Specialist Surgical Practice* series has attempted to incorporate, where appropriate, **evidence-based practice in surgery**, which has been highlighted in the text and relevant references. A detailed chapter on evidence-based practice in surgery, written by Kathryn Rigby and Jonathan Michaels, has been included in the volume *Core Topics in General and Emergency Surgery*, to which the reader is referred for further information on assessing levels of evidence. We are grateful to them for providing this summary for each volume.

Critical appraisal for developing evidence-based practice can be obtained from a number of sources, the most reliable being randomised controlled clinical trials, systematic literature reviews, meta-analyses and observational studies. For practical purposes three grades of evidence can be used, analogous to the levels of 'proof' required in a court of law:

1. **Beyond reasonable doubt** – such evidence is likely to have arisen from high-quality randomised controlled trials, systematic reviews, or high-quality synthesised evidence such as decision analysis, cost-effectiveness analysis or large observational data sets. The studies need to be directly applicable to the population of concern and have clear results. The grade is analogous to burden of proof within a crimimal court and may be thought of as corresponding to the usual standard of 'proof' within the medical literature (i.e. $P<0.05$).
2. **On the balance of probabilities** – in many cases a high-quality review of literature may fail to reach firm conclusions owing to conflicting or inconclusive results, trials of poor methodological quality or a lack of evidence in the population to which the guidelines apply. In such cases it may still be possible to make a statement as to the best treatment on the 'balance of probabilities'. This is analogous to the decision in a civil court where all the available evidence will be weighed up and the verdict will depend upon the balance of probabilities.
3. **Not proven** – insufficient evidence upon which to base a decision or contradictory evidence.

Depending on the information available three grades of recommendation can be used:

a. strong recommendation, which should be followed unless there are compelling reasons to act otherwise;
b. a recommendaton based on evidence of effectiveness but where there may be other factors to take into account in decision-making, for example the user of the guidelines may be expected to take into account patient preferences, local facilities, local audit results or available resources;
c. a recommendation made where there is no adequate evidence as to the most effective practice, although there may be reasons for making a recommendation in order to minimise cost or reduce the chance of error through a locally agreed protocol.

 The text and references that are considered to be associated with reasonable evidence are highlighted in this volume with a 'scalpel code', leaving the reader to reach his or her own conclusion.

Editor's note

The first two editions of this volume in the *Companion to Specialist Surgical Practice* series were put together and edited by Professor John Farndon. The first edition was a joint edition comprising breast and endocrine disease but, with the increasing specialisation in breast disease, the second edition featured a separate volume on breast disease. Both were successful – in the case of the volume *Breast Surgery* because Professor Farndon managed to produce a very balanced and comprehensive series of chapters dealing with all aspects of breast disease. Following his sudden and untimely death, with some apprehension I agreed to take on the task of editing the third edition. I hope that those who owned and read the first two editions feel that this new edition has remained true to Professor Farndon's aims and objectives.

This third volume has been comprehensively rewritten. With an increasing number of surgeons wishing to be pure breast surgical specialists, they are becoming involved in all aspects of patients' care from diagnosis through to palliative care. Although the book concentrates largely on breast cancer, a new chapter on benign disease has been added. Benign disease is sometimes forgotten in such texts and yet the overwhelming majority of patients attending breast clinics have benign disease. Their management is not always optimal and there is a limited volume of literature on which to base current practice. This chapter summarises current knowledge in many areas and provides a framework for the management of these patients, many of whom have difficult and challenging problems. There have been significant advances in our abilities to diagnose breast cancer before operation with the advent of improved imaging and more sophisticated pathological techniques, including the routine use of immunohistochemistry for hormone receptor and growth factor receptor assays. These are reflected in new chapters on these topics. As over two-thirds of patients are now candidates for breast conserving surgery this is now covered in more detail in a separate chapter. To reflect the increasing interest of trainees in oncoplastic procedures there are many more chapters dealing with technical aspects of oncoplastic breast surgery. These chapters have been written by the leading lights and proponents in this field and I am grateful for their contributions. Other chapters cover oncology, medico-legal aspects, new clinical trials and palliative care.

With breast cancer continuing to increase in frequency by almost 25% every decade, it is imperative that those managing patients are fully trained and well informed. I hope that this volume will provide trainees in surgery and consultants alike with the wide-ranging knowledge and perspective of breast disease that is now necessary for the specialist breast surgeon.

J. Michael Dixon BSc, MB, ChB, MD, FRCS, FRCS(Ed), FRCP
Honorary Senior Lecturer, Clinical and Surgical Sciences (Surgery), University of Edinburgh, and Consultant Surgeon, Edinburgh Breast Unit, Western General Hospital

Acknowledgements

First of all I would like to acknowledge the authors, some of whom I have hassled and bullied and all of whom have produced consistently high-quality work. This book could not have been produced without the diligent help of Mrs Jan Mauritzen, my PA in the Edinburgh Breast Unit, and Sheila Black, Project Development Manager at Elsevier. I would like to thank my colleagues in the Edinburgh Breast Unit for their continued patience and encouragement. Being both an academic and a full-time consultant breast surgeon has only been possible with their support. Finally, I would like to pay tribute to all the men and women who pass through breast clinics throughout the world and in particular those who are unfortunate enough to be diagnosed with breast cancer. The way they deal with their disease and cope with all that we do to them is our inspiration. We must and need to strive to do better for them.

JMD

One

The role of imaging in breast diagnosis including screening and excision of impalpable lesions

A. Robin M. Wilson and
R. Douglas Macmillan

INTRODUCTION

Breast cancer is a major health problem. Worldwide it has an increasing incidence, with over 1 million newly diagnosed cases each year, and is the commonest cancer to affect women and is the commonest cause of cancer death in women. Breast cancer mortality in the UK is among the highest in the world, with approximately 28 deaths per 100 000 women per annum. This equates to around 35 000 new breast cancers diagnosed and 14 500 deaths attributable to breast cancer each year. Approximately 1 in 9 women in the UK will develop breast cancer at some time during their life.[1]

Strategies for diagnosing and managing breast cancer are based on our current understanding of breast disease epidemiology. Around 5% of breast cancer is hereditary, mainly associated with the *BRCA1* and *BRCA2* gene defects. This type of breast cancer tends to occur in younger women. The remaining 95% of breast cancer is sporadic and its incidence increases with age. Breast cancer is very rare under the age of 35 years and over 80% of breast cancer occurs in women over the age of 50. The causes of sporadic breast cancer are largely believed to be environmental factors. Recognised risk factors include early menarche, late menopause, nulliparity and long-term use of the contraceptive pill and hormone replacement therapy (HRT). Less than 1% of breast cancer occurs in men.

As there is a poor understanding of the causes of breast cancer, primary prevention is currently not a realistic or achievable option. It is known that earlier diagnosis of breast cancer is more likely to result in a favourable outcome. Tumour size at diagnosis and lymph node stage are the best predictors of outcome. Regardless of tumour type or grade, the smaller a breast cancer is at the time of diagnosis, the more likely it is that it has not spread beyond the breast. As a result the current strategy for reducing breast cancer mortality is to seek diagnosis as early as possible.

 Early detection and improvements in treatment have led to a 30% reduction in breast cancer mortality in the UK in all age groups over the past 20 years.[2]

Early diagnosis is achieved by encouraging women to present as early as possible to breast clinics when they develop breast symptoms and through pre-emptive breast cancer screening. Breast imaging is fundamental to both.

IMAGING IN SYMPTOMATIC BREAST PRACTICE

Based on mortality statistics from the 1980s and 1990s, the UK does not have the highest incidence of breast cancer but it has had the highest death rate.

Recognising that breast cancer diagnosis and treatment required significant improvement, in 1995 the UK Department of Health published guidelines for improving outcomes in breast cancer. These guidelines were updated in 2002 by the National Institute for Clinical Excellence (NICE).[3] The guidelines emphasise the following three key issues in breast cancer care:

- accurate and timely diagnosis;
- appropriate treatment decided by accurate staging of disease;
- appropriate follow-up of patients undergoing treatment.

Imaging is required at all three stages of this process, and mammography and ultrasound have a pivotal role to play. Around 200 specialist breast units in the NHS deal with the diagnosis of symptomatic breast problems. About 60% of breast cancer is detected by symptomatic breast referral clinics. These clinics follow national protocols that define the triple test, i.e. the combination of clinical assessment, imaging (mammography and ultrasound) and needle cytology or core biopsy, as the required standard. 'One-stop' clinics are recommended at which all the necessary tests required to make a diagnosis, including needle biopsy, are performed at one clinic visit. In order to achieve the earliest possible diagnosis of symptomatic breast cancer, women are encouraged through a variety of health promotion methods to present to these clinics as soon as possible when they develop any change in their breasts.

BREAST IMAGING TECHNIQUES

Mammography

X-ray mammography has been the basis of breast imaging for more than 30 years. The sensitivity of mammography for breast cancer is age dependent. The denser the breast, the less effective this method is for detecting early signs of breast cancer. Breast density tends to be higher in younger women and increased density obscures early signs of breast cancer. The sensitivity of mammography for breast cancer in women over 60 years of age approaches 95%, while mammography can be expected to

detect less than 50% of breast cancers in women under 40 years of age.[4]

Mammography uses ionising radiation to obtain an image and therefore should only be used where there is likely to be a clinical benefit. Consensus is that the benefits of mammography in women over the age of 40 years are likely to far outweigh any oncogenic effects of repeated exposure. Screening of women over the age of 40 by mammography is accepted practice. However, in symptomatic practice there is rarely an indication for performing mammography in women under the age of 35 unless there is a strong clinical suspicion of malignancy. In many centres, all women over the age of 35 presenting to breast clinics undergo mammography as a routine. Practice is changing and ultrasound is being increasingly used for the assessment of women with focal breast symptoms in this age range. Mammography is routine in all women in the screening age group attending symptomatic clinics who have not had a screening mammogram in the past year.

Most mammography in the UK is carried out using conventional analogue X-ray films. Film/screen mammography has been refined over the years and has now reached the limits of this technology. Film/screen mammography is a difficult technique to maintain at the quality levels required for optimal diagnosis because of the narrow latitude of operation of these systems and because it requires labour-intensive quality-control measures to maintain the necessary diagnostic standards. The future of mammography lies in digital acquisition of the image.[5-9] Major benefits have been predicted from acquiring mammograms in direct digital format.[9] The resolution required for digital mammography has only recently become available. Compared with conventional mammography, the predicted benefits of full-field digital mammography include better imaging of the dense breast, the application of computer-aided detection and a number of logistical advantages providing potential for more efficient mammography services.[10,11] The much wider dynamic range of digital mammography means that visualisation of the entire breast density range on a single image is easily achievable. In the clinical setting, comparative studies have shown that digital mammography performs as well as film/screen mammography.[5-7]

Mammography is the basis of stereotactic breast biopsy. Stereotactic biopsy can be carried out using a dedicated prone biopsy table or by using an add-on device to a conventional upright mammography unit. This technique is used for biopsy of impalpable lesions that are not clearly visible on ultrasound (e.g. microcalcifications).

Ultrasound

High-frequency (≥10 MHz) ultrasound is a very effective diagnostic tool for the investigation of focal breast symptoms.[12] Ultrasound does not involve ionising radiation and is a very safe imaging technique. It has a high sensitivity for breast pathology and also a very high negative predictive value.[13]

High-resolution ultrasound easily distinguishes between most solid and cystic lesions and can differentiate benign from malignant lesions with a high degree of accuracy. However, in most circumstances, solid lesions seen on ultrasound require needle sampling for accurate diagnosis.

Ultrasound is the technique of choice for the further investigation of focal symptomatic breast problems at all ages. Under 35 years of age, when the risk of breast cancer is very low, it is usually the only imaging technique required. Over 35, when the risk of breast cancer begins to increase, it is often used in conjunction with mammography. Ultrasound is less sensitive than mammography for the early signs of breast cancer and is therefore not used for population screening. However, ultrasound does increase the detection of small breast cancer in women who have a dense background pattern on mammography.[4] In the screening setting, there is currently insufficient evidence of any mortality benefit and insufficient resources to allow for routine ultrasound screening of women with dense mammograms.[14] Ultrasound is the technique of first choice for biopsy of both palpable and impalpable breast lesions visible on scanning.

Ultrasound is being increasingly used to assess the axilla in women with breast cancer. Axillary nodes that show abnormal morphology can be accurately sampled by fine-needle aspiration (FNA) or needle core biopsy.

Up to 50% of patients with axillary metastatic disease can be diagnosed using this method, avoiding the need for node sampling or sentinel node biopsy in women with pathologically proven nodal involvement.[15]

Doppler ultrasound adds little to breast diagnosis and is not widely used. Three-dimensional ultrasound of the breast is said to increase the accuracy of biopsy and the detection of multifocal disease but again is not widely available. Elastography is a new application of ultrasound technology that allows the accurate assessment of the stiffness of breast tissue. It is being evaluated at present and may prove to be a useful tool in excluding significant abnormalities, for instance in assessment of asymptomatic abnormalities detected by ultrasound screening.

Magnetic resonance mammography

Magnetic resonance imaging (MRI) is now widely available. However, magnetic resonance mammography (MRM) of the breast requires dedicated breast coils and these are much less widely available. In order to image the breast the patient is scanned prone and injection of intravenous contrast is required. MRM is the most sensitive technique for detection of breast cancer, approaching 100% for invasive cancer and 80% for ductal carcinoma in situ (DCIS), but it has a high false-positive rate. Rapid acquisition of images facilitates assessment of signal enhancement curves that can be helpful in distinguishing benign and malignant disease. However, significant overlap in the enhancement patterns usually means that needle sampling is required. Magnetic resonance-guided breast biopsy is now available in a few centres but most breast lesions seen on MRM that are larger than 10 mm can be seen on ultrasound if they are clinically significant.

MRM is likely to prove the best method for screening younger women (under 40 years) at increased risk of breast cancer but, because of cost, it is unlikely to be used for general population screening.[16–19]

MRM is the best technique for imaging women with breast implants. It is also of benefit in identifying recurrent disease where conventional imaging and biopsy have failed to exclude recurrence. Provided it is carried out more than 18 months after surgery, MRI will accurately distinguish between scarring and tumour recurrence. MRI is being increasingly used to examine women for multifocal disease prior to conservation surgery, although the lack of evidence of efficacy means that it is not routine in this clinical setting. MRI of the axilla will demonstrate axillary metastatic disease but its sensitivity is not sufficient for it to replace surgical staging of the axilla. For advanced breast cancer, MRI is the technique of choice for assessing spinal metastatic disease.

Computed tomography

Computed tomography (CT) has no role in primary imaging of the breast. CT is used to diagnose and stage systemic spread of breast cancer and to assess response of metastatic disease to treatment, particularly lung, pleural and liver metastases.

Isotope imaging

Breast scintigraphy is not widely used because of its lack of sensitivity compared with other techniques. It is used in a few centres to stage the breast prior to surgery and to assess response to treatment. Scintigraphy is widely used to diagnose and assess the presence of skeletal metastatic disease.

Positron emission scintigraphy, particularly when combined with CT, is a new technology that may have a role in future in staging breast cancer and monitoring response to treatment. At present, it is regarded as a research tool and its specific uses and indications are still being evaluated.

BREAST CANCER SCREENING

Aim

The aim of breast screening is to reduce mortality through early detection. Randomised controlled trials and case–control studies carried out between the 1960s and 1980s demonstrated that population screening by mammography can be expected to

reduce overall breast cancer mortality by around 25% and by 35–40% in those who participate.

The validity of these trials was questioned in 2000–2002 but subsequent reviews by the Swedish combined trials group and a World Health Organisation International Agency for Research on Cancer committee of experts have reaffirmed the mortality benefit of mammographic screening and determined that criticisms of the mammographic screening trials were unjustified.[20–25]

The mortality benefit of screening is greatest in women aged 55–70 years.[22,23] The mortality benefit of screening women aged between 40 and 55 is approximately 20%. Screening women under the age of 40 has not been shown to provide any mortality benefit.[22,23]

Population screening

Breast screening has been introduced in many countries over the past 20 years. In most countries, screening is recommended in all women aged 40 and over but in countries that provide population-based screening, women of 50 and over are specifically targeted. Breast cancer screening was introduced in the UK in 1987 and provides screening by invitation, free at the point of delivery, to all women between the ages of 50 and 70.[1] Women over 70 can attend but are not invited. Over 70% of the invited population need to attend for a significant overall mortality benefit to be achieved. Women under the age of 50 are not offered screening in the UK unless they are at increased risk.

Method and frequency

The screening method is two-view mammography; clinical examination of the breast and breast self-examination have not been shown to contribute to mortality reduction through early detection and so are not included.[9,26,27]

Women are invited every 3 years. There has been some concern that this screening interval is too long. Mammography can be expected to detect breast cancer approximately 2 years before it becomes clinically apparent. The frequency of mammographic screening is determined by the lead-time of breast cancer. Based on the average growth time of breast cancer according to age, this means that mammographic screening should ideally be carried out yearly in women aged 40–50, every 2 years in women aged 50–60 and every 3 years thereafter. However, the breast screening frequency trial completed in 1995 did not show any predicted benefit for women aged 50–64 screened every year compared with those screened every 3 years.[28] Screening once every 3 years can be expected to detect approximately two-thirds of breast cancer that will arise during the 3-year screening interval. One-third of breast cancers will present in the interval between screens, so-called interval cancers. Half of these present in the third year after screening.

Factors affecting the effectiveness of screening

HRT increases breast density and in a proportion of women this treatment reduces the sensitivity of mammography for breast cancer.[9,27–35] Up to 25% of women taking combined estrogen/progestogen preparations continuously show increased density on mammography. This effect is significantly less with other HRT preparations. The use of HRT has been shown to significantly reduce the sensitivity and specificity of mammographic screening. HRT also increases the risk of developing breast cancer.[29]

Quality assurance

Breast screening programmes should have in-built quality assurance and the NHS Breast Screening Programme is subject to comprehensive quality assessment and all 100 screening units across the country have to comply with nationally defined standard guidelines. There are national targets for screening set by a central Department of Health Advisory Committee (**Table 1.1**).

The screening process

Women invited for screening attend either a static or mobile screening unit where two-view mammography is performed. The images are then double read within a few days. The vast majority of

women (95%) are informed by letter within 2 weeks of attendance that their mammograms show no evidence of breast cancer. Those women in the appropriate age range will be invited for screening 3 years later. They are advised to contact their general practitioner as soon as possible if they become aware of any change in their breasts in the meantime.

The screening process includes a fully integrated multidisciplinary assessment process for all screen-detected mammographic abnormalities; screening programmes should ideally retain responsibility through to definitive diagnosis. Approximately 5% of women screened are recalled for further assessment of a problem identified at screening. Some women are recalled for further assessment of a clinical sign or symptom identified at the time of screening but the vast majority of women are recalled because of a mammographic abnormality.

The most important cancers detected at screening are high-grade DCIS, as most cases of this type will progress to grade 2 or 3 invasive breast cancer within the following 3 years, and grade 2 and 3 invasive breast cancers under 10 mm in diameter, as at this size these tumours are much less likely to have metastasised.[36,37]

The common types of mammographic abnormality and their positive predictive value for cancer are shown in **Table 1.2**. Well-defined masses are almost always benign and do not require recall, whereas ill-defined masses and spiculated lesions always require further assessment (**Figs 1.1** and **1.2**). Clustered microcalcifications account for a high proportion of recalls that result in needle biopsy. More than 20% of screen-detected breast cancer is DCIS, mostly high or intermediate grade, and most of this type of cancer is detected by the presence of clustered microcalcifications (**Fig. 1.3**). Invasive cancer is usually represented on mammography by either an ill-defined or spiculated mass. It is essential to detect these lesions at small size as they more commonly represent grade 2 or 3 invasive cancer.

Three-quarters of women recalled simply require further imaging (mammography and/or ultrasound) and clinical assessment before being reassured and discharged. The remaining 25% will undergo a needle biopsy procedure in order to diagnose

Table 1.1 • NHS Breast Screening Programme: screening targets, September 2003

Objective	Criteria	Minimum standard	Target
To maximise the number of eligible women who attend for screening	Percentage of eligible women who attend for screening	• ≥70% of invited women to attend for screening	• 80%
To maximise the number of cancers detected	(a) Rate of invasive cancers detected in eligible women	• Prevalent screen ≥2.7 per 1000 • Incident screen ≥3.1 per 1000	• Prevalent screen >3.6 per 1000 • Incident screen ≥4.2 per 1000
	(b) Rate of cancers detected that are in situ carcinoma	• Prevalent screen ≥0.4 per 1000 • Incident screen ≥0.5 per 1000	
	(c) Standardised detection ratio	• ≥0.85	• ≥1.0
To maximise the number of small invasive cancers	Rate of invasive cancers less than 15 mm in diameter detected in eligible women invited and screened	• Prevalent screen ≥1.5 per 1000 • Incident screen ≥1.7 per 1000	• Prevalent screen >2.0 per 1000 • Incident screen ≥2.5 per 1000
To achieve optimum image quality	(a) High-contrast spatial resolution	• ≥12 lp/mm	
	(b) Minimal detectable contrast: 5–6 mm detail 0.5 mm detail 0.25 mm detail	• ≤1.2% • ≤5% • ≤8%	• ≤0.8% • ≤3% • ≤5%
	(c) Aim film density	• 1.5–1.9	
To limit radiation dose	Mean glandular dose per film for a standard breast at clinical settings	• ≤2.5 mGy	
To minimise the number of women undergoing repeat examinations	Number of repeat examinations	• <3% of total examinations	• <2% of total examinations
To minimise the number of women screened who are referred for further tests*	(a) Percentage of women who are referred for assessment	• Prevalent screen <10% • Incident screen <7%	• Prevalent screen <7% • Incident screen <5%
	(b) Percentage of women screened who are placed on early recall	• <0.5%	• ≤0.25%
To ensure that the majority of cancers, both palpable and impalpable, receive a non-operative tissue diagnosis of cancer	Percentage of women who have a non-operative diagnosis of cancer by cytology or needle histology after a maximum of two visits	• ≥80%	• >90%

Table 1.1 • (*cont.*) NHS Breast Screening Programme: screening targets, September 2003

Objective	Criteria	Minimum standard	Target
To minimise the number of unnecessary operative procedures	Rate of benign biopsies	• Prevalent screen <3.6 per 1000 • Incident screen <2.0 per 1000	• Prevalent screen <1.8 per 1000 • Incident screen <1.0 per 1000
To minimise the number of cancers in the women screened presenting between screening episodes	Rate of cancers presenting in screened women: (a) in the 2 years following a normal screening episode (b) in the third year following a normal screening episode	*Expected standard* • 1.2 per 1000 women screened in the first 2 years • 1.4 per 1000 women screened in the third year	
To ensure that women are recalled for screening at appropriate intervals	Percentage of eligible women whose first offered appointment is within 36 months of their previous screen	• >90%	• 100%
To minimise anxiety for women awaiting the results of screening	Percentage of women who are sent their result within 2 weeks	• >90%	• 100%
To minimise the interval from the screening mammogram to assessment	Percentage of women who attend an assessment centre within 3 weeks of attendance for the screening mammogram	• >90%	• 100%
To minimise diagnostic delay for women who are diagnosed non-operatively	Proportion of women for whom the time interval between non-operative biopsy and result is 1 week or less	• ≥90%	• 100%
To minimise the delay for women who require surgical assessment	Proportion of women for whom the time interval between the decision to refer to a surgeon and surgical assessment is 1 week or less	• >90%	• 100%
To minimise any delay for women who require treatment for screen-detected breast cancer	Percentage of women who are admitted for treatment within 2 months of their first assessment visit	• >90%	• 100%

Table 1.2 • Positive predictive value (PPV) for malignancy of mammographic signs

Sign	PPV (%)
Well-defined mass	<1
Ill-defined mass	35–50
Spiculated mass	50–90
Architectural distortion	20–40
Asymmetric density	<2
Clustered microcalcifications	15

around 6 cancers per 1000 women screened. Interval follow-up of uncertain mammographic findings is discouraged, the emphasis being on obtaining a definitive diagnosis by the use of image-guided breast biopsy, with an achievable standard of over 90% of breast cancers diagnosed prior to first surgery. Despite advances in breast needle biopsy techniques a small proportion of women still require open surgical biopsy for diagnosis (up to 0.25% of women screened).

The performance of the NHS Breast Screening Programme in 2003 is shown in **Table 1.3**. The screening programme is predicted to produce a 25% reduction in mortality (1750 cancers per year) directly attributable to early detection through screening by the year 2010.

Adverse effects

Receiving an invitation for screening and attending for mammography are not associated with any significant anxiety. However, recall for further assessment does cause measurable anxiety, although this has largely subsided after 3 months.

The numbers of women who undergo open surgical biopsy for what proves to be benign disease should be kept to a minimum. Considerable training and investment in equipment has resulted in a fourfold decline in benign surgical biopsies generated through the screening programme. False-positive recall and benign surgical biopsy are both more likely in younger women.

Overdiagnosis refers to the detection via screening of breast cancers that require treatment but which would never have threatened the life of the woman. There is considerable debate about what proportion

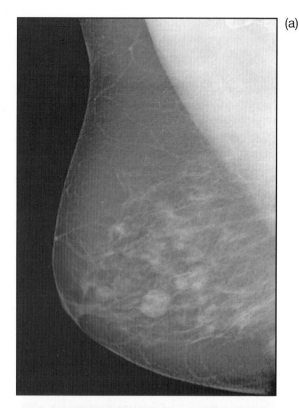

(a)

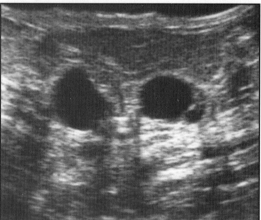

(b)

Figure 1.1 • **(a)** Digital mammogram showing well-defined masses, the typical appearance of simple breast cysts. **(b)** Ultrasound image showing typical features of simple cysts, i.e. well-circumscribed anechoic masses with distal acoustic enhancement.

if any of screen-detected breast cancers fall into this category. It is likely that most low-grade DCIS and some special low-grade invasive cancers do represent overdiagnosis, and detection of these results in unnecessary treatment and unnecessary

Table 1.3 • NHS Breast Screening Programme: results 2003

	2001/2002	2002/2003
Total number of women invited	1 752 526	1 873 470
Acceptance rate	75.5%	74.7%
Number of women screened (invited)	1 323 968	1 400 039
Number of women screened (self-referral)	137 549	123 752
Total number of women screened	1 461 517	1 541 794
Number of women recalled for assessment	77 911	79 441
Percentage of women recalled for assessment	5.3%	5.2%
Number of benign surgical biopsies	1930	1843
Number of cancers detected	10 003	10 467
Cancers per 1000 women screened	6.8	7.5
Number of in situ cancers detected	2132	2375
Number of cancers less then 15 mm	4159	4877
Standardised detection ratio (invited only)	1.22	1.32

From NHS Breast Screening Programme Annual Review 2004. Available at http:\\www.cancerscreening.nhs.uk

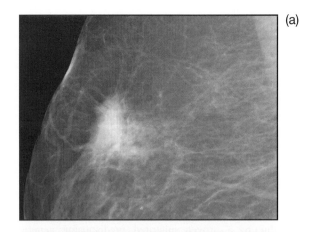

(a)

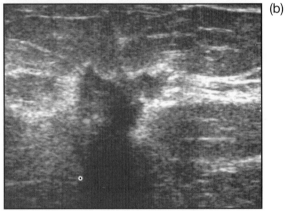

(b)

Figure 1.2 • **(a)** Digital mammogram showing a spiculated mass in the right breast. The appearances are typical of an invasive carcinoma. The mass contains microcalcifications and there is evidence of skin tether. **(b)** Ultrasound image showing the typical features of an invasive carcinoma with an irregular mass with intraduct tumour extension and causing acoustic shadowing.

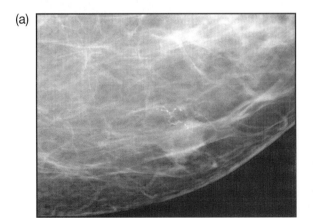

(a)

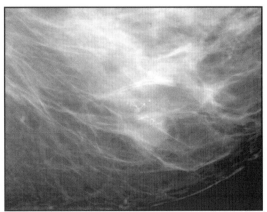

(b)

Figure 1.3 • Digital mammograms showing a cluster of casting microcalcifications in the lower inner quadrant of the left breast. The appearances are typical of high-grade ductal carcinoma in situ.

morbidity associated with knowledge of the diagnosis of cancer. The consensus view is that overdiagnosis applies to no more than 10% of screen-detected breast cancer and that at this level this does not negate the overall mortality benefit of breast screening. Women attending for screening must be fully informed about both the likely positive and negative effects of screening.

Screening women at increased risk

Women at increased risk of developing breast cancer due to a proven inherited predisposing genetic mutation, family history (with no proven genetic mutation), previous radiotherapy (e.g. mantle radiotherapy for Hodgkin's lymphoma) or benign risk lesions (atypical hyperplasia, lobular carcinoma in situ) may be selected for screening at young age. Whether it is possible to identify other substantially increased risk groups by summating various other epidemiological factors (e.g. age at menarche, body mass index, age at first pregnancy, alcohol intake) continues to be debated. The cut-off point at which clinical management of a woman is altered is often referred to as moderate risk. This risk group has various definitions but is commonly interpreted as including those with an absolute risk of at least 5% by age 50 and 17% over a lifetime. Such cut-offs are useful as guidelines for specialist referral but most risk factors require clinical interpretation before a risk management policy is discussed.

Unfortunately, the underlying problem with screening young women at increased risk of breast cancer is that no screening test has yet been shown to reduce mortality in such women. Screening is this group is therefore a management option for which an exact benefit cannot be quoted to an individual woman. Screening should not be offered to those who fall below the moderate-risk cut-off.

METHODS OF SCREENING YOUNG WOMEN AT INCREASED RISK: MAMMOGRAPHY

A national evaluation study of mammographic screening for young women with a family history of breast cancer is being conducted (FH01 study). The study compares screening in women aged 40–44 who are at least moderate risk with the control arm of the age trial (population-based trial of screening women in their forties as yet unreported). Mammography has a greater positive predictive value in young women at high risk compared with age-matched controls but lacks sensitivity. This may be a particular problem in women with *BRCA1* mutations.[19,38–41] *BRCA1*-related breast cancer is usually high grade and often has a 'pushing' margin. It rarely presents with associated DCIS. The mammographic features are therefore usually of a mass lesion with no associated microcalcification and no architectural distortion (**Fig. 1.4a**). Such cancers usually present symptomatically as interval cases. *BRCA2*-related cancers are more similar to sporadic cases and may be more likely to be detected by mammography. Ultrasound screening significantly improves sensitivity when there is a dense mammographic background pattern but has lower positive predictive value and has not been shown to be a useful screening modality. Ultrasound features of *BRCA1* cancers are often benign or indeterminate (**Fig. 1.4b**). If mammographic screening is selected, it should be repeated annually in women under age 50.

METHODS OF SCREENING YOUNG WOMEN AT HIGH RISK: MRM

There is evidence that MRM is the most sensitive method of imaging young women but has significant resource implications.[38,42] The specificity of MRM has been a concern, although with second-look recall (after which many potentially abnormal findings may resolve), targeted ultrasound and the slowly increasing availability of MRI-guided biopsy this may be less of a problem than initially thought. The MARIBS study evaluating MRI in addition to mammography and several other studies have shown that MRI may be the most sensitive screening test for young high-risk women, but it is arguable whether the prognosis of cancers detected is sufficiently influenced to make this an option that can be recommended.

AGE TO START SCREENING IN YOUNG WOMEN AT INCREASED RISK

The age for starting screening should be based on risk rather than the age of affected relatives. For women at moderate risk, screening should start at age 40. This can seem paradoxical if the reason

(a)
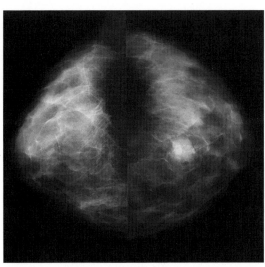
(b)
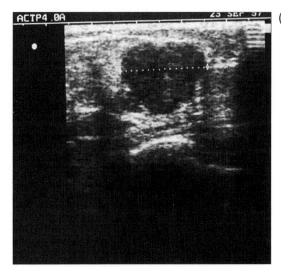

Figure 1.4 • **(a)** Conventional mammogram showing a circumscribed mass in the central part of the left breast. **(b)** Ultrasound image of the same mass. Core biopsy showed an invasive carcinoma.

moderate risk has been established is because there is one first-degree relative affected in their thirties. However, if no other affected relatives can be identified, then the individual only just qualifies as moderate risk and the emphasis of management should be on reassurance rather than screening. For women at high risk, screening may be started at age 30–35. Again, the definition of high risk is variable but a common definition would be a greater than 8% risk by age 50 or a greater than 30% lifetime risk. Such high-risk women should ideally be managed in a specialist setting. Women must be advised about the limitations of screening at young age.

IMAGE-GUIDED BREAST BIOPSY

Needle biopsy is highly accurate in determining the nature of most breast lesions.[43–46] Patients with benign conditions avoid unnecessary surgery; carrying out open surgical biopsy for diagnosis should be regarded as a failure of the diagnostic process. For patients who prove to have breast cancer, needle biopsy provides accurate understanding of the type and extent of disease so ensuring that patients, and the doctors treating them, are able to make informed treatment choices. Needle biopsy not only provides accurate information on the nature of malignant disease, such as histological type and

grade, but also facilitates pretreatment assessment of tumour biology.

Which biopsy technique?

The current methods available for breast tissue diagnosis are FNA for cytology, needle core biopsy for histology, vacuum-assisted mammotomy (VAM) and open surgical biopsy.

FNA VERSUS NEEDLE CORE BIOPSY

There has been much debate about the comparative benefits of FNA and core biopsy,[43–46] but 14G 22-mm automated core biopsy provides significantly better sensitivity, specificity and positive predictive value. Results with core biopsy are particularly superior to FNA in stereotactic biopsy of microcalcifications and architectural distortions.

The overall better performance achievable with core biopsy compared with FNA is illustrated in the performance of the NHS Breast Screening Programme in the UK. In 1994, using FNA as the primary diagnostic technique, fewer than 10% of 90 units were able to achieve the target of 70% preoperative diagnosis of cancer. By 2003, most units had converted to automated core biopsy and all units achieved the minimum standard and the majority exceeded the expected standard of more then 90% preoperative diagnosis.[1]

VACUUM-ASSISTED MAMMOTOMY

The predominant reasons for not achieving an accurate diagnosis by needle biopsy are sampling error and failure to retrieve sufficient representative material. These problems have been largely addressed by the development of larger directional core techniques that yield significantly greater volumes of tissue.[47–49]

VAM is proving to be a very successful method for improving the diagnostic accuracy of borderline breast lesions and lesions at sites in the breast difficult to biopsy using other techniques. VAM has been shown to understage both in situ and invasive cancer approximately half as often as conventional core biopsy (typically 10% vs. 20%).[50,51] The VAM technique has a higher sensitivity because it allows sampling of lesions at sites that are difficult to biopsy using either FNA or core biopsy and because the amount of tissue harvested is at least five times greater per core specimen.

The indications for VAM include:

- very small mass lesions;
- architectural distortions;
- failed 'conventional' core biopsy;
- small clusters of microcalcifications;
- papillary and mucocele-like lesions;
- diffuse non-specific abnormality;
- excision of benign lesions;
- sentinel node sampling.

Core biopsy and VAM are now the recommended techniques for sampling calcifications and mammographic architectural distortions.[52] For calcifications it is imperative that there is proof of representative sampling with specimen radiography. If calcification is not demonstrated on the specimen radiograph and the histology is benign, then management cannot be based on this result as there is a high risk of sampling error; the procedure must either be repeated or open surgical biopsy carried out.

Guidance techniques for breast needle biopsy

Ultrasound guidance is the technique of choice for biopsy of both palpable and impalpable breast lesions; it is less costly, easy to perform and more accurate than freehand or other image-guided techniques.[43]

Ultrasound provides real-time visualisation of the biopsy procedure and visual confirmation of adequate sampling. Between 80 and 90% of breast abnormalities will be clearly visible on ultrasound and amenable to biopsy using this technique. For impalpable abnormalities not visible on ultrasound, stereotactic X-ray-guided biopsy is required. A few lesions are only visible on MRI and require magnetic resonance-guided biopsy.[53] A number of different approaches have been developed for this procedure using both closed and open magnets. FNA, core biopsy and VAM may all be used for magnetic resonance-guided sampling.

The negative predictive value of combined normal mammography and ultrasound is extremely high; where there is a clinically palpable abnormality and mammography and ultrasound are entirely normal, the likelihood of malignancy is low (<1%). However, in these circumstances it remains prudent in the presence of a localised clinical abnormality to carry out freehand biopsy to exclude the occasional diffuse malignant process, such as classical lobular carcinoma or low-grade DCIS, that may be occult on both mammography and ultrasound.

For stereotactic procedures it is prudent to mark the biopsy site for future reference. Gel pellets or cellulose can be placed during the procedure to mark the biopsy site. These markers have the advantage of being visible on ultrasound so that repeat biopsy or localisation for surgery can be subsequently performed under ultrasound rather than X-ray guidance. These markers dissolve and are reabsorbed in a few weeks, leaving a small metal marker in case delayed X-ray identification of the biopsy site is required.

Number of samples

A simple rule for satisfactory sampling using needle techniques is to obtain sufficient material to achieve a diagnosis.[52,54] For ultrasound-guided core biopsy, a diagnosis may be possible on a single core. Showing on ultrasound that the needle has passed through the centre of the abnormality and by examining the sample with the naked eye, it is usually possible to confirm whether a satisfactory sample has been obtained. It is unnecessary to obtain multiple cores as a matter of routine but, as some lesions are heterogeneous, sensitivity does increase with more extensive sampling of a lesion. The number of core specimens obtained should reflect the nature of the abnormality being sampled. For ultrasound-guided biopsy where there is a suspicion of carcinoma, it is recommended that a minimum of two core specimens are obtained.

As stereotactic biopsy is used for abnormalities that are difficult to define on ultrasound and are therefore more difficult to sample, a minimum of five core specimens should be obtained. Ensuring that calcification is present in at least three separate cores and/or five separate flecks of calcification are retrieved from the area of suspicion will provide accurate diagnosis.

When there is still diagnostic uncertainty, 8G VAM can be used to obtain larger tissue volumes (approximately 300 mg per core). An 8G mammotomy probe is preferred for therapeutic removal of breast lesions such as fibroadenomas.

Biopsy results

It is important that the result of needle breast biopsy is always correlated with the clinical and imaging findings before clinical management is discussed with the patient. This is best achieved by reviewing each case at prospective multidisciplinary meetings.[43]

SURGERY FOR CLINICALLY OCCULT BREAST LESIONS

Wire-guided excision

The number of impalpable, clinically occult breast lesions detected by screening is increasing. Accurate localisation techniques are required to facilitate their surgical excision. The hooked wire is the most commonly employed technique and has proved very reliable but does have inherent associated problems. There are various designs of localisation wire in common use. All have some form of anchoring device such as a hook with a splayed or barbed tip. The wire is deployed under stereotactic or ultrasound guidance within a rigid over-sheath cannula, which is then removed once positioning is satisfactory (**Fig. 1.5**). The patient is then transferred to the operating theatre with the wire in situ. Most wires are very flexible and when the cannula is

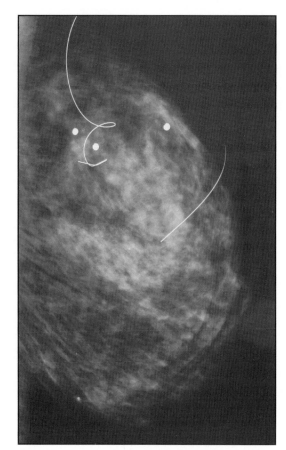

Figure 1.5 • Conventional mammogram showing a Nottingham wire marking a small impalpable mass.

removed the wire may assume a quite circuitous course, especially after stereotactic insertion when the breast is released from compression. This may lead to difficulty in any resheathing of the wire with the cannula in theatre. In order to achieve resheathing the wire needs to be pulled gently and as straight as possible. In a very fatty breast in which there is no solid lesion or the wire has not transfixed the lesion, care must be taken to avoid displacing the wire. Wire kinking can also occur if the over-sheath is forced over the wire. The purpose of the over-sheath is to enable palpability of the wire tip by ballottement. This can be difficult in fibrous breasts or for lesions deep in the breast. After resheathing, a cosmetically considered incision is placed near to the tip of the wire and an excision performed. Accurate wire placement is essential and ideally the shortest possible length of wire should be within

(a)

(b)

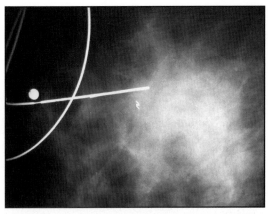

Figure 1.6 • **(a)** Ultrasound showing a cluster of gel pellets placed at the site of a previous stereotactic biopsy. The clear visibility of the pellets facilitates ultrasound localisation for surgery of abnormalities that would normally require X-ray localisation. **(b)** Mammogram after ultrasound localisation in the same case showing accurate placement of the marker wire.

the breast. In recent practice this has been greatly facilitated by the use of radio-opaque markers placed at the time of initial stereotactic biopsy such that wire localisation can be performed under ultrasound guidance (**Fig. 1.6**). In addition, for superficial lesions a skin marker may be more appropriate.

Although lesions may be clinically occult prior to surgery, most mass lesions will be palpable intra-operatively. Procedures that can be surgically more challenging are wide local excisions for DCIS with no mass lesion. In such cases, where the distribution of disease is often more eccentric, careful excision planning is necessary. Inserting more than one wire and even bracketing the lesion with three or four wires can occasionally be useful.

If the procedure is being performed to establish a diagnosis, a small representative portion of the lesion is excised through a small incision, so leaving a satisfactory cosmetic result if the lesion proves to be benign (the European surgical quality assurance guidelines require such diagnostic surgical excision specimens to weigh less than 30 g). For diagnostic excisions of very small lesions, a therapeutic wide excision may (after discussion with the patient) be considered appropriate, as the resulting cosmetic effect of removing an extra rim of tissue may be insignificant. Protocols vary for therapeutic excisions, but in general the lesion should be excised with a 10-mm macroscopic margin of normal tissue. Intraoperative specimen radiography is essential, both to check that the lesion has been removed and,

if cancer has been diagnosed, to ensure that adequate wide local excision has been achieved.

Some surgeons experienced in this imaging technique have also used intraoperative ultrasound. Not only can excision be guided but the margins of a wide local excision specimen can also be imaged intraoperatively.

Radioisotope occult lesion localisation

Radioisotope occult lesion localisation (ROLL) has been advocated as an alternative to the hooked-wire technique.[55] ROLL was first described by the Milan group using ^{99m}Tc-labelled human macro-aggregate albumin, check scintigraphy and a hand-held gamma probe to guide surgical excision. The Nottingham method has modified the Milan technique and uses radio-opaque contrast injected with the radiolabel and immediate check mammography (**Fig. 1.7**). Subsequently some centres have combined ROLL with sentinel node biopsy. ROLL uses essentially the same equipment as sentinel node biopsy. It has been described using macroaggregate (which does not migrate from the injection site) or low-molecular-weight colloid (which does migrate and is normally used for sentinel node biopsy). In both situations it is radiolabelled with ^{99m}Tc and injected directly into the lesion. The threshold of the signal processor on the gamma detector is then

(a)
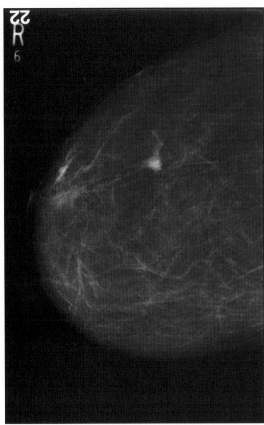

(b)
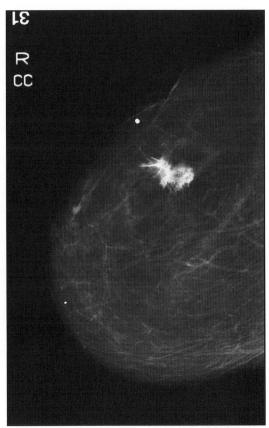

Figure 1.7 • **(a)** Mammogram of the right breast showing a small impalpable cancer. **(b)** Mammogram after injection of radionuclide mixed with X-ray contrast confirming satisfactory localisation (ROLL).

adjusted so that an audible signal is only heard when the probe is directly over the lesion. The probe then directs excision intraoperatively.

In a randomised trial of ROLL versus wire localisation, 2% of ROLL patients had a failed technique due to intraductal injection of radiolabelled colloid and dye that gave a ductogram appearance on check mammography in both cases.[56,57] As the radio-opaque dye is absorbed rapidly, both cases were successfully converted to wire localisation. The main differences between ROLL and wire guidance were that both surgeons and radiologists found ROLL easier to perform overall and patients found ROLL less painful. There was no significant difference in accuracy of marking, operating time, mean specimen weight, intraoperative re-excision or

second therapeutic operation. Other studies have suggested that obtaining clear margins may be significantly easier with ROLL. In essence there is little to choose between ROLL and wire localisation, although we prefer ROLL in the localisation of non-mass lesions (e.g. DCIS).

There are various methods described for combining ROLL with sentinel node biopsy.[58–60] Low-molecular-weight colloid can be injected at a different site, at the same site with a different radiolabel, or into the tumour. With intratumoral injection of ^{99m}Tc nanocolloid, only one injection is required and high success rates have been reported. Combined with radio-opaque contrast, this modification of the Nottingham method has proved successful.

• **Key points**

- Breast imaging is an essential part of modern multidisciplinary breast diagnosis.
- Mammography is the technique of choice for population breast screening.
- Screening is targeted at women aged 50–70 years and can be expected to reduce mortality through early detection by 30%.
- The aim should be to achieve as near as possible 100% non-operative diagnosis of breast problems.
- Both palpable and impalpable breast lesions are best sampled under image guidance.
- Automated core biopsy is the sampling technique of first choice.
- Ultrasound is the guidance technique of first choice.
- Digital stereotactic core biopsy should be reserved for sampling lesions not visible on ultrasound.
- A 14G core biopsy can provide a definitive diagnosis in more than 90% of cases and should be the preferred method.
- Mammotomy can provide the diagnosis in most of the remainder.
- Stereo-guided vacuum-assisted mammotomy (VAM) is particularly effective for small clusters of indeterminate microcalcifications and calcifications in sites difficult to access with core biopsy.
- VAM is an effective and well-tolerated sampling device for breast diagnosis and can also be used to completely excise benign lesions.
- All breast needle biopsy results should be discussed at prospective multidisciplinary meetings where the pathology results are correlated with the clinical and imaging findings.
- Accurate image-guided localisation and skills in wide local excision are required for the surgical treatment of impalpable breast lesions.

REFERENCES

1. NHS Cancer Screening Programmes. Available at http:\\www.cancerscreening.nhs.uk/breastscreen/index.html

   Full, detailed, up-to-date information on the performance of the NHS Breast Screening Programme, with PDF downloads available for quality assurance guidelines and annual reports.

2. Blanks RG, Moss SM, McGahan CE et al. Effects of NHS breast screening programme on mortality from breast cancer in England and Wales, 1990–8: comparison of observed with predicted mortality. Br Med J 2000; 321:1724–31.

   Review of 8 years' data on breast screening performance with discussion on the contributions of screening and improved treatment to reducing breast cancer mortality.

3. National Institute for Clinical Excellence. Guidance on cancer services. Improving outcomes in breast cancer: manual update. London: National Institute for Clinical Excellence, 2002. Available at http:\\www.nice.org.uk

   NICE recommendations for the provision of breast cancer services in England.

4. Kolb TM, Lichy J, Newhouse JH. Comparison of the performance of screening mammography, physical examination, and breast US and evaluation of factors that influemce them: an analysis of 27,825 patient evaluations. Radiology 2002; 225:165–75.

5. Lewin JM, Hendrick RE, D'Orsi CJ et al. Comparison of full-field digital mammography with screen-film mammography for cancer detection: results of 4945 paired examinations. Radiology 2001; 218:873–80.

6. Lewin JM, D'Orsi CJ, Hendrick RE et al. Clinical comparison of full-field digital mammography with screen-film mammography for detection of breast cancer. Am J Roentgenol 2002; 179:671–7.

7. Skaane P, Young K, Skjennald A. Comparison of film-screen mammography and full-field mammography with soft-copy reading in a population-based screening program: the Oslo II study. Radiology 2002; 225:267.

8. James JJ. The current status of digital mammography. Clin Radiol 2004; 59:1–10.

9. Committee on technologies for the early detection of breast cancer. Mammography and beyond: developing technologies for the early detection of breast cancer. Washington, DC: National Academy Press, 2001.

10. Legood R, Gray A. A cost comparison of full-field digital mammography with film-screen mammography in breast cancer screening. NHSBSP Equipment Report 0403. Sheffield: NHS Breast Screening Programme Publications, 2004.

11. Gur D, Sumkin JH, Rockette HE et al. Changes in breast cancer detection and mammography recall rates after the introduction of a computer-aided detection system. J Natl Cancer Inst 2004; 96:185–190.

12. Wilson ARM, Teh W. Mini Symposium: Imaging of the breast. Ultrasound of the breast. Imaging 1998; 9:169–85.

13. Lister D, Evans AJ, Burrell HC et al. The accuracy of breast ultrasound in the evaluation of clinically benign discrete breast lumps. Clin Radiol 1998; 53:490–2.

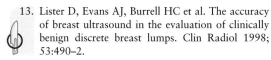

Prospective observations on the relative value of ultrasound compared with mammography in the assessment of clinically benign breast lumps.

14. Teh W, Wilson ARM. The role of ultrasound in breast cancer screening: a consensus statement for the European Group for Breast Cancer Screening. Eur J Cancer 1998; 34:449–50.

15. Damera A, Evans AJ, Cornford EJ et al. Diagnosis of axillary nodal metastases by ultrasound guided core biopsy in primary operable breast cancer. Br J Cancer 2003; 89:1310–13.

Prospective audit showing the value of axillary ultrasound and core biopsy in the preoperative detection of axillary metastatic disease.

16. Kuhl CK, Schmutzler RK, Leutner CC et al. Breast MR imaging screening in 192 women proved or suspected to be carriers of a breast cancer susceptibility gene: preliminary results. Radiology 2000; 215:267–79.

17. Warner E, Plewes DB, Shumak RS et al. Comparison of breast magnetic resonance imaging, mammography, and ultrasound for surveillance of women at high risk for hereditary breast cancer. J Clin Oncol 2001; 19:3524–31.

18. Stoutjesdijk MJ, Boetes C, Jager GJ et al. Magnetic resonance imaging and mammography in women with a hereditary risk of breast cancer. J Natl Cancer Inst 2001; 93:1095–102.

19. Brekelmans CTM, Seynaeve C, Bartels CCM et al. Effectiveness of breast cancer surveillance in BRCA1/2 gene mutation carriers and women with high familial risk. J Clin Oncol 2001; 19:924–30.

20. Olsen O, Gotzsche PC. Cochrane review on screening for breast cancer with mammography. Lancet 2001; 358:1340–2.

21. Olsen O, Gotzsche PC. Systematic review of screening for breast cancer mammography. Available at http://image.thelancet.com/lancet/extra/fullreport.pdf

22. WHO handbook on cancer prevention, 7th edn. Lyons: IARC Press, 2002.

A comprehensive review of all the available data on the effectiveness of breast cancer screening in reducing breast cancer mortality.

23. Nystrom L, Andersson I, Bjurstam N et al. Long-term effects of mammographic screening: update overview of the Swedish randomised trials. Lancet 2002; 359:909–19.

Long-term follow-up of the combined Swedish trials showing significant mortality benefit after more than 20 years.

24. Tabar L, Vitak B, Tony HH et al. Beyond randomised controlled trials: organised mammographic screening substantially reduces breast carcinoma mortality. Cancer 2001; 91:1724–31.

25. Duffy S, Tabar L, Chen HH et al. The impact of organised mammographic screening on breast carcinoma mortality in seven Swedish counties. Cancer 2002; 95:458–69.

26. Hackshaw AK, Paul EA. Breast self-examination and death from breast cancer: a meta-analysis. Br J Cancer 2003; 88:1047–53.

27. Smith RA, Saslow D, Sawyer KA et al. American Cancer Society guidelines for breast cancer screening: update 2003. CA Cancer J Clin 2003; 53:141–69.

28. Breast Screening Frequency Trial Group. The frequency of breast cancer screening: results from the UKCCCR randomized trial. Eur J Cancer 2002; 38:1458–64.

29. Million Women Study Collaborators. Breast cancer and hormone replacement therapy in the Million Women Study. Lancet 2003; 362:419–27.

Report of significantly increased risk of breast cancer in women taking HRT in the UK.

30. Perrson I, Thurfjell E, Holmberg I. Effect of estrogen and estrogen–progestin replacement regimes on mammographic breast parenchymal density. J Clin Oncol 1997; 15:3201–7.

31. Sendag F, Cosan Terek M, Ozsener S et al. Mammographic density changes during different postmenopausal hormone replacement therapies. Fertil Steril 2001; 76:445–50.

32. Evans A. Hormone replacement therapy and mammographic screening. Clin Radiol 2002; 57:563–4.

33. Litherland JC, Stallard S, Hole D, Cordiner C. The effect of hormone replacement therapy on the sensitivity of screening mammograms. Clin Radiol 1999; 54:285–8.

34. Kavanagh AM, Mitchell H, Giles GG. Hormone replacement therapy and accuracy of mammographic screening. Lancet 2000; 355:270–4.

35. Litherland JC, Evans AJ, Wilson ARM. The effect of hormone replacement therapy on recall rate in

the National Health Breast Screening Programme. Clin Radiol 1997; 52:276–9.

36. Evans AJ, Pinder SE, Ellis IO et al. Screen detected ductal carcinoma in situ (DCIS): over-diagnosis or obligate precursor of invasive disease? J Med Screen 2001; 8:149–51.

    Discussion of the likely importance to mortality reduction of the detection of high-grade DCIS through mammographic screening.

37. Evans AJ, Burrell HE, Pinder SE et al. Detecting which invasive cancers at mammographic screening saves lives? J Med Screen 2001; 8:86–90.

    Data indicating the importance of finding higher-grade invasive cancers at small size if screening is to have a significant impact on mortality reduction.

38. Robson M. Breast cancer surveillance in women with hereditary risk due to BRCA1 or BRCA2 mutations. Clin Breast Cancer 2004; 5:260–8.

39. Tilanus-Linthorst M, Verhoog L, Obdeijn I-M et al. A BRCA1/2 mutation, high breast density and prominent pushing margins of a tumour independently contribute to a frequent false-negative mammography. Int J Cancer 2002; 102:91–5.

40. Warner E, Plewes DB, Hill KA et al. Surveillance of BRCA1 and BRCA2 mutation carriers with magnetic resonance imaging, ultrasound, mammography, and clinical breast examination. JAMA 2004; 292:1317–25.

41. Hamilton LJ, Evans AJ, Wilson ARM et al. Breast imaging findings in women with BRCA1- and BRCA2-associated breast cancer. Clin Radiol 2004; 59:895–902.

42. Kriege M, Brekelmans CTM, Boetes C et al. Efficacy of MRI and mammography for breast cancer screening in women with a familial or genetic predisposition. N Engl J Med 2004; 351:427–37.

43. Teh W, Wilson ARM. Definitive non-surgical breast diagnosis: the role of the radiologist. Clin Radiol 1998; 53:81–4.

44. Britton PD. Fine needle aspiration or core biopsy. Breast 1999; 8:1–4.

    A review of the published data showing the increased sensitivity and positive predictive value of core biopsy compared with FNA for breast diagnosis.

45. Britton PD, McCann J. Needle biopsy in the NHS Breast Screening Programme 1996/7: how much and how accurate? Breast 1999; 8:5–11.

46. Vargas HI, Agbunag RV, Khaikhali I. State of the art of minimally invasive breast biopsy: principles and practice. Breast Cancer 2000; 7:370–9.

47. Heywang-Kobrunner SH, Schaumloffel U, Viehweg P et al. Minimally invasive stereotaxic vacuum core breast biopsy. Eur Radiol 1998; 8:377–85.

48. Brem RF, Schoonjans JM, Sanow L, Gatewood OM. Reliability of histologic diagnosis of breast cancer with stereotactic vacuum-assisted biopsy. Am Surg 2001; 67:388–92.

49. Parker SH, Klaus AJ, McWey PJ et al. Sonographically guided directional vacuum-assisted breast biopsy using a handheld device. Am J Roentgenol 2001; 177:405–8.

50. Kettritz U, Rotter K, Murauer M et al. Stereotactic vacuum biopsy in 2874 patients: a multicenter study. Cancer 2004; 100:245–51.

51. Brenner RJ, Bassett LW, Fajardo LL et al. Stereotactic core needle breast biopsy: a multi-institutional prospective trial. Radiology 2001; 218:866–72.

    Two large series reporting the additional diagnostic accuracy of VAM.

52. Bagnall MJC, Evans AJ, Wilson ARM et al. When have mammographic calcifications been adequately sampled at needle core biopsy? Clin Radiol 2000; 55:548–53.

53. Kuhl CK, Morakkabati N, Leutner CC et al. MR imaging-guided large-core (14-gauge) needle biopsy of small lesions visible at breast MR imaging alone. Radiology 2001; 220:31–9.

54. Fishman JE, Milikowski C, Ramsinghani R et al. US-guided core-needle biopsy of the breast: how many specimens are necessary? Radiology 2003; 226:779–82.

55. Luini A, Zurrida S, Paganelli G et al. Comparison of radioguided excision with wire localisation of occult breast lesions. Br J Surg 1999; 86:522–5.

56. Rampaul RS, Bagnall M, Burrell H et al. Radio-isotope for occult lesion localisation: results from a prospective randomised trial of ROLL versus wire guidance in occult lesions of the breast. Br J Surg 2004; 91:1575–7.

57. Rampaul RS, Burrell H, Macmillan RD, Evans AJ. Intraductal injection of the breast: a potential pitfall of radioisotope occult lesion localisation. Br J Radiol 2002; 76:425–6.

58. Patel A, Pain SJ, Britton P et al. Radioguided occult lesion localisation (ROLL) and sentinel node biopsy for impalpable invasive breast cancer. Eur J Surg Oncol 2004; 30:918–23.

59. Tanis PJ, Deurloo EE, Valdes Olmos RA et al. Single intralesional tracer dose for radio-guided excision of clinically occult breast cancer and sentinel node. Ann Surg Oncol 2001; 8:850–5.

60. Gray RJ, Giuliano R, Dauway EL et al. Radio-guidance for nonpalpable primary lesions and sentinel lymph node(s). Am J Surg 2001; 182:404–6.

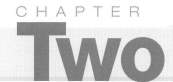

Two

Pathology and biology of breast cancer

Rajendra S. Rampaul, Sarah E. Pinder,
John F.R. Robertson and Ian O. Ellis

INTRODUCTION

Management of women with breast carcinoma has undergone significant changes over the past 20 years. We have come to understand and recognise the importance of the pathology and biology of breast cancer in influencing diagnosis, prognosticating patients, selecting primary and adjuvant treatment, formulating follow-up protocols, and providing counselling and reassurance. Screening programmes and public education have accounted for a major shift in the quantity and biology of the breast carcinomas detected today. Cancers are now of smaller size and more often lymph node negative. We are thus increasingly required to discriminate risk accurately in order to ensure judicious use of adjuvant systemic therapies.

Current data suggest that up to 70% of patients diagnosed today may not need systemic adjuvant treatment. We have demonstrated clearly that certain types of primary breast cancer have such an excellent prognosis without adjuvant treatment that they could be considered chronic rather than lethal diseases. There is an increasing emphasis on the use of prognostic factors in managing patients with breast cancer.

The three main reasons for the use of prognostic factors are to identify:

1. patients whose prognosis is so good that adjuvant systemic treatment after local surgery would not be cost beneficial;
2. patients whose prognosis is poor enough to warrant a more intensive adjuvant approach to therapy; and
3. patients whose tumours are likely to respond, or be resistant, to a particular type of therapy.

This chapter deals with the pathological prognostic factors that are important to the modern-day surgeon.

TRADITIONAL FACTORS

Lymph node stage

In surgical practice, lymph node stage has been the factor used most consistently as a guide to therapy. It is a time-dependent factor: the longer the tumour has been growing, the more likely that lymph nodes are involved by spread. Involvement of local and regional lymph nodes by metastatic carcinoma is one of the most important prognostic factors in breast cancer.[1,2] However, when used as the sole predictive factor, lymph node stage is incapable of defining either a cured group or one with close to 100% mortality from breast cancer.[3]

The clinical assessment of nodal status (as in the TNM classification) is unreliable.[4,5] Palpable nodes may be enlarged because of benign reactive changes while nodes bearing tumour deposits can be impalpable. Thus histological examination of excised axillary lymph nodes must be carried out in all patients with primary operable breast cancer. It is well known that patients who have histologically confirmed lymph node involvement have a significantly poorer prognosis than those without nodal metastases.[3,6–9] The 10-year survival is reduced from 75% for patients with no nodal involvement to 25–30% for those with metastatic disease.

The greater the number of nodes involved, the worse the prognosis.[9–11]

The level of nodal involvement may provide further useful information; metastasis to the higher-level nodes in the axilla, particularly those at the apex (level III), carries a worse prognosis.[12,13] Additionally, studies suggest that overall survival decreases as the number of nodes involved increases.[11,14,15]

Optimal management of the axilla is currently a topic of ongoing debate among surgeons and radiation oncologists.[15] All agree on the importance of obtaining prognostic information but it is important that this be achieved with as little morbidity (e.g. sensory nerve damage, lymphoedema, pain, restriction of shoulder movement) as possible. Some units favour full axillary clearance,[16,17] whereas others prefer a more limited low axillary sample or level I dissection.[18,19] One option is for patients to undergo a four-node axillary sample.

This has been shown to provide accurate prognostic information[20] and has an extremely low rate of lymphoedema; of 1275 patients, only 0.04% suffered symptomatic lymphoedema.[21]

Sampling can also provide similar prognostic information to that obtained in patients who undergo axillary clearance.[22–24]

A refinement of lymph node sampling is provided by the recently developed technique of sentinel lymph node biopsy. The concept, first introduced in 1977 by Cabanas[25] in relation to the lymphatic drainage of penile cancer, relies on the fact that if metastatic spread occurs it will first involve the sentinel node and thus biopsy of this node or nodes will provide an accurate determination of lymph node stage. In breast cancer the current method is to use blue dye and radioisotope. Several studies have examined the validity of this technique.[26] Ongoing randomised trials are examining its role in identifying those patients who have a positive sentinel node but may require no further axillary treatment, as well as those who are best treated by completion axillary dissection or are candidates for axillary radiotherapy following a positive sentinel node biopsy.

From a pathological perspective, there are unresolved questions about how best to assess the sentinel node.

Several studies have shown that the mean number of sentinel nodes is around 2–2.5.[26]

Because there are only a small number of sentinel lymph nodes and because they are one of the most important determinants of prognosis, the challenge for pathologists is to process this tissue optimally. Several methods have been studied: routine paraffin sections, intraoperative cytology and frozen section, immunohistochemistry (IHC), and more intensive methods such as serial sectioning and molecular methods such as polymerase chain reaction (PCR) and reverse transcriptase PCR.

Recently, a European working group for breast screening pathology has formulated working guidelines for the assessment and pathological work-up of sentinel lymph nodes in breast cancer. From the literature reviewed, the committee found that it is not possible as yet to determine the significance of micrometastasis or isolated tumour cells. It suggests that approximately 18% of patients have further nodal (non-sentinel node) metastases. False-negative rates are most often determined by IHC. However, at present it is recommended that such an intensive work-up is not justified on a population level. The committee suggests multilevel assessment and, where resources permit, intraoperative assessment.[27]

Tumour size

Tumour size is a time-dependent prognostic factor that has been shown in many studies to influence outcome.[3,6,7,10] In the short term, population screening with mammography will detect cancers that are different in their biological behaviour and size from those that present symptomatically (of a larger size). Patients with smaller tumours have a better long-term survival than those with larger tumours (**Fig. 2.1**). Estimation of tumour size has assumed particular importance since the introduction of population screening. The term 'minimally invasive carcinoma' (MIC) has been used to identify small tumours with a very good prognosis. In most studies the frequency of axillary lymph node metastasis in MIC is 15–20%[6,28,29] compared with over 40% in tumours measuring 15 mm or more.[30] During the prevalent round of breast screening even more favourable results are obtained, with the rate of axillary lymph node metastasis ranging from 0 to 15%.[31–34] The Nottingham Tenovus Primary Breast Cancer Study (NTPBCS) has generated data that suggest the cut-off point of 10 mm is not necessarily the best discriminator for MIC because life-table analysis of survival curves has shown no difference between tumours measuring up to 9 mm and those measuring 10–14 mm. This indicates that 15 mm may be a more realistic watershed in defining small invasive carcinomas with a good prognosis. It is clear that pathological tumour size is a valuable prognostic factor and it has become an important quality assurance measure for breast screening programmes.[33,35–38] It is also used partly to judge the ability of radiologists to detect small impalpable invasive carcinomas on mammograms.

Differentiation

At the end of the 19th century, Juan Hassiman[39] was the first to suggest a correlation between the microscopic appearance of tumours and their degree of malignancy. Modern pathologists have also recognised that invasive carcinomas can be divided according to their degree of differentiation. There are two ways to achieve this: (i) by allocating a histological type based on the architectural pattern of the tumour; and (ii) by assigning a grade of differentiation based on semiquantitative evaluation of structural characteristics.

Certain histological types of invasive carcinoma carry a favourable prognosis. Tubular,[40] mucinous,[41] invasive cribiform,[42] medullary,[43] infiltrating lobular[44] and tubulo-lobular[45] types, together with rare tumour types such as adenoid cystic carcinoma, adenomyoepithelioma and low-grade and squamous carcinoma, have all been reported to have a more favourable outcome than invasive carcinoma of no special type (ductal NST). Assessment of histological type provides important prognostic information in breast cancer. However, this effect has been shown

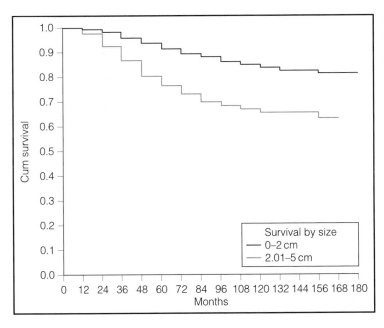

Figure 2.1 • Overall survival by size. (Data derived from the Nottingham Tenovus Primary Breast Cancer Study.)

to be relatively small when evaluated in multivariate analysis.[46] When compared with histological grade and type, differentiation may prove to be more useful in increasing our understanding of the biology of breast cancer.[47] Bloom and Richardson[48] made a useful contribution by adding numerical scoring to the method devised by Patey and Scarfe,[49] although the former system did not provide clear guidance on cut-off points. The Nottingham method was therefore devised in order to provide greater objectivity than was originally available.[50] It is now the recommended method for use in the NHS Breast Screening Programme[51] and is also approved by the European Community Breast Screening Pathology Group[38] and by the Director of Anatomical and Surgical Pathology in the USA.[52]

In the Nottingham method, three histological features are evaluated in combination: glandular (tubule) formation, nuclear polymorphism and an accurate mitotic count. There is a highly significant correlation with long-term prognosis (**Fig. 2.2**); patients with a grade 1 tumour have an 85% chance of surviving 10 years after diagnosis, whereas in patients with grade 3 tumours this is reduced to 45%. It has now been shown conclusively that the Nottingham method, with its more objective criteria, has excellent reproducibility when used by experienced pathologists.[53,54]

Lymphovascular invasion

The presence of tumour emboli in vascular spaces has emerged as an important prognostic factor.[55,56] Several studies have now shown that the presence of lymphovascular invasion correlates closely with local and regional lymph node involvement,[56,59] and it has been suggested that lymphovascular invasion can provide prognostic information as powerful as lymph node stage.[57] Reproducibility has been a limiting factor in its widespread adoption and routine clinical assessment. In our study of lymphovascular invasion, the issue of reproducibility was specifically addressed. Of the 1704 cases examined, a subset of 400 cases was examined by two or more pathologists. Analysis of interobserver variation showed overall agreement of 77% and overall agreement in the classification of lymphovascular invasion of 85.8%. Other studies have reported a similarly high concurrence among pathologists.[58–60] Therefore, although the assessment of lymphovascular invasion may be regarded as subjective, there is good evidence that a high degree of concurrence can be obtained as long as strict criteria are adhered to, essential for improving reproducibility. Lymphovascular invasion is considered a valuable surrogate for lymph node stage in cases where nodes have not been removed for examination.

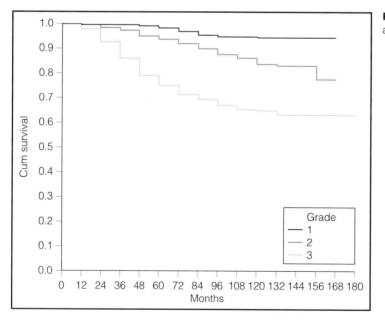

Figure 2.2 • Overall survival according to grade.

Even in patients whose axillary nodes are tumour-free on histological examination, there is a correlation between the presence of lymphovascular invasion and early recurrence.[57,61]

Miscellaneous factors

There are a number of other morphological characteristics of breast carcinoma that have been proposed as prognostic factors. However, they are less important than those already discussed.

TUMOUR NECROSIS

This is a relatively common phenomenon and can be seen occasionally as a central sharply demarcated area. It is seen most often in ductal NST carcinomas and appears to occur most frequently in those with high histological grade.[61,62] A small number of studies have evaluated the prognostic significance of tumour necrosis but the results are conflicting. Some of these data suggest that the presence of necrosis may be a poor prognostic feature; however, for this to become a useful prognostic factor, reproducible criteria for the definition of necrosis must be devised. In addition, necrosis must be tested in multivariate analysis against established factors, especially grade, with which it appears to be closely correlated.

STROMAL FIBROSIS

Stromal fibrosis is found in invasive carcinoma of the breast in varying amounts. The prognostic significance is uncertain and the presence of stromal fibrosis has been associated with a favourable prognosis.[63,64]

MOLECULAR PREDICTIVE FACTORS

The morphological prognostic factors currently in use in the routine assessment of clinical breast cancer are described above. Morphological factors are excellent predictors for survival but are unable to predict response to systemic treatments.[65] The use of strategies ranging from hormonal therapy to chemotherapy and now to novel receptor-directed therapies and vaccines depends on the expression of a range of hormonal and growth factors (estrogen/progesterone receptor, HER-2, EGFR) that not only guide treatment but also monitor response and detect

relapse. It is envisaged that molecular predictive factors could help tailor an individual's adjuvant therapy and provide information based on a genetic fingerprint to help select all aspects of care in the near future.

Estrogen receptor/progesterone receptor

Steroid receptors demonstrate an interesting irony of breast cancer. They create fertile ground for the development and metastasis of the transformed cell yet their expression and signalling pathways can be used as treatment targets. Knowledge of the expression of steroid receptors and of subcellular regulatory pathways is one of the classic examples of the use of experimental medicine to further the diagnosis and treatment of breast cancer. The degree of estrogen receptor (ER) expression is used to predict an individual's response to tamoxifen. ER and progesterone receptor (PR) are steroid receptors located in the cell nucleus. Hormones are considered to diffuse, or be transported, into the nucleus. Genes regulated by steroid receptors are involved in controlling cell growth and the current belief is that these effects are most relevant to the ER: genes regulated by the ER influence the behaviour and treatment of breast cancer. Elucidation of the downstream effect of genes influenced by hormone receptors has led to the inclusion of these genes in high-density oligonucleotide array panels. This should better define those pathways that are endocrine responsive and may lead to improved therapies with reduced adverse effects and greater potential for cure.

In unselected patients, approximately 30% will respond to endocrine therapy.

Response is seen in 50–60% of patients with ER-positive tumours compared with few if any responses in patients with truly ER-negative tumours.[66]

It has been suggested that prediction of response can be further refined by combining ER and PR assays and that ER/PR-positive tumours carry a 78% response rate while ER/PR-negative tumours respond rarely if at all. Because of its close relationship with histological grade, ER is not of independent prognostic significance.[3,66,68]

METHODS FOR MEASURING ER AND PR

There are a multitude of assay methods available, although in clinical practice most rely on two distinct strategies. The first is based on ligand binding methods (i.e. radiolabelled steroid ligand is used to detect the receptor), whereas the second relies on the recognition of the receptor protein by specific antibodies. Several studies have examined the correlation between assay and outcome/response and while at present there is no clear benefit to any one method, some studies have suggested that IHC may have a slight advantage.[69,70] Furthermore, IHC is easier to perform, ensures that only ER in malignant invasive cancer is considered and is currently the most commonly used method.

INTERPRETATION OF ASSAYS

The optimal way to score IHC for ER and PR remains controversial. At Nottingham we use an 'H' score ('histo' score), which is calculated by multiplying the frequency of positivity and the intensity of staining. An alternative scoring system adds the percentage of cells stained (score 0–5) to the intensity (score 0–3), as in the Allred scale (score 0–8); others estimate the percentage of positively stained tumour nuclei. It is important to appreciate that all these methods of interpretation are subjective and, at best, semiquantitative. In the histopathological report, ER/PR status has a clearly defined role as a predictive factor for the response of systemic endocrine therapy. ER and PR should be assessed on all invasive and non-invasive breast tumour specimens. As these assays have become simpler and less costly, it is hoped that they will be available for all patients. Progress still needs to be made in the areas of standardisation of assay technique, objectivity and reproducibility.

Histopathology of patients with *BRCA1* and *BRCA2* mutations

Patients with a genetic predisposition to breast cancer as a result of mutations in the breast cancer susceptibility genes *BRCA1* and *BRCA2* are of great clinical interest. Identification of histological features that may indicate a genetic predisposition would be useful in providing an insight into the function of these genes and may aid in identifying those in whom screening for these abnormalities would be useful. There is general agreement that *BRCA1*-related cancers are more frequently medullary carcinomas, atypical medullary carcinomas or high-grade invasive ductal carcinomas (compared with patients without this genetic alteration). Cancers associated with *BRCA1* mutations have a significantly higher mitotic rate, a larger proportion of tumour with a continuous pushing margin, and more lymphocytic infiltration than sporadic breast cancers. These are also less likely to be positive for ER and PR and are often more aneuploid, have a high S-phase fraction and show greater accumulation of p53 protein than do sporadic breast cancers.[71–76] However, it is important to appreciate that none of these features, alone or in combination, can be used to uniquely identify a cancer as *BRCA1*. Pathological features reported in *BRCA2*-related breast cancer have been less consistent.

Marcus et al.[71] noted a significantly higher proportion of tubulo-lobular cancers in *BRCA2* mutation carriers than in other patients. However, it has been reported in another study that tubular carcinomas are less common in *BRCA2* mutation carriers.[73]

Ames et al.[76] investigated the histological phenotypes of breast carcinoma in women aged less than 40 years with and without *BRCA1* and *BRCA2* germline mutations. It was found that the pleomorphic variant of invasive lobular carcinoma was related to *BRCA2* mutations. Others have reported that *BRCA2*-related cancers tend to be of high histological grade,[73,77] whereas others have not noted a significant difference in grade when *BRCA2*-related cancers are compared with controls.[78]

Type 1 growth factor receptors

Activation of a growth factor receptor was first linked to human cancer with the identification of the homology between the viral oncogene v-*erbB* and epidermal growth factor receptor (EGFR).[79] Sequence similarity to the *ERBB1* gene encoding EGFR resulted in the isolation of the human orthologue *neu* (erbB-2, HER-2).[80–82] Screening of genomic DNA and mRNAs with probes derived from these *ERBB* genes allowed isolation of two additional relatives of the human *ERB1* gene. They were subsequently named *ERBB3* (*HER3*) and *ERBB4* (*HER4*). There are four known receptors in the type 1 growth factor receptor family (HER-1, HER-2, HER-3, HER-4) and 11 ligands have been identified. The family works in a coreceptor dimerisation type activation pathway.

The first two members of this family have been extensively studied in breast cancer. There are limited data on the role of HER-3 and HER-4 as well as the ligands related to this family. This family of signalling molecules are currently of immense clinical interest as the first two members are models upon which novel bioreceptor targets are being developed (e.g. Iressa, Tarveca and Herceptin).

EGFR

EGFR is a 170-kDa transmembrane glycoprotein encoded by a gene on 7q21. EGFR expression has been well studied in breast cancer. However, because of major differences in study design, assays used and other confounding factors such as influence of adjuvant therapy, there is no consensus on its prognostic value. With the development of tyrosine kinase inhibitors (TKIs) and EGFR-directed biotherapies, there is now a growing impetus not only to standardise assays for detecting EGFR but also to accurately delineate its prognostic and predictive potential.

Methods of testing

Several techniques directed at DNA, RNA, protein (including functionally active protein) or serum can be employed to identify EGFR expression in breast cancer. Of all such methods, IHC is the most practical. The detection of EGFR by IHC has the same advantages as the detection of HER-2 by IHC, i.e. reproducibility, ease of interpretation and low cost compared with other techniques; more importantly, it can be employed on archival tissue. Nonetheless, lack of standardisation has led to differences in cut-offs, assay optimisation and types of antibody employed and these make inferences from different studies difficult. Protein levels can also be quantified by Western analysis or enzyme immunoassay, although the architecture of tissue is lost in these procedures and there may be contamination with normal tissue cells or ductal carcinoma

in situ. The technique of radioimmunohistochemistry (R-IHC) has been employed by Robertson et al.[83] In this study eight EGFR-expressing cell lines and 50 breast cancer specimens were analysed by IHC (EGFR1), R-IHC and LB assay (mouse EGF). EGFR was detected in 38% by LB, 48% by IHC and 92% by R-IHC. Compared with IHC, LB was found to correlate poorly with R-IHC. Up to 52% of EGFR-negative cases by IHC were shown to be positive by R-IHC. Recently, Eberhard et al.[85] examined a panel of antibodies and Western blot applications in a series of breast cancer specimens and three cell lines (A431, SKBr3 and MCF). Although the study was designed to assess only the sensitivity of such assays and not the prognostic value of EGFR, the authors were able to clearly demonstrate the necessity of using controls such as cell lines as results from IHC are assay dependent.

Serum EGFR levels have also been examined in patients with breast carcinoma, although these studies are few[84,85] and have used either Elisa or enzyme immunoassay technology. Because of the paucity of relevant data, it is difficult to draw conclusions about the clinical value of serum EGFR testing at present except to say that EGFR is detectable in the serum of patients.

Prognostic and predictive value

The prognostic value of EGFR in breast cancer has been examined in several large studies but there is no consensus on its prognostic value. This lack of clarity has been attributed to several factors: lack of standard assays (monoclonal vs. polyclonal), lack of cut-offs for positivity and great variation in study design (size, follow-up and influence of adjuvant therapy).[86]

Klijn et al.[87] reviewed data from over 5000 patients who were examined for EGFR status using various methods. Findings from this extensive review demonstrated great heterogeneity in study design, levels of cut-offs and, importantly, differences in prognostic value. Recently, Tsutsui et al.[88] reported on a large series of 1029 (with adjuvant therapy) and found EGFR to be of independent prognostic value irrespective of nodal status. However, Ferrero et al.[89] and Rampaul et al.[90] (without adjuvant therapy) showed EGFR to be of no prognostic value (these latter series also used grade and longer follow-up).

The predictive value of this marker for hormone resistance or responsiveness is better defined. EGFR-positive tumours are considered more resistant to endocrine therapy, whereas EGFR-negative tumours (more likely ER positive) are often sensitive to endocrine manipulation. Although some studies have been able to demonstrate EGFR status as a predictor of tamoxifen failure, others have shown response rates as high as 80%,[91] there are also conflicting results from well-designed level II studies[92] that have shown no value of EGFR in predicting the efficacy of tamoxifen in high-risk postmenopausal women.

Perhaps the most exciting use of EGFR status, and indeed the impetus for clinicians and scientists alike, is its putative role in better defining those who may respond to novel EGFR-directed therapies.

HER-2

Methods of testing

The various anti-HER-2 antibodies in use today differ with respect to epitope specificity, binding affinity and cross-reactivity with other non-HER-2 proteins. Differences in methodology and patient selection and the relationships observed in these early studies typify the problems currently encountered in recommendations for HER-2 testing strategies, and have led to conflicting data regarding prognostic and predictive characteristics. The interpretation of data can also be operator dependent and influenced by the type of assay used.

Southern blot,[93,94] slot blot,[95,96] dot blot analyses,[96,97] PCR,[98,99] in situ hybridisation[100] and fluorescence in situ hybridisation (FISH)[96] can be used to evaluate gene amplification. Northern blot analysis,[94] slot blot analysis and in situ hybridisation[95] can be used to determine mRNA overexpression, whereas Western blot analysis,[94] immunoassays[101] and IHC are employed to assess protein overexpression.[94,102–104]

Western blotting can detect HER-2 protein overexpression in both tumour cytosols and archival material but the technique is cumbersome and impractical for routine specimens. A dilution effect can be seen, as contamination of the tumour sample with non-tumour tissue can dilute HER-2 protein expression. Southern and slot blotting are similarly hampered by tumour cell DNA being diluted by DNA from benign breast tissue and

Box 2.1 Simple algorithm for HER-2 testing

Standardised validated immunohistochemistry (IHC) assay	
IHC score	**Result**
0 and 1+	Negative
2+	Borderline
3+	Positive
Fluorescence in situ hybridisation (FISH) assay	
FISH ratio	**Result**
<2.0, not amplified	Negative
>2.0, amplified	Positive

inflammatory cells, resulting in underestimation of gene amplification.

Now that the National Institute for Clinical Excellence has endorsed the use of trastuzumab for the treatment for metastatic breast cancer, there is a need to formalise testing guidelines for determining HER-2 status. Pinder and Ellis[105] have recently published updated guidelines for HER-2 testing and recommend a simple algorithm (**Box 2.1**). The debate about which test best predicts response to trastuzumab (IHC vs. FISH) is ongoing. (For an in-depth review on HER-2 testing and other clinical applications, see Rampaul et al.[106])

Prognostic significance and association with other prognostic factors

The seminal work by Slamon et al. in 1987 showed that *HER2* gene amplification independently predicted overall survival and disease-free survival in a multivariate analysis in node-positive patients.[93]

Since then, most large studies have confirmed this relationship in multivariate analysis.[107] Thus it is now well established that there is a significant correlation between HER-2 overexpression/amplification and poor prognosis for patients with nodal metastasis.[8–11,93] At present, there is no consensus on the prognostic value of HER-2 in node-negative breast cancer, a group most often diagnosed by screening programmes and one which could potentially benefit from appropriate adjuvant therapy for selected patients.

Rilke et al.[108] have reported on the prognostic significance of HER-2 expression and its relationship with other prognostic factors. They examined specimens from 1210 consecutive patients treated between 1968 and 1971 at a single institution (National Cancer Institute of Milan) who received no systemic adjuvant therapy and who were followed up for 20 years. Overexpression of HER-2 was found in 23% and showed a negative impact on survival in node-positive but not node-negative patients. Larger tumour size and higher grade (poor prognostic factors) were found to be correlated with HER-2 overexpression. Analysis of HER-2 with regard to the presence of lymphoplasmacytic infiltrate (LPI) (favourable prognosis) and nodal status demonstrated that in node-negative LPI-negative patients, HER-2 overexpression showed the same level of correlation with poor prognosis as in those patients with nodal metastasis. However, in patients with node-negative LPI-positive disease, HER-2 overexpression correlated with good prognosis. Some studies have reported a prognostic value for HER-2 in node-negative patients in selected subgroups,[109–114] whereas others have shown no correlation.[115,116]

Mirza et al. published a systematic review of prognostic factors in node-negative disease ($N = 200$, median follow-up >5 years). Conclusions for HER-2 included a lack of standardisation of assays and no association with survival.[117] However, HER-2 status was shown to be of independent prognostic significance in two large studies with long-term follow-up.[118,119] These findings will need to be prospectively validated by an independent dataset before being considered for use in the routine setting for prognostication.

There is at present no agreement on the association between HER-2 and other prognostic factors. Several studies have found no association between HER-2 status and increasing tumour size,[93,120,121] yet some have found a correlation.[108,110,116,122–125] Most studies have failed to find an association between patient age at diagnosis and HER-2 status.[93,113,116,126,127] Similar inconsistencies have been reported for aneuploidy, grade and proliferation index.[108,121,127]

Prediction of response to therapy

Hormonal therapy Transfection of normal breast cancer cells with the *HER2* gene has been shown to result in acquisition of estrogen-independent growth that is insensitive to tamoxifen.[128,129]

A number of clinical studies, using various endpoints such as increased risk for aggressive disease, time to relapse, more rapid spread to other tissues and disease-free or overall survival, have reported an association between HER-2 positivity and resistance to hormonal therapy.[130–134] Some reports have described specific resistance to tamoxifen in HER-2-overexpressing tumours.[132,133,135] The 20-year update of the Naples GUN Trial[132] found that HER-2 overexpression not only predicted resistance to tamoxifen but also that HER-2-positive patients had a worse outcome on tamoxifen therapy compared with those untreated.

Several studies have also shown that HER-2 overexpression confers a reduction in response rates to hormonal therapy. Metastatic breast cancer that overexpressed HER-2 [measured by high plasma levels of extracellular domain (ECD)] demonstrated a substantial reduction in response rate to hormonal therapy.[130] Other studies have failed to find an association or even a trend between HER-2 status and response to hormonal therapy.[136–138] Elledge et al. examined the response to tamoxifen in 205 tumours with ER positivity. In HER-2-positive compared with HER-2-negative patients, they found no significant evidence for a poorer response, time to treatment failure or survival.[137] In a more recent study, the relationship between HER-2 overexpression and response to tamoxifen was examined in the adjuvant setting in 741 (650 ER positive, 91 ER negative/PR positive) of 1572 patients in the Cancer and Leukemia Group B (CALGB) 8541 trial who had HER-2 measured.[138] Tamoxifen significantly improved response, disease-free survival and overall survival irrespective of HER-2 status. However, tamoxifen was not randomised within this trial and all patients received one of three regimens of doxorubicin. Thus there are limitations in the interpretation of these data.

Chemotherapy HER-2 status may be predictive of response to cyclophosphamide, methotrexate and 5-fluorouracil (CMF) therapy, although most of these studies were based on archival material obtained from retrospective analysis using multiple techniques and scoring methods. Initial studies examined regimens containing CMF, the results from these analyses demonstrating a reduced benefit from CMF therapy in HER-2-positive compared with HER-2-negative patients.[131,135] However, more recent studies do not support this.

A potential relationship between HER-2 status and response to anthracycline-based chemotherapy, usually doxorubicin combined with cyclo-phosphamide and 5-fluorouracil (CAF), has been addressed in several studies. In the first analysis of an interaction between expression of HER-2 and adjuvant therapy with doxorubicin-containing regimens using results from the CALGB study, Muss et al. found that tumours that overexpressed HER-2 responded well to dose-intensive CAF.[138]

Recently, additional studies have confirmed these results.[139,140] The NSABP B-11 study[139] was originally designed to compare regimens of L-phenylalanine mustard plus 5-fluorouracil with or without doxorubicin. In this trial the addition of doxorubicin improved outcome in patients with HER-2-positive tumours to the same extent as that seen in patients with HER-2-negative tumours. These data suggest a significant interaction between HER-2 overexpression and chemosensitivity to anthracyclines.

However, several studies have demonstrated no predictive value in response to anthracycline-based therapy.[141-143] Nevertheless, it is important to note that most of these had fewer patients than those showing a positive predictive value. In the study by Clahsen et al.,[141] patients received only one cycle of perioperative chemotherapy rather than the standard four or more cycles. Thus HER-2 over-expression may indicate a relative sensitivity to optimal versus suboptimal anthracycline dosage.

The predictive potential of HER-2 overexpression for response to other forms of treatment has been investigated in several studies, although the results are not definitive and further studies are required before conclusions can be drawn.

GENOMICS AND PROTEOMICS

Sequencing of the entire human genome has now been successfully completed. Cancer development is driven by the accumulation of DNA changes within this genome. DNA repair defects lead to genome-wide genetic instability and this can drive further cancer progression. **Genomics** (the study of the human genome) and **proteomics** (the analysis of the protein complement of the genome) are two branches of molecular biology that will have a major role in understanding, diagnosing, prognosticating and potentially providing therapeutic targets in breast cancer.

Genomics

MECHANISMS OF GENETIC ABERRATION

The genetic message provides the fingerprint for normal cellular processes and morphological/phenotypic expression. When this message is altered, it forms the nidus for the development and progression of cancer. These alterations can be caused by DNA mutations, chromosomal aberrations, epigenetic modification and protein interactions. DNA muta-tions can lead to a change in gene function. These mutations are often due to base substitutions and can directly cause a stop codon. As a result the gene is only partly transcribed and functional protein production is terminated. Chromosomal instability can often be due to DNA modification, mutation and viral genome integration. Chromosomal aber-rations lead to altered genes and gene expression; these aberrations can result in aneuploid (60–90 chromosomes) or near-diploid nuclei (46 chromo-somes). In solid tumours virtually all rearrangements are unbalanced, which results in a net loss or gain in certain parts of the chromosome. Using screen-ing, current losses and gains can be identified. This information can be used to investigate regions of overlap to reveal the genes involved. Gene expression can be silenced by epigenetic modification. The DNA code remains intact but the accessibility of this DNA for transcription is impaired; this process often occurs through DNA mutilation. Epigenetic modification silences genes directly by interfering with the binding of transcription factors or indirectly by changing the chromatin structure around the gene. Global hypomethylation is characteristic of the genome of a cancer cell. However, some sequences can be hypermethylated, such as CpG islands, and these tend to lie around the transcription start sites of approximately half of all human genes. DNA hypomethylation has been shown to correlate with chromosome instability.

The remodelling of chromatin architecture is essential for gene transcription and gene expression,[142] thus explaining the significance of quantitative chromatin changes.[143–145]

MOLECULAR DNA TECHNIQUES

Loss of heterozygosity can be used to identify chromosomal regions where allelic losses are more frequent. In one study,[146] a panel of 150 polymorphic microsatellite markers scattered throughout the whole genome was used to identify such regions. Data obtained were correlated with clinicopathological features and this showed that four specific loci correlated with lymph node metastasis (11q23–24, 13q12, 17p13.3 and 22q13). Microsatellites can also be used to check the ability of cells to repair DNA replication errors. Microsatellite instability can be employed to identify both genetic and epigenetic modification. It has been shown that both genetic and epigenetic alterations of *hMSH2* and *hMLH1* contribute to genomic instability and tumour genesis in sporadic breast cancer prognosis.

Comparative genomic hybridisation

Chromosomal comparative genomic hybridisation (CGH) can be used to identify the loss of one or both copies of a given gene as well as regions of amplification. In addition, the technique provides in one experiment information on the number of copies of each chromosome region throughout the whole genome. There have been several studies using CGH in breast carcinoma[147,148] and those with clinical follow-up have led to the identification of genetic changes that can be related to prognosis. However, the resolution of chromosomal CGH is limited to approximately 10 Mb. This limitation makes it difficult to link copy number changes to the genes involved. Another limitation of this technique is the need to perform karyotyping for target identification in every experiment.

Microarray CGH

Array CGH does not require a normal metaphase spread but rather an array of DNA fragments (100 bp to 100 kb) and their precise chromosomal locus. This approach can provide resolutions up to 1 Mb. Albertson et al. used this technique to map the recurrent breast cancer amplicon at chromosome 20q12.3. They were able to demonstrate that

what was previously described as a single amplicon is in fact two distinct amplicons (ZNF217 and CYP24). A novel amplicon at 17q21.3, which is implicated in the amplification and overexpression of the *HOXB7* gene in breast cancer, has been recently characterised using array CGH.[149]

Gene expression cDNA array

In gene expression profiling, each gene is usually represented by each element (created with a cDNA or oligonucleotide for the gene studied); with high-density oligonucleotide cDNA microarray technology, many thousands of gene-specific mRNAs can be examined in parallel in a single tissue sample.

The principle of gene expression cDNA array is similar to that of array CGH except that it uses oligonucleotides. Large-scale expression analysis has proved a valid strategy in developing gene expression profiles (or signatures) and these are useful in classifying tissues into pathologically prognostic subgroups.

In breast cancer, cDNA arrays have been useful in identifying distinct gene expression patterns, e.g. 'basal type' (ER positive, c-erbB-2 negative: good outcome) and 'luminal type' (ER negative, c-erbB-2 positive: worse outcome).[69] cDNAs have been used to distinguish cancers with *BRCA1*/*BRCA2* mutations[150–152] and to determine ER status,[153] lymph node status[154,155] and prognostic subgroups in node-negative breast cancer.[156] These recent studies demonstrate the ability of cDNA to have a direct use in clinical practice.[150]

Proteomics

Proteomics is quickly evolving to provide critical supportive information to data generated by genomic approaches in high-throughput formats such as array CGH, cDNA arrays and whole-genome approaches to identify low penetrance genes. The genetic code does not indicate which proteins are expressed or, if they are expressed, whether they are functional. Post-translational modifications such as glycosylation or phosphorylation will enable us to not only identify phenotypic differences between normal and malignant cells but also to subclassify within malignancies.

Several proteomic techniques are in use, again almost exclusively within the remit of the research laboratory, e.g. two-dimensional polyacrylamide gel electrophoresis, surface-enhanced laser desorption ionisation and matrix-associated laser desorption ionisation–time of flight. There are excellent reviews on the methodologies of these techniques.[157]

Tissue microarray deserves a special mention here. The technique allows for a composite slide of up to 1000 cores of tissue to be included in one paraffin block (**Fig. 2.3**; see Plate 1, facing p. 116). The advantages are obvious in screening for novel protein expression.

However, there are concerns about whether cores are representative samples, and indeed this aspect has not been well researched. Only one study has examined a large sample size of corresponding whole sections and correlated these with the tissue microarrays.[158]

This technology and its application has been extensively covered in a recent review.[159]

Clinical use of genomics and proteomics

In the future, it is envisaged that gene expression profiles may be able to guide decisions on the choice of hormonal or chemotherapeutic agent for each individual. Presently, one of the best examples of the use of genomics and proteomics in clinical practice is the use of HER-2 expression/amplification to select patients for trastuzumab therapy. Such profiles are useful for identifying prognostically significant genes, which some studies have demonstrated can perform better than traditional markers.[148,156]

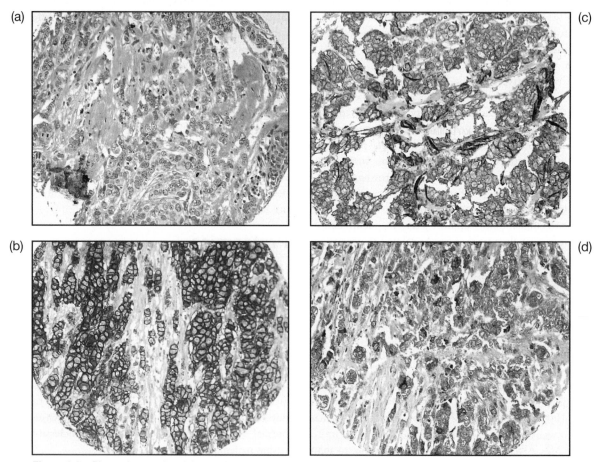

Figure 2.3 • Photomicrographs of tissue microarray discs: staining is for receptors of the erbB family.

Perou et al.[150] used cDNA arrays with 800 genes to examine 65 breast biopsies. They were able to correctly identify primary clusters with the following characteristics: ER positive and a luminal cell pattern of gene expression; ER negative with a myoepithelial cell pattern of gene expression; and HER-2 positive. A fourth group clustered with normal tissue.

In metastatic disease, expression patterns can be used to establish the primary lesion in patients with more than one primary. Proteomics have begun to assume a role in the monitoring of response and prediction of both resistance and relapse in patients treated with novel biodirected therapies.[160]

Transcription profiling has also been shown to accurately differentiate breast cancers with germ-line mutations in *BRCA1/BRCA2* from those without such mutations. Such findings, if validated in other studies, open the way for molecular pheno-typing in high-risk families.

The most convincing study to date has been reported by van't Veer et al.[152] Expression profiles of 117 primary breast cancers were compared with known prognostic factors and matched with 5 years of follow-up data. A total of 25 000 genes were used to generate expression profiles, which separated the tumours into two groups: 34% of group 1 and 70% of group 2 developed distant metastasis. From the 25 000 gene set, 70 had the greatest accuracy in predicting recurrent disease. Multivariate analysis with grade, size, vascular invasion, age and ER showed the poor-prognosis microarray profile to be an independent predictor of recurrent disease. This approach was further tested in 295 patients and again use of gene profiling was able to accurately identify a poor-prognosis group.[150,152]

CLINICAL USE OF PROGNOSTIC FACTORS IN PATIENT MANAGEMENT

Prognosis in breast cancer depends on the presence of disease spread and on the inherent aggressiveness or virulence of the tumour. The latter depends on a number of intrinsic biological characteristics, some of which have already been evaluated, such as morphological features, growth rate and hormone responsiveness. Accurate prognostication is now required on an individual patient basis and this can only be achieved by using a prognostic index that includes both time-dependent and biological factors. The best way to obtain such an index is to take potential factors that have been shown to have some value in univariate analysis and submit them to multivariate analysis. This has been the approach in deriving the Nottingham Prognostic Index (NPI),[3,68,161] which is based on three factors using the following formula:

NPI = pathological tumour size (cm) × 0.2 + lymph node stage (1, 2 or 3) + histological grade (1, 2 or 3)

Arbitrary cut-off points of 2.4, 3.4, 4.4, 5.4 and 6.4 are used to divide patients into six prognostic groups: excellent (EPG), good (GPG), moderate (MPG) I and II, poor (PPG) and very poor (VPG) (**Tables 2.1–2.3, Figs 2.4** and **2.5**).

The NPI provides extremely powerful prognostic information within the NTPBCS and has been able to demonstrate its utility and reproducibility in studies from other centres. In this respect, Henson et al. in a retrospective analysis of prognostic data in over 22 000 women from the SEER Programme of the National Cancer Institute in the USA confirmed that a combination of lymph node stage and histological grade improved prediction of prognosis. In a similar way to the NTPBCS, Chevallier et al.[162] have identified 'young' age, tumour size and histological grade as factors which added to lymph

Table 2.1 • Nottingham Prognostic Index showing percentage in each prognostic group

	1980–86	1990–99
EPG	12	14
GPG	19	21
MPGI	29	28
MPGII	24	22
PPG	11	11
VPG	5	4

See text for explanation of prognostic groups.

Table 2.2 • Differences in 10-year survival for each prognostic group

	10-year survival (%)	±95% CL	P (log rank)
EPG	96	2	0.14
GPG	93	4	<0.0001
MPGl	82	4	0.0007
MPGII	75	4	<0.0001
PPG	53	8	0.003
VPG	39	12	
All groups	80	2	

See text for explanation of prognostic groups.

node stage in the prediction of recurrence; these factors were used to divide lymph node-negative patients into three prognostic groups.

One of the strengths of the NPI is the fact that it has been verified prospectively in the NTPBCS.[3,161] Further confirmation of its value has been provided by its validation in two large multicentre studies involving nearly 11 000 patients in total.[163,164] Furthermore, in both studies histological grading was carried out by general hospital pathologists, confirming its robustness as a prognostic factor. Such studies demonstrate the inherent power of the pathological factors used in the NPI, which has become the most widely used index for the management of patients with breast cancer in the UK.

CONTENTS OF THE FINAL SURGICAL PATHOLOGY REPORT: THE MINIMUM DATASET

The Royal College of Pathologists minimum dataset for breast cancer was originally developed in recognition that certain histopathological features of both in situ and invasive carcinoma are directly related to clinical outcome and may therefore be important in deciding the most appropriate treatment, including extent of surgery and use and choice of adjuvant therapy. In addition, histopathological features can be used to monitor breast screening programmes, the success of which is reflected by more favourable prognostic features of the cancers detected and also changing patterns of disease, particularly identified by cancer registries.

The minimum set of data should be used by pathologists reporting all breast cancers, both screen detected and those presenting symptomatically. The Royal College of Pathologists minimum dataset has been approved by the NHS Breast Screening Programme, the European Commission Working Group, the British Association of Surgical Oncologists, the British Breast Group and the United Kingdom Association of Cancer Registries (**Fig. 2.6**).

Table 2.3 • Relative risk reduction (RRR) by Nottingham Prognostic Index

	1980–86	±95% CL	1990–99	±95% CL	RRR (death)	%ARR (death)
EPG	88	6	96	2	0.67	8
GPG	72	8	93	4	0.75	21
MPGl	61	6	82	4	0.54	21
MPGII	42	6	75	4	0.57	35
PPG	14	8	53	8	0.45	39
VPG	12	10	39	12	0.31	27
All groups	55		80		0.56	25

See text for explanation of prognostic groups.
ARR, absolute risk reduction.

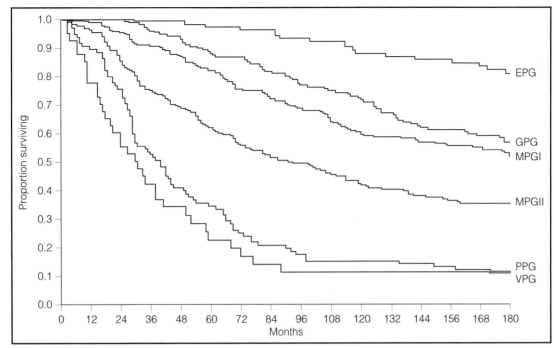

Figure 2.4 • Survival by Nottingham Prognostic Index (1980–86). See text for explanation of abbreviations.

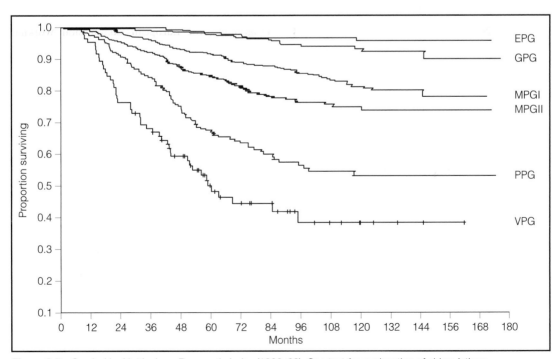

Figure 2.5 • Survival by Nottingham Prognostic Index (1990–99). See text for explanation of abbreviations.

Breast cancer histopathology minimum dataset.

Surname........................Forenames..........................Date of birth............

Sex...... Hospital............ Hospital No............ NHS No............

Date of receipt........................ Date of reporting .... Report No......................

Side: [ ] Right [ ] Left   Pathologist................. Surgeon ....

Specimen type: [ ] Diagnostic localisation biopsy   [ ] Diagnostic open biopsy

[ ] Therapeutic excision   [ ] Mastectomy

Specimen weight ....g

Axillary procedure: [ ] Lymph node sample [ ] Axillary clearance [ ] Sentinel node biopsy

----

Non-invasive malignant lesion [ ] Not present

[ ] Ductal,high grade   [ ] Ductal,intermediate grade   [ ] Ductal,low grade

Growth pattern(s): [ ] Solid   [ ] Cribriform [ ] Micropapillary [ ] Papillary

[ ] Apocrine   [ ] Flat/ clinging   [ ] Other

Size (pure DCIS only)..........................mm

[ ] Paget's disease of the nipple

[ ] Lobular neoplasia

Microinvasion: [ ] Not present [ ] Present [ ] Possible

Invasive carcinoma   [ ] Not present

Grade: [ ] ^{I} [ ]^{II} [ ]^{III} [ ] Not assessable

[ ] Ductal / no specific type (NST)   [ ] Tubular carcinoma   [ ] Lobular carcinoma

[ ] Mucinous carcinoma   [ ] Medullary type carcinoma

[ ] Mixed (please tick component types present)   [ ] Not assessable

[ ] Other primary carcinoma (please specify)...

[ ] Other malignant tumour (please specify)...

Maximum diameter of invasive tumour ....mm

Whole size of tumour (to include DCIS extending >1mm beyond invasive area)............mm

Vascular invasion (blood or lymphatic) [ ] Present   [ ] Possible   [ ] Not seen

----

For DCIS and invasive carcinoma

Excision margins: [ ] Reaches margin [ ] Uncertain   [ ] Does not reach margin

Nearest (surgically relevant) margin ....mm

Axillary nodes received: [ ] Yes [ ] No Number positive........... Total number...........

Other nodes received: [ ] Yes [ ] No Number positive........... Total number...........

Site of the nodes..

Estrogen receptor status: [ ] Positive   [ ] Negative   [ ] Not known

Figure 2.6 • Breast cancer histopathology minimum dataset.

REFERENCES

1. Breast Cancer Trialists' Collaborative Group. Systemic treatment of early breast cancer by hormonal, cytotoxic or immunotherapy. Lancet 1992; 339:1–15.

2. Robertson JFR, Bates K, Pearson D et al. Comparison of two oestrogen receptor assays in the prediction of the clinical course of patients with advanced breast cancer. Br J Cancer 1992; 65:727–30.

3. Galea MH, Blamey RW, Elston CW et al. The Nottingham Prognostic Index in primary breast cancer. Breast Cancer Res Treat 1992; 22:207–19.

4. Robertson JFR, Ellis IO, Pearson D et al. Biological factors of prognostic significance in locally advanced breast cancer. Breast Cancer Res Treat 1994; 29:259–64.

5. National Co-ordinating Group for Breast Screening Pathology. Pathology reporting in breast screening pathology, 2nd edn. Sheffield: NHSBSP Publications no. 3, 1995.

6. Carter GL, Allen C, Henson DE. Relation of tumour size, lymph node status, and survival in 24,740 breast cancer cases. Cancer 1989; 63:181–7.

7. Elston CW, Gresham GA, Rao GS et al. The Cancer Research Campaign (Kings/Cambridge) trial for early breast cancer: pathological aspects. Br J Cancer 1982; 45:655–69.

8. Fisher ER, Sass R, Fisher B et al. Pathologic findings from the National Surgical Adjuvant Project for breast cancer (protocol no 4). Discrimination for tenth year treatment failure. Cancer 1984; 53:712–23.

9. Neville AM, Bettelheim R, Gelber RD et al. Predicting treatment responsiveness and prognosis in node-negative breast cancer. J Clin Oncol 1992; 10:696–705.

10. Hartman WH. Minimal breast cancer: an update. Cancer 1984; 53:681–4.

11. Rampaul RS, Evans AJ, Ellis IO et al. Long term regional recurrence and survival after axillary nodal sampling for breast cancer (abstract). Eur J Cancer 2003; 1:23.

12. Clark GM. Integrating prognostic factors. Breast Cancer Res Treat 1992; 22:187–91.

13. Bedwani R, Vana J, Rosner D et al. Management and survival of female patients with 'minimal' breast cancer: as observed in the long-term and short-term surveys of the American College of Surgeons. Cancer 1981; 47:2769–78.

14. Shukla HS, Melhuish J, Mansel RE, Hughes LE. Does local therapy affect survival rates in breast cancer? Ann Surg Oncol 1999; 6:455–60.

15. Macmillan RD, Rampaul RS, Lewis S, Evans AJ. Preoperative ultrasound-guided node biopsy and sentinel node augmented node sample is best practice. Eur J Cancer 2004; 40:176–8.

16. Rosen PP, Groshen S. Factors influencing survival and prognosis in early breast carcinoma (T1N0M0–T1N1M0). Assessment of 644 patients with median follow up of 19 years. Surg Clin North Am 1990; 70:937–62.

17. Beahrs OH, Shapiro S, Smart C et al. Summary report of the working group to review the National Cancer Institute–American Cancer Society Breast Cancer Demonstration Detection Projects. J Natl Cancer Inst 1979; 62:641–709.

18. Gibbs NM. Comparative study of the histopathology of breast cancer in a screened and unscreened population investigated by mammography. Histopathology 1985; 9:1307–18.

19. Tabar L, Duffy SW, Krusemo UB. Detection method, tumour size and node metastases in breast cancers diagnosed during a trial of breast cancer screening. Eur J Cancer Clin Oncol 1987; 23:959–62.

20. Rampaul RS, Pinder SE, Elston CW, Ellis IO. Prognostic and predictive factors in primary breast cancer and their role in patient management: the Nottingham Breast Team. Eur J Surg Oncol 2001; 27:229–38.

21. Rampaul RS, Mullinger K, Macmillan RD et al. Incidence of clinically significant lymphoedema as a complication following surgery for primary operable breast cancer. Eur J Cancer 2003; 39:2165–7.

22. Frisell J, Eklund G, Hellström L, Somell A. Analysis of interval breast carcinomas in a randomized screening trial in Stockholm. Breast Cancer Res Treat 1987; 17:219–25.

23. Royal College of Radiologists. Quality assurance guidelines for radiologists. Sheffield: NHSBSP Publication no. 15, 1990.

24. Royal College of Radiologists. Quality assurance guidelines for radiologists. Sheffield: NHSBSP Publication no. 15, 1997.

25. Cabanes PA, Salmon RJ, Vilcoq JR et al. Value of axillary dissection in addition to lumpectomy and radiotherapy in early breast cancer. Lancet 1992; 339:1245–8.

26. Mansel RE, Goyal A, Newcombe RG. Internal mammary node drainage and its role in sentinel lymph node biopsy: the initial ALMANAC experience. Clin Breast Cancer 2004; 5:279–84.

27. Cserni G, Amendoeira I, Apostolikas N et al. Discrepancies in current practice of pathological evaluation of sentinel nodes in breast cancer. Results of a questionnaire based survey by the European Working Group for Breast Screening Pathology. J Clin Path 2004, 57:695–701.

28. O'Dwyer PJ. Axillary dissection in primary breast cancer: the benefits of node clearance warrant reappraisal. Br Med J 1992; 302:360–1.

29. Blamey RW. Clinical aspects of malignant disease. In: Elston CW, Ellis IO (eds) Systemic pathology: the breast, 3rd edn. London: Churchill Livingstone, 1998; pp. 501–13.

30. Henson DE, Ries L, Freedman LS, Carriaga M. Relationship among outcome stage of disease and histologic grade for 22,616 cases of breast cancer. Breast Cancer Res Treat 1991; 22:207–19.

31. Kutianawala MA, Sayed M, Stotter A et al. Staging the axilla in breast cancer: an audit of lymph-node retrieval in one UK regional centre. Eur J Surg Oncol 1998; 24:280–2.

32. Steele RJC, Forrest APM, Gibson T. The efficacy of lower axillary sampling in obtaining lymph node status in breast cancer: a controlled randomized trial. Br J Surg 1985; 72:368–9.

33. Dixon JM, Dillon P, Anderson TJ, Chetty U. Axillary sampling in breast cancer: an assessment of its efficacy. Breast 1998; 7:206–8.

34. Cabanas RM. An approach for the treatment of penile carcinoma. Cancer 1977; 39:456–66.

35. Morton DL, Wen D-R, Wong JH et al. Technical details of intraoperative lymphatic mapping for early stage melanoma. Arch Surg 1992; 127:392–9.

36. Alex JC, Weaver DL, Fairbank JT et al. Gamma probe guided lymph node localisation in malignant melanoma. Surg Oncol 1993; 2:303–8.

37. Giuliano AE, Kirgan DM, Guenther JM, Morton DL. Lymphatic mapping and sentinel lymphadenectomy for breast cancer. Ann Surg 1994; 220:391–401.

38. Albertini JJ, Lyman GH, Cox C et al. Lymphatic mapping and sentinel node biopsy in the patient with breast cancer. JAMA 1996; 276:1818–22.

39. Carstens PHB, Greenberg RA, Francis D, Lyon H. Tubular carcinoma of the breast. A long-term follow-up. Histopathology 1985; 9:271–80.

40. Veronesi U, Zurrida S, Galimberti V. Consequences of sentinel node in clinical decision making in breast cancer and prospect for future studies. Eur J Surg Oncol 1998; 24:93–5.

41. Dixon M. Sentinel node biopsy in breast cancer. Br Med J 1998; 317:295–6.

42. McMasters KM, Giuliano AE, Ross MI et al. Sentinel-lymph node biopsy for breast cancer: not yet the standard of care. N Engl J Med 1998; 339:990–5.

43. McIntosh SA, Puroshotham AD. Lymphatic mapping and sentinel node biopsy in breast cancer. Br J Surg 1998; 85:1347–56.

44. Anderson TJ. The challenge of sentinel lymph node biopsy. Histopathology 1999; 35:82–4.

45. Goyal A, Newcombe RG, Mansel RE. Clinical relevance of multiple sentinel nodes in patients with breast cancer. Br J Surg 2005; 92:438–42.

46. Rosen PP, Groshen S, Saigo S et al. Pathological prognostic factors in stage I (T1N0M0) and stage II (T1N1M0) breast carcinoma: a study of 644 patients with median follow-up of 18 years. J Clin Oncol 1989; 7:1239–51.

47. Parker C, Rampaul RS, Pinder SE et al. E-cadherin as a prognostic indicator in primary breast cancer. Br J Cancer 2001; 85:1958–63.

48. Rosz PP. Tumor emboli in intramammary lymphatics in breast carcinoma: pathological criteria for diagnosis and clinical significance. Pathol Annu 1983; 18:215–32.

49. Davis BW, Gelber R, Goldhirsh A et al. Prognostic significance of peritumoral vessel invasion in clinical trials of adjuvant therapy for breast cancer with axillary node metastases. Hum Pathol 1985; 16:1212–18.

50. Roses DF, Bell DA, Fotte TJ et al. Pathologic predictors of recurrence in stage 1 (T1N0M0 and T2N0M0) breast cancer. Am J Clin Pathol 1982; 78:817–20.

51. O'Rourke S, Galea MH, Euhus D et al. An audit of local recurrence after simple mastectomy. Br J Surg 1994; 81:386–9.

52. Fisher ER, Palekar AS, Gregorio RM et al. Pathologic findings from the National Surgical Adjuvant Project for breast cancers (protocol no 4). IV. Significance of tumour necrosis. Hum Pathol 1978; 9:523–30.

53. Carter D, Elkins RC, Pipkin RD et al. Relationship of necrosis and tumour border to lymph node metastases and 10 year survival in carcinoma of the breast. Am J Surg Pathol 1978; 2:39–46.

54. Parham DM, Hagen N, Brown RA. Morphometric analysis of breast carcinoma: association with survival. J Clin Pathol 1988; 41:173–7.

55. Underwood JCE. A morphometric analysis of human breast carcinoma. Br J Cancer 1972; 26:234–7.

56. Parfrey NA, Doyle CT. Elastosis in benign and malignant breast disease. Hum Pathol 1985; 16:674–6.

57. Sistrunk WE, MacCarty WC. Life expectancy following radical amputation for carcinoma of the breast: a clinical and pathological study of 218 cases. Ann Surg 1922; 75:61–9.

58. NIH Consensus Development Conference. Steroid receptors in breast cancer. Cancer 1980; 46:2759–963.

59. Haybittle JL, Blamey RW, Elston CW et al. A prognostic index in primary breast cancer. Br J Cancer 1982; 45:361–6.

60. Ellis IO, Bell J, Todd J et al. Evaluation of immuno-reactivity with monoclonal antibody NCRC-II in breast carcinoma. Br J Cancer 1987; 56:295–9.

61. Devine PL, McKenzie IFC. Mucins: structure, function, and association with malignancy. Bioessays 1992; 14:619–25.

62. Poller DN, Hutchings CE, Galea M et al. p53 protein expression in human breast cancer: relationship to expression of epidermal growth factor, C-erbB-2 protein overexpression, and oestrogen receptor. Br J Cancer 1992; 66:583–8.

63. Harris AL. What is the biological, prognostic, and therapeutic role of the EGF receptor in human breast cancer? Breast Cancer Res Treat 1994; 29:1–2.

64. Lovekin C, Ellis IO, Locker A et al. C-erbB-2 oncoprotein in primary and advanced breast cancer. Br J Cancer 1991; 63:439–43.

65. Barnes DM, Dublin EA, Fisher CJ et al. Immunohistochemical detection of p53 protein in mammary carcinoma: an important new independent indicator of prognosis? Hum Pathol 1993; 24:469–76.

66. Walker RA, Senior PV, Jones JL et al. An immunohistochemical and in situ hybridization study of c-myc and c-erbB-2 expression in primary human breast carcinomas. J Pathol 1989; 158:97–105.

67. Walker RA, Camplejohn RS. DNA flow cytometry of human breast carcinomas and its relationship to transferrin and epidermal growth factor receptors. J Pathol 1986; 150:37–42.

68. Dowle CS, Owainati A, Robins A et al. The prognostic significance of the DNA content of human breast cancer. Br J Surg 1987; 74:133–6.

69. Elston CE, Ellis IO. Pathologic factors in primary operable breast cancer. In: Elston CW, Ellis IO (eds) The Breast, 3rd edn. Edinburgh: Churchill Livingstone, 1998; pp. 1209–12.

70. Snead DRJ, Goulding H, Pinder SE et al. Is combined progesterone and oestrogen receptor (PR and ER) status better than ER alone in predicting hormone sensitivity in breast cancer? J Pathol 1997; 181:5A.

71. Marcus JN, Watson P, Page DL. Hereditary breast cancer. Pathobiology, prognosis and BRCA1 and BRCA2 linkage. Cancer 1996; 77:967–709.

72. Marcus JN, Page DL, Watson P et al. BRCA1 and BRCA2 hereditary breast cancer phenotypes. Cancer 1997; 80:543–556.

73. Breast Cancer Linkage Consortium. Pathology of familial breast cancer: differences between breast cancer in carriers of BRCA1 or BRCA2 mutations and sporadic cases. Lancet 1997; 349:1505–7.

74. Robson M, Gilewski T, Haas B et al. BRCA-associated breast cancer in young women. J Clin Oncol 1998; 16:1642–9.

75. Karp SE, Tonin PN, Begin LR et al. Influence of BRCA1 mutations on nuclear grade and oestrogen receptor status of breast carcinoma in Ashkenazi Jewish women. Cancer 1997; 80:435–41.

76. Armes JE, Egan AJM, Southey MC et al. The histologic phenotypes of breast carcinoma occurring before age 40 in women with and without BRCA1 or BRCA2 germline mutations. Cancer 1998; 83:2335–9.

77. Agnarsson BA, Jonasson JG, Bjornsdottir IB et al. Inherited BRCA2 mutation associated with high grade breast cancer. Breast Cancer Res Treat 1998; 47:121–7.

78. Marcus JN, Watson P, Page DL et al. BRCA2 hereditary breast cancer phenotype. Breast Cancer Res Treat 1997; 44:275.

79. Downward J, Yarden Y, Mayes E et al. Close similarity of epidermal growth factor receptor and v-erb-B oncogene protein sequences. Nature 1984; 307:521–7.

80. Coussens L, Yang Feng TI, Liao YC et al. Tyrosine kinase receptor with extensive homology to EGF receptor shares chromosomal location with neu oncogene. Science 1985; 230:1132–9.

81. King CR, Kraus MH, Aaronson SA. Amplification of a novel v-erb-B related gene in a human mammary carcinoma. Science 1985; 229:974–6.

82. Yamamoto T, Ikawa S, Akiyama T et al. Similarity of protein encoded by the human c-erbB-2 gene to epidermal growth factor receptor. Nature 1986; 319:230–4.

83. Robertson KW, Reeves JR, Lannigan AK et al. Radioimmunohistochemistry of epidermal growth factor in breast cancer. Arch Pathol Lab Med 2001; 126:177–81.

84. Kumar RR, Meenakshi A et al. Enzyme immunoassay of human epidermal growth factor. Hum Antibodies 2001; 10:143–7.

85. Eberhard DA, Huntzicker E, Anderson S et al. Epidermal growth factor receptor immunohistochemistry: assay selection and amplification to breast cancers (abstract). Proc Am Soc Clin Oncol 2002: abs. 1791.

86. Rampaul RS, Pinder SE, Nicholson RI, Gullick WJ et al. Clinical value of epidermal growth factor receptor expression in primary breast cancer. Adv Anat Path (in press).

87. Klijn JGM, Berns PMJ, Schmitz PI et al. The clinical significance of epidermal growth factor receptor in human breast cancer: a review of 5232 patients. Endocr Rev 1992; 13:3–17.

88. Tsutsui S, Ohno S, Murakami S et al. Prognostic value of epidermal growth factor and its relationship to the ER status of 1029 patients with breast cancer. Breast Cancer Res Treat 2002; 71:67–75.

89. Rampaul RS, Pinder SE, Robertson JF et al. EGFR expression in operable breast cancer: is it of prognostic significance? Clin Cancer Res 2004; 10:2578.

90. Ferrero JM, Ramaioli A, Largillier R et al. Epidermal growth factor receptor expression in 780 breast cancer patients: a reappraisal of the prognostic value based on an eight-year median follow-up. Ann Oncol 2001; 12:835–41.

91. Nicholson RI, McCelland RA, Gee JMW et al. Epidermal growth factor receptor expression in breast cancer. Association with response to endocrine therapy. Breast Cancer Res Treat 1994; 29:117–25.

92. Knoop A, Bentzen SM, Nielsen MM et al. Value of epidermal growth factor receptor, HER-2, p53 and steroid receptors in predicting the efficacy of tamoxifen in high risk postmenopausal breast cancer patients. J Clin Oncol 2001; 19:3376–84.

93. Slamon DJ, Clark GM, Wong SG et al. Human breast cancer: correlation of relapse and survival with amplification of the HER-2/neu oncogene. Science 1987; 235:177–82.

94. Slamon DJ, Godolphin W, Jones LA et al. Studies of the Her-2 proto-oncogene in human breast and ovarian cancer. Science 1989; 244:707–12.

95. Naber SP, Tsutsumi Y, Yin S et al. Strategies for the analysis of oncogene overexpression. Studies of the neu oncogene in breast carcinoma. Am J Clin Pathol 1990; 94:125–36.

96. Kallioniemi OP, Kallioniemi A, Kurisu W et al. ERBB2 amplification in breast cancer analysed by fluorescence in situ hybridization. Proc Natl Acad Sci USA 1992; 89:5321–5.

97. Seshadri R, Figaira FA, Horsfall DJ et al. Clinical significance of Her-2/neu oncogene amplification in primary breast cancer. J Clin Oncol 1993; 11:1936–42.

98. Gramlitch TL, Cohen C, Fritsch C et al. Evaluation of Cerb-2 amplification in breast carcinoma by differential polymerase chain reaction. Am J Clin Pathol 1994; 101:493–9.

99. Youngson BJ, Anelli A, Van Zee KJ et al. Micro-dissection and molecular genetic analysis of Her-2 in breast carcinoma. Am J Surg Pathol 1995; 19:1354–8.

100. Smith KL, Robbins PD, Dawkins HJ et al. Cerb-2 amplification in breast cancer: detection in formalin-fixed, paraffin embedded tissue by in situ hybridization. Hum Pathol 1994; 25:413–18.

101. Dittadi R, Brazzale A, Pappagallo G et al. ErbB 2 assay in breast cancer: possible improved clinical information using a quantitative method. Anticancer Res 1997; 17:1245–7.

102. Singleton TP, Niehans GA, Gu F et al. Detection of Cerb 2 activiation in paraffin- embedded tissue by immmunohistochemistry. Hum Pathol 1992; 23:1141–50.

103. Kerns BJ, Jordan PA, Huper G et al. Assessment of C erb-2 amplification by immunohistochemistry in paraffin-embedded breast cancer. Mod Pathol 1993; 6:673–8.

104. Press MF, Hung G, Godolphin W et al. Sensitivity of Her-2/neu antibodies in archival tissue samples: potential source of error in immunohistochemical studies of oncogene expression. Cancer Res 1994; 54:2771–7.

105. Pinder SE, Ellis IO. Recommendations for HER-2 testing. Immunocytochemistry 2003; 2:6–9.

106. Rampaul RS, Pinder SE, Robertson JF, Ellis IO. HER-2 expression in breast cancer: methods of detection. Crit Rev Oncol Hematol 2002; 43:231–44.

107. Ross JS, Fletcher JA. The HER-2/neu oncogene in breast cancer: prognostic factor, predictive factor, and target for therapy. Stem Cells 1998; 16:413–28.

108. Rilke F, Colnaghi MI, Cascinelli N et al. Prognostic significance of Her-2/neu expression in breast cancer and its relationship to other prognostic factors. Int J Cancer 1991; 49:44–9.

109. Collan Y, Haapasalo H. The value of mitotic counting in the assessment of prognosis and proliferation in human tumours. J Pathol 1991; 163:361–2.

110. Borg Å, Tandon AK, Sigurdsson H. Her2/neu amplification predicts poor survival in node-positive breast cancer. Cancer Res 1990; 50:4330–7.

111. Wright C, Angus B, Nicholson S et al. Expression of c erb B-2 oncoprotein: a prognostic indicator in human breast cancer. Cancer Res 1989; 49:2087–90.

112. Dati C, Muraca R, Tazartes O et al. c-erbB-2 and ras expression levels in breast cancer are correlated and show a co-operative association with unfavorable clinical outcome. Int J Cancer 1991; 47:833–8.

113. Borg Å, Baldetorp B, Fernö M et al. ERBB2 amplification is associated with tamoxifen resistance in steroid-receptor positive breast cancer. Cancer Lett 1994; 81:137–44.

114. Paik S, Hazan R, Fisher ER et al. Pathologic findings from the National Surgical Adjuvant Breast and Bowel Project: prognostic significance of erbB-2 protein overexpression in breast cancer. J Clin Oncol 1990; 8:103–12.

115. Bianchi S, Paglierani M, Zampi G et al. Prognostic significance of CerbB-2 expression in node negative breast cancer. Br J Cancer 1993; 67:625–9.

116. Clark GM, McGuire WL. Follow-up study of HER-2/neu amplification in primary breast cancer. Cancer Res 1991; 51:944–8.

117. Rampaul RS, Pinder SE, Elston CW et al. Prognostic significance of HER-2 in node negative breast cancer (abstract). Eur J Cancer 2001; 37:5.

118. Mirza AN, Mirza NQ, George V, Eva SS. Prognostic factors in node negative breast cancer: a review of studies with sample size more than 200 and follow-up more than 5 years. Ann Surg 2002; 235:10–26.

119. Volpi A, Nanni O, De Paola F et al. HER-2 expression and cell proliferation: prognostic markers in patients with node-negative breast cancer. J Clin Oncol 2003; 14:2708–12.

120. Yamashita J, Ogawa M, Sakai K. Prognostic significance of three novel biologic factors in a clinical trial of adjuvant therapy for node-negative breast cancer. Surgery 1995; 117:601–8.

121. Molina R, Ciocca DR, Tandon AK et al. Expression of HER-2/neu oncoprotein in human breast cancer: a comparison of immunohistochemical and Western blot techniques. Anticancer Res 1992; 12:1965–71.

122. Van de Vijver MJ, Peterse JL, Mooi WJ et al. Neu-protein over-expression in breast cancer. Association with comedo-type ductal carcinoma in situ and limited prognostic value in stage II breast cancer. N Engl J Med 1988; 319:1239–45.

123. Borg Å, Baldetorp B, Fernö M et al. ERBB2 amplification in breast cancer with a high rate of proliferation. Oncogene 1991; 6:137–43.

124. Arguello F, Baggs RB, Eskenazi AE et al. Vascular anatomy and organ-specific tumor growth as critical factors in the development of metastases and their distribution among organs. Int J Cancer 1991; 48:583–90.

125. Schonborn I, Zschiesche W, Spitzer E et al. C-erbB2 overexpression in primary breast cancer: independent prognostic factor in patients at high risk. Breast Cancer Res Treat 1994; 29:287–95.

126. Benz CC, Scott GK, Sarup JC et al. Estrogen-dependent, tamoxifen- resistant tumorigenic growth of MCF-7 cells transfected with Her-2/neu. Breast Cancer Res Treat 1992; 24:85–95.

127. Pietras RJ, Arboleda J, Reese DM et al. Her-2 tyrosine kinase pathway targets oestrogen receptor and promotes hormone-independent growth in human breast cancer cells. Oncogene 1995; 10:2435–46.

128. PathVysion Her-2 package insert. Downers Grove, Ill: Vysis, iNc, 1998.

129. Berns EMJJ, Foekens JA, van Staveren IL et al. Oncogene amplification and prognosis in breast cancer: relationship with systemic treatment. Gene 1995; 159:11–18.

130. Bianco AR, De Laurentis M, Carlomagno C et al. 20 year update of the Naples GUN trial of adjuvant breast cancer therapy: evidence of interaction between c-erb-2 expression and tamoxifen efficacy. Proc Am Soc Clin Oncol 1998; 17:97A.

131. Newby JC, Johnston SRD, Smith I et al. Expression of epidermal growth factor and C-erb-2 during the development of tamoxifen resistance in human breast cancer. Clin Cancer Res 1997; 3:1643–1651.

132. Nicholson RI, McCelland RA, Finlay P et al. Relationship between EGF-R, C-erb-2 protein expression and Ki67 immunostaining in breast cancer and hormone sensitivity. Eur J Cancer 1993; 29A:1018–23.

133. Giai M, Roagna R, Ponzone R et al. Prognostic and predictive relevance of C-erb-2 and ras expression in node positive and negative breast cancer. Anticancer Res 1994; 14:1441–50.

134. Archer SG, Eliopoulos SA, Spandidos D et al. Expression of ras p21, p53 and C-erb-2 in advanced breast cancer and response to first line hormonal therapy. Br J Cancer 1995; 72:1259–66.

135. Elledge RM, Green S, Ciocca D et al. Her-2 expression and response to tamoxifen in oestrogen receptor-positive breast cancer: a Southwest Oncology Group Study. Clin Cancer Res 1998; 4:7–12.

136. Muss H, Berry D, Thor A et al. Lack of interaction of tamoxifen (T) use and ErbB-2/HER-2/neu (H) expression in CALGB 8541: a randomized adjuvant trial of three different doses of cyclophosphamide, doxorubicin and fluorouracil (CAF) in node-positive primary breast cancer (BC). Proc Am Soc Clin Oncol 1999; 18:68a.

137. Paik S, Bryant J, Park C et al. ErbB-2 and response to doxorubicin in patients with axillary lymph node positive, hormone receptor-negative breast cancer. J Natl Cancer Inst 1998; 90:1361–70.

138. Ravin PM, Green S, Albain V et al. Initial report of the SWOG biological correlative study of CerbB-2 expression as a predictor of outcome in a trial comparing adjuvant CAF with tamoxifen (T) alone. Proc Am Soc Clin Oncol 1998; 17:97a.

139. Clahsen PC, van de Velde CJ, Duval C et al. P53 protein accumulation and response to adjuvant chemotherapy in pre-menopausal women with node-negative early breast cancer. J Clin Oncol 1998; 16:470–9.

140. Niskanen E, Blomqvist C, Franssila K et al. Predictive value of C-erb-2, p53, cathepsin-D and histology of the primary tumour in metastatic breast cancer. Br J Cancer 1997; 76:917–22.

141. Untch M, Thomssen C, Kahlert D et al. Lack of C-erb-2 overexpression predicts better response to dose intensification of anthracycline-based chemotherapy in high risk breast cancer. Presented at the San Antonio Breast Cancer Conference, 12–15 December 1998, Abstract no. 110.

142. Klochendler-Yeivin A, Yaniv M. Chromatin modifiers and tumour suppression. Biochim Biophys Acta 2001; 1551:M1–M10.

143. Baak JPA, Vooiji GP, Brugal G. Nuclear image cytometry: quantitation of chromatin pattern, steroid receptor content and Ki-67. In: Baale JPA (ed.) Manual of quantitative pathology in cancer diagnosis and prognosis. Heidelberg: Springer-Verlag, 1991; pp. 232–43.

144. Palcic B, Garner DM, MacAulay CE. Image cytometry and chemoprevention in cervical cancer. J Cell Biochem 1995; 23(suppl.):43–54.

145. Mommers EC, Poulin N, Sangulin J et al. Nuclear cytometry changes in breast carcinogenesis. J Pathol 2001; 193:33–9.

146. Nagahata T, Hirano A, Utada Y et al. Correlation of allelic losses and clinicopathologic factors in 504 primary breast cancers. Breast Cancer 2002; 9:208–15.

147. Hermsen MAJA, Baak JPA, Weiss J et al. Genetic analysis of 513 lymph node negative breast carcinomas by CGH and relation to clinical, pathologic, morphometric and DNA cytometric prognostic factors. J Pathol 1998; 186:356–62.

148. Janssen EAM, Baak JPA, Guervos MA et al. Lymph node negative breast cancer: specific chromosomal aberrations are strongly associated with high mitotic activity and predict outcome more accurately than grade, tumour diameter and oestrogen receptor. J Pathol 2003; 201:556–61.

149. Hyman E, Kauraniemi P, Hautaniemi S et al. Impact of DNA amplification on gene expression patterns in breast cancer. Cancer Res 2002; 62:6240–5.

150. Perou CM, Sorlie T, Eisen MB et al. Molecular portraits of human breast tumours. Nature 2000; 406:747–52.

151. Hedenfalk I, Duggan D, Chen Y et al. Gene expression profiles in hereditary breast cancer. N Engl J Med 2001; 344:539–48.

152. van't Veer LJ, Dai H, van de Vijer MJ et al. Expression profiling predicts outcomes in breast cancer. Breast Cancer Res 2002; 5:57–8.

153. Gruvberger S, Ringner M, Chen Y et al. Oestrogen receptor status in breast cancer is associated with remarkably distinct gene expression profiles. Cancer Res 2001; 61:5979–84.

154. West M, Blanchette C, Dressman H et al. Predicting the clinical status of human breast cancer by using gene expression profiles. Proc Natl Acad Sci USA 2001; 98:11462–7.

155. Ahr A, Kam T, Solbach S et al. Identification of high risk breast cancer by gene expression profiling. Lancet 2002; 359:131–2.

156. van de Vijver MJ, He YD, van't Veer LJ et al. A gene expression signature as a predictor of survival in breast cancer. N Engl J Med 2002; 347:1999–2009.

157. Aebersold R, Mann M. Mass spectrometry-based proteomics. Nature 2003; 422:198–207.

158. Rampaul RS, Pinder SE, Blamey RW et al. Evaluation of a high throughput approach to assess HER-2 using tissue microarray and ACIS technology. Breast Cancer Res Treat 2001; 54:4.

159. Rampaul RS, Pinder SE, Robertson JF et al. Tissue microarray technology: still a dress rehearsal? Adv Anat Path (in press).

160. McCelland CM, Gullick WJ. Identification of surrogate markers for determining drug activity using proteomics. Biochem Soc Trans 2003; 31:1488–90.

161. Todd JH, Dowle C, Williams MR et al. Confirmation of a prognostic index in primary breast cancer. Br J Cancer 1987; 56:489–92.

162. Chevallier B, Mossen V, Dauce JP et al. A prognostic score in histological node negative breast cancer. Br J Cancer 1990; 61:436–40.

163. Brown JM, Benson EA, Jones M. Confirmation of a long term prognostic index in breast cancer. Breast 1993; 2:144–7.

164. Balslev I, Axesson CK, Zedelev K et al. The Nottingham Prognostic Index applied to 9,149 patients from the studies of the Danish Breast Cancer Cooperative Group (DBCG). Breast Cancer Res Treat 1994; 32:281–90.

Three

Ductoscopy and the intraductal approach to breast cancer

William C. Dooley

The intraductal approach to breast cancer diagnosis was recognised early by cytologists such as George Papanicolau.[1] Unfortunately, few breast cancers could be diagnosed from the few microlitres of cell-poor fluid that could be elicited from most women's breasts.[2] In the 1960s, Wrench, Petrakis and King from the University of California began a series of studies on women in the San Francisco region to determine if the presence of nipple fluid or its cytological characteristics could predict future breast cancer risk.[3] They have now published data based on more than 30 years of follow-up on more than 7000 women and have shown that the relative risk of being able to express nipple fluid was 1.88 greater for the development of cancer in the following decade than in women who had no fluid expressed. Further, if there was cytological atypia in that fluid, the relative risk increased to 4.9 for the development of breast cancer within a decade. This is interesting because other series of cytological or histological breast epithelial atypia have shown that the risk for subsequent breast cancer development falls rapidly in the second and third decade after initial detection. Fine needle aspiration studies from Fabian and Kimler showed similar levels of risk associated with cellular atypia.[4] Dupont and Page both defined the current histological criteria for atypical ductal hyperplasia (ADH) and its natural history with a series of papers in the 1980s.[5,6] Each

of these series demonstrates an increased risk of breast cancer development associated with epithelial atypia in breast ducts independent of sampling method and has shown the same time-dependent nature of that elevated risk. In spite of this elegant body of medical work, little of these findings have affected the daily practice of breast care.

Frustrated with the poor results of mammographic screening in East Asian oriental populations, Japanese surgeons such as Okazaki began investigating the use of ductoscopy in the early 1990s.[7-9] Endoscope technologies had greatly improved optics and decreased the diameter needed for both illumination and image capture. Early studies on Japanese patients with bloody nipple discharge using a solid rigid scope less than 2 mm in diameter showed that it was possible to identify the cause of the discharge but the scopes were fragile and expensive and rarely advanced more than 3 cm into the breast. Persistence with this technology and improved optics and designs has produced sub-millimetre multifibre scopes and the addition of a working channel allowed greater success, as reported in the mid-1990s in studies from the Orient.[10-14] The technique of ductal endoscopy for the evaluation and management of symptomatic nipple discharge using endoscopy then spread to Korea and Hong Kong. The oriental approach has several drawbacks. First, the scopes are usually rigid, with the camera mounted as a heavy object at the end of a delicate optical fibre. The torque caused by such a long lever arm makes manipulating the scope around tight turns in the breast difficult. Second, the working channel has been used primarily to instill air into the ductal system. This does not relax the smooth muscle of the ductal walls and affords little distension for investigation of more distal branches. It also causes sharp bright boundaries between the fluid and air interface, causing optical distortion and degraded images secondary to light reflection. In spite of these difficulties, oriental investigators have moved to cyst endoscopy and other uses beyond investigating nipple discharge.[15–17]

In the USA, early attempts with submillimetre scopes were unsuccessful in patients with central tumors but in these attempts saline was used to distend the ductal system.[18] Cells recovered from this saline showed promise, and results from cytology improved compared with those from simple nipple aspiration or expression. Combining this experience with the prior data of Wrench and Petrakis, an attempt was made to develop a method of cannulating fluid-producing ducts and maximising the recovery of ductal cells shed into the duct lumen. Recent data from the NSABP P-01 study suggested that high-risk patients with ductal atypia had the greatest reduction in future breast cancer incidence with tamoxifen treatment.[19] Increasing cell yield from nipple aspiration was necessary in order to have a viable screen for ADH. The initial ductal lavage study enrolled women with prior contralateral breast cancer or who were high risk by the Gail model and had normal mammograms and physical examinations.[20] The majority (85%) produced fluid from at least one duct per breast. Atypia was present in 24% of the patients who successfully had a fluid-producing duct cannulated and lavaged with saline. At least 7% of this atypia was severe and bordered on malignancy. Subsequent series of severely atypical cells detected by lavage suggest that 50–70% of the atypia is from a mammographically occult malignancy. Future studies will determine the natural history of lavage-detected atypia, will allow assessment of changes seen with chemoprevention agents and how this reduces future breast cancer, and will document the rates and causes of false-positive atypia such as from duct papillomas.

Finding malignant cells, which can be repeatedly lavaged from a single ductal orifice with negative clinical and radiographic findings in the breast, is surprising but documented. After a number of imaging techniques such as ductography, magnetic resonance imaging (MRI) and ultrasound failed to identify the occult source of these malignant cells, it was decided to apply the oriental approach of duct endoscopy. The lavage experience had taught us how to relax the smooth muscle of the ducts and produce maximal distension of the ductal system using local anaesthetic topically prior to saline distension. Using this major variation, patients with concerning atypia, where imaging had failed to identify the source, were endoscoped. It soon became clear that the technique was successful at identifying not only the source of the atypia but often identified tumours with an extensive intraductal component in some early-stage breast cancers.[21] Papers from a number of American investigators now show benefit of ductoscopy in the investigation of symptomatic nipple discharge and discharge or elicitable fluid from a cancerous breast.[22–26] New biopsy technologies to direct minimal access biopsy either through the scope or in conjunction with other devices are being developed and tested in pilot settings.

Current technology can identify a group of high-risk women with epithelial atypia. What percentage of atypia is missed? This cannot be answered since this is really the first attempt to screen for atypia and there are no data with which to compare. Ductoscopy is a viable option for the identification of intraluminal defects that either cause symptomatic nipple discharge or give rise to severe cytological atypia on nipple aspiration or ductal lavage. Much is said of the power of MRI to screen for multifocal breast cancer. Unfortunately, it images primarily invasive cancer because of its increased blood flow and grossly underestimates low-grade ductal carcinoma in situ (DCIS), which is often a problem in breast conservation in early-stage breast cancer. My current series show that ductoscopy of breast cancer patients undergoing lumpectomy yields far more evidence of the extent of any proliferative disease than MRI. Further, the assumption of most MRI studies is that multiple lesions make mastectomy necessary. In all the cases seen so far of multifocality in my ductoscopy series, all tumours appear connected to the same duct orifice at the nipple. The operative surgeon can work out the anatomy of the ductal system and plan a cosmetically satisfactory lumpectomy, achieving clear margins at the first operation in the vast majority of cases.[24]

Advances in the laboratory will drive the future of these technologies. For the first time we have the ability to sample premalignant ductal epithelium and monitor its response to prevention strategies while optimal samples can be obtained for molecular investigations.[27] Just as the polyp model of colon cancer progression developed because of the experience with clinical gastrointestinal endoscopy, the same increase in our understanding of the evolution of breast cancer can be anticipated with the new intraductal approaches. For the intraductal approach to have value beyond the highest risk patients, molecular markers will need to be identified that can be measured in simple nipple aspirates. Those with 'molecular risk markers' can be screened through lavage and endoscopy, proceeding to intraductal biopsy for premalignant and early malignant lesions prior to radiographic image detection. It will then be possible to merge prevention and treatment as the development and progression of these lesions can be monitored endoscopically.

SPECIAL TECHNICAL CONSIDERATIONS

The difficulty of all intraductal technologies is achieving initial access to the lactiferous sinus without puncturing the ductal system. The key, whether using the ductal lavage catheter or a prolene suture as a soft guidewire, is timing. The sphincter of each duct in the papilla has a type of 'anal wink' when expressing fluid. It is open for only a fraction of a second when expressing fluid and successful cannulation of a duct occurs when the catheter or prolene suture is introduced during this brief relaxation of the sphincter. In women with symptomatic spontaneous discharge, the sphincter opens more widely for longer intervals and is therefore much easier to cannulate. Cannulating the minimally fluid-producing duct associated with a peripheral subcentimetre breast cancer is much more

difficult. Initially, the nipple should be thoroughly cleaned with a facial exfoliant until all keratin and sebaceous plugs are removed from its surface. Next, the breast should be lubricated with hand lotion and massaged deeply from the periphery to the centre to move any fluid into the lactiferous sinuses. Kneading of the breast in a manner similar to that of kneading bread should be performed in a centripetal fashion. These first two steps are the most important and often the most neglected in achieving success with any of the intraductal technologies. Lastly, radial compression of each lactiferous sinus will identify the fluid-producing orifice. As soon as an orifice is identified, stop expressing fluid until you are ready to cannulate. With cannulating tool in hand, re-express fluid while slowly distracting the nipple upward. Cannulation should occur at the time fluid first appears on the nipple surface. If you fail, then do not empty the sinus of fluid before trying again. I strongly advise using tapered 2-0 prolene since it is too soft to penetrate most duct walls and will not advance even in the presence of minimal resistance. All harder objects must be used with great caution.

Once in the duct, a 26 or 24G Angiocath and a Seldinger technique can be used, with the prolene as a guidewire. Progressive dilation will allow objects of up to 1 mm external diameter to be placed into the ductal system with ease. Injection of 3–5 mL of buffered local anaesthetic into the ducts comes next. It is important to wait for 2–5 minutes for relaxation of the ductal walls to occur before starting saline distension. Success in the cannulation technique can readily be measured by assessing the cellularity of ductal lavage samples. If the lactiferous sinus is perforated, then the samples will have few epithelial cells (<100). If the ducts are intact (and even if normal), the cell counts will be greater than 1000 cells.

Patients with spontaneous nipple discharge are the easiest to cannulate and endoscope. Further, because of chronic fluid production, the ducts are often larger and it is easier to manipulate the scope into the breast. For the first several cases I would suggest obtaining preoperative ductography (a galactogram). Until you learn how to manipulate through some of the lengthy papillomas, it can be very disconcerting to insert a scope and find yourself in a yellow kelp forest of papilloma without a central lumen. Starter cases are those with 1–1.5 cm of normal duct before any lesion is found. This way you can gain access to the duct and become oriented before pathological findings distort landmarks. After success with cases of spontaneous discharge, patients with central DCIS with or without invasive cancer should be tackled next. The spectrum of visual findings associated with malignant and premalignant breast disease can then be identified and the surgeon's expertise at recognition of differing pathological lesions rapidly improves (**Figs 3.1–3.4**; see Plates 2–5, facing p. 116).

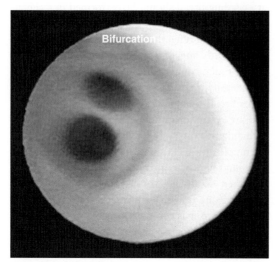

Figure 3.1 • Bifurcation.

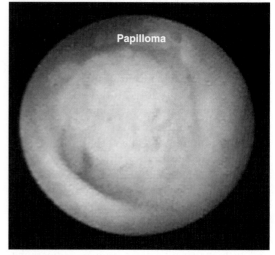

Figure 3.2 • Papilloma.

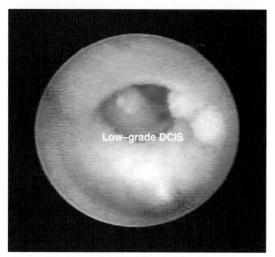

Figure 3.3 • Low-grade ductal carcinoma in situ.

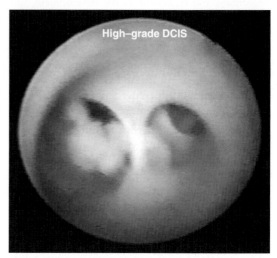

Figure 3.4 • High-grade ductal carcinoma in situ.

Key points

- The majority of non-obstructing malignant and premalignant breast diseases are associated with fluid production.
- Cytological analysis of fluid produced in high-risk women can identify subgroups at high short-term risk of breast cancer development.
- Direct ductal endoscopy with submillimetre endoscopes is now feasible and can offer value beyond simple investigation of symptomatic nipple discharge.
- The rapid evolution of intraductal technology and techniques will add considerably to our understanding of the biological progression to breast cancer and its prevention and treatment.

REFERENCES

1. Papanicolaou GN, Holmquist DG, Bader GM, Falk EA. Exfoliative cytology of the human mammary gland and its value in the diagnosis of cancer and other diseases of the breast. Cancer 1958; 11:377–409.

2. Sartorius OW, Smith HS, Morris P et al. Cytologic evaluation of breast fluid in the detection of breast disease. J Natl Cancer Inst 1977; 59:1073–8.

3. Wrensch MR, Petrakis NL, King EB et al. Breast cancer incidence in women with abnormal cytology in nipple aspirates of breast fluid. Am J Epidemiol 1992; 135:130–41.

    Classic paper on risk assessment.

4. Fabian CJ, Kimler BF, Zalles CM et al. Short-term breast cancer prediction by random periareolar fine-needle aspiration cytology and the Gail risk model. J Natl Cancer Inst 2000; 92:1217–27.

    Classic paper on risk assessment.

5. Dupont WD, Page DL. Risk factors for breast cancer in women with proliferative breast disease. N Engl J Med 1985; 312:146–51.

    Original description of ADH.

6. Dupont WD, Parl FF, Hartmann WH et al. Breast cancer risk associated with proliferative breast disease and atypical hyperplasia. Cancer 1993; 71:1258–65.

7. Okazaki A, Okazaki M, Asaishi K et al. Fiberoptic ductoscopy of the breast: a new diagnostic procedure for nipple discharge. Jpn J Clin Oncol 1991; 21:188–93.

    Original paper on ductoscopy.

8. Okazaki A, Okazaki M, Hirata K, Tsumanuma T. Progress of ductoscopy of the breast. [In Japanese] Nippon Geka Gakkai Zasshi 1996; 97:357–62.

9. Okazaki A, Hirata K, Okazaki M et al. Nipple discharge disorders: current diagnostic management and the role of fiberductoscopy. Eur Radiol 1999; 9:583–90.

10. Shen KW, Wu J, Lu JS et al. Fiberoptic ductoscopy for patients with nipple discharge. Cancer 2000; 89:1512–19.

11. Shao ZM, Liu Y, Nguyen M. The role of the breast ductal system in the diagnosis of cancer (review). Oncol Rep 2001; 8:153–6.

12. Matsunaga T, Ohta D, Misaka T et al. Mammary ductoscopy for diagnosis and treatment of intraductal lesions of the breast. Breast Cancer 2001; 8:213–21.

13. Shen KW, Wu J, Lu JS et al. Fiberoptic ductoscopy for breast cancer patients with nipple discharge. Surg Endosc 2001; 15:1340–5.

14. Yamamoto D, Shoji T, Kawanishi H et al. A utility of ductography and fiberoptic ductoscopy for patients with nipple discharge. Breast Cancer Res Treat 2001; 70:103–8.

15. Yamamoto D, Ueda S, Senzaki H et al. New diagnostic approach to intracystic lesions of the breast by fiberoptic ductoscopy. Anticancer Res 2001; 21:4113–16.

16. Makita M, Akiyama F, Gomi N et al. Endoscopic classification of intraductal lesions and histological diagnosis. Breast Cancer 2002; 9:220–5.

17. Tamaki Y, Miyoshi Y, Noguchi S. Application of endoscopic surgery for breast cancer treatment. [In Japanese] Nippon Geka Gakkai Zasshi 2002; 103:835–8.

18. Love SM, Barsky SH. Breast-duct endoscopy to study stages of cancerous breast disease. Lancet 1996; 348:997–9.

19. Fisher B, Costantino JP, Wickerham DL et al. Tamoxifen for prevention of breast cancer: report of the National Surgical Adjuvant Breast and Bowel Project P-1 Study. J Natl Cancer Inst 1998; 90:1371–88.

    Chemoprevention.

20. Dooley WC, Ljung B-M, Veronesi U et al. Ductal lavage for detection of cellular atypia in women at high risk for breast cancer. J Natl Cancer Inst 2001; 93:1624–32. Ductal lavage.

21. Dooley WC. Endoscopic visualization of breast tumors. JAMA 2000; 284:1518.

    American endoscopy.

22. Khan SA, Baird C, Staradub VL, Morrow M. Ductal lavage and ductoscopy: the opportunities and the limitations. Clin Breast Cancer 2002; 3:185–91; discussion 192–5.

23. Dietz JR, Crowe JP, Grundfest S et al. Directed duct excision by using mammary ductoscopy in patients with pathologic nipple discharge. Surgery 2002; 132:582–7; discussion 587–8.

24. Dooley WC. Routine operative breast endoscopy during lumpectomy. Ann Surg Oncol 2003; 10:38–42.

    American endoscopy.

25. Dooley WC. Routine operative breast endoscopy for bloody nipple discharge. Ann Surg Oncol 2002; 9:920–3.

    American endoscopy.

26. Dooley WC. Ductal lavage, nipple aspiration, and ductoscopy for breast cancer diagnosis. Curr Oncol Rep 2003; 5:63–5.

27. Evron E, Dooley WC, Umbricht CB et al. Detection of breast cancer cells in ductal lavage fluid by methylation-specific PCR. Lancet 2001; 357:1335–6.

    First paper on molecular identification of cancer from lavage/endoscopy samples.

CHAPTER

Four

Breast-conserving surgery: the balance between good cosmesis and local control

J. Michael Dixon

INTRODUCTION

The aim of local treatment of breast cancer is to achieve long-term local disease control with the minimum of local morbidity. The majority of women presenting symptomatically to breast clinics or who are diagnosed with breast cancer through screening programmes have small breast cancers, which are suitable for breast-conserving surgery. The major advantages of breast-conserving treatment are as follows:

- breast-conserving treatment produces an acceptable cosmetic appearance in the majority of women;[1]
- breast-conserving treatment results in lower levels of psychological morbidity, with less anxiety and depression and improved body image, sexuality and self-esteem, compared with mastectomy;[2,3]
- two systematic reviews have shown equivalence in terms of disease outcome for breast-conserving treatment and mastectomy.[4,5]

One of these reviews (search date 1995) analysed data from six randomised controlled trials that compared breast conservation treatment with mastectomy.[4] A meta-analysis of data from five of these six trials involving 3006 women found no significant difference in the risk of death at 10 years (odds ratio 0.91, 95% CI 0.78–1.05). The sixth randomised trial used different protocols. In the second systematic review, nine randomised controlled trials involving 4981 women randomised to mastectomy or breast-conserving treatment were included in the analysis.[5] A meta-analysis of these nine trials found no significant difference in the risk of death over 10 years: the relative risk reduction for breast-conserving surgery compared with mastectomy was 0.02 (95% CI –0.05 to +0.09).[5] There was also no difference in the rates of local recurrence in the six randomised controlled trials involving 3006 women where data were available: the relative risk reduction for mastectomy versus breast-conserving surgery was 0.04 (95% CI –0.04 to +0.12).[4]

Originally it was thought that local therapy had little influence on overall survival but it is becoming clear that local therapy is responsible, at least in part, for some patients developing metastatic disease.[6–8] It is important therefore to ensure that only appropriate patients are selected for breast-conserving treatment, and for those patients who have this treatment the aim is to minimise local recurrence while at the same time achieving a good cosmetic outcome.

SELECTION OF PATIENTS FOR BREAST CONSERVATION

Single cancers clinically measuring 4 cm or less, without signs of local advancement, can usually be managed by breast-conserving treatment (**Box 4.1**). Different units have different size criteria and many units have a cut-off for breast-conserving surgery of tumours measuring 3 cm or less clinically. Increasing tumour size does not mean increasing local recurrence rates and this approach is illogical. Clinical tumour size overestimates actual tumour size. There is a much better correlation between pathological tumour size and the size measured on imaging, with ultrasound assessment being more accurate than mammographic measurements. It is the balance between tumour size as assessed by imaging and breast volume that determines whether a patient is suitable for breast-conserving surgery. Patients with tumours clinically measuring larger than 4 cm can be treated by breast-conserving surgery if the patient has large breasts. Conversely, in a patient with small breasts, excision of even a small tumour may produce an unacceptable cosmetic result. Options for patients with tumours considered too large, relative to the size of the breast, for breast-conserving treatment include neoadjuvant systemic therapy to shrink the tumour, an oncoplastic procedure (see Chapter 5) involving transfer of tissue into the breast, or surgery to the opposite breast to obtain symmetry.[9,10]

Patients with multiple tumours in the same breast are not good candidates for breast-conserving treatment because they have a high incidence of in-breast recurrence[11,12] and so are best treated by mastectomy, combined in appropriate patients with immediate reconstruction. Patients seen on mammography to have two tumours very close to each other or those with multifocal disease identified only by the pathologist can undergo breast-conserving treatment providing that all disease is excised and margins of excision are clear.[12] Patients with bilateral small cancers can be treated by bilateral breast conservation. The rates of breast-conserving surgery vary significantly between countries and within countries. These rates are probably more influenced by the views of the surgeon than the availability of radiotherapy equipment. Failure to offer breast-conserving surgery to suitable and appropriate patients is becoming a medicolegal

Box 4.1 • Indications and contraindications for breast-conserving surgery

Indications
T1, T2 (<4 cm), N0, N1, M0
T2 >4 cm in large breasts
Single clinical and mammographic lesion
Contraindications
T4, N2 or M1
Patients who prefer mastectomy
Clinically evident multifocal/multicentric disease
Relative contraindications
Collagen vascular disease
Large or central tumours in small breasts
Women with a strong family history of breast cancer or BRCA1 and BRCA2 mutation carriers

issue. The exact reasons why a patient who fulfils the criteria for breast-conserving surgery is treated by mastectomy should be recorded legibly in the patient's notes.

Clinical and pathological factors have until recently influenced selection of patients for breast-conserving surgery because of their perceived impact on local recurrence. These include young age (under 35–39 years), the presence of an extensive in situ component associated with an invasive tumour, grade 3 histology and widespread lymphatic/vascular invasion.[13,14] These are considered in detail below.

BREAST-CONSERVING SURGERY

Two surgical procedures have been extensively studied: quadrantectomy and wide local excision. Quadrantectomy is based on the belief that the breast is organised into segments, with each segment draining into its own major duct, and that invasive cancer spreads down the duct system towards the nipple.[15] The evidence is that both of these premises are incorrect. A single major subareolar can drain large areas of the breast. Studies have also shown that both invasive and non-invasive disease are no more likely to extend toward the nipple than in any other direction.[14] The effectiveness of quadrantectomy relates to the large amount of tissue excised around the tumour rather than to the removal of a cancer and its draining duct.[16] One of the early studies of breast-conserving treatment randomised patients to lumpectomy or quadrantectomy. A significantly greater number of patients who had lumpectomy had incomplete local excisions.[17] Not surprisingly therefore local recurrence was greater after lumpectomy than after the more extensive quadrantectomy, although survival was no different.[15] Other non randomised studies have shown similar rates of local recurrence in both quadrantectomy and wide local excision, providing margins of excision are clear.[16] The reason why quadrantectomy is no longer advocated is that it produces a significantly poorer cosmetic outcome than wide local excision.[18] The consensus view is that the majority of patients having breast-conserving surgery can be adequately treated by wide local excision and do not require either a segmental or quadrantic excision.[13,19]

Special technical details: wide local excision

The aim of wide local excision is to remove all invasive and any ductal carcinoma in situ with a 1-cm macroscopic margin of normal surrounding breast tissue. Controversy has surrounded which incisions give the best cosmetic results. The predominant orientation of collagen fibres in the skin was described by Langer[20] and these skin crease lines around the breast are essentially circular (**Fig. 4.1**). Subsequent work by Kraissl[21] demonstrated that lines of maximum resting skin tension run in a more transverse orientation across the breast (**Fig. 4.1**). In general, scars that are parallel both to the lines of maximum resting skin tension and to the orientation of collagen fibres are quickest to heal and produce the best cosmetic incisions, with least hypertrophy and keloid formation. Incisions at right angles to both the orientation of collagen fibres and to the lines of maximum resting skin tension, such as radial incisions in the upper outer quadrant, produce the most cosmetically unacceptable scars. A knowledge of Langer's lines and Kraisl's lines thus allows a surgeon to make incisions that enhance the cosmetic outcome of breast-conserving surgery. Usually an incision to excise a cancer is placed directly over the lesion. Using circumareolar incisions to excise a cancer some distance away from the nipple is not generally recommended because if re-excision is required this procedure can be difficult through such an incision. Excising skin directly overlying a cancer is only necessary if the carcinoma is very superficial and/or the skin is tethered. The cosmetic result after breast-conserving surgery is influenced by the amount of

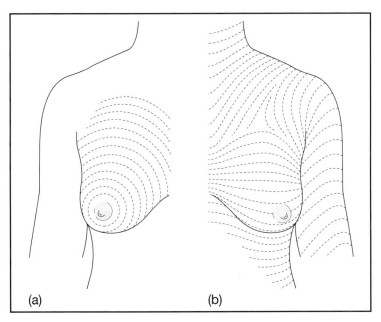

Figure 4.1 • The direction of **(a)** Langer's lines and **(b)** lines of maximum resting skin tension in the breast (so-called dynamic lines of Kraissl).

(a)   (b)

skin excised, with poor results being obtained in those patients who have most skin removed.[22] Routine excision of skin when performing a wide excision is discouraged by current guidelines and cannot be justified.[13] Limiting the length of incision is important, as longer incisions produce significantly poorer cosmetic outcomes. In a patient who has a previous incomplete excision it is usual to narrowly excise the previous scar.

Having made the skin incision, the skin and subcutaneous fat is dissected off the breast tissue. Care should be taken when elevating skin not to dissect into the subcutaneous fat as thin skin flaps give a poor postoperative cosmetic result. Having elevated skin flaps 1–2 cm beyond the edge of the cancer, the fingers of the non-dominant hand are placed over the palpable cancer and the breast tissue is divided beyond the fingertips, the line of incision being 1 cm beyond the limit of the palpable mass. Having divided breast tissue beyond the posterior edge of the cancer, the deep aspect of the tumour can be palpated and breast tissue under the cancer divided. If the lesion is superficial, it is not necessary to remove full thickness of breast tissue. In the majority of patients, however, it is necessary to continue dissection through breast tissue down to the pectoral fascia to ensure there is an adequate margin deep to the cancer. Having reached this fascia, the breast tissue and cancer is dissected from the fascia. It is not necessary to excise pectoral fascia unless it is tethered to the tumour or the tumour is involving it. If a carcinoma is infiltrating one of the chest wall muscles, then a portion of the affected muscle should be removed beneath the tumour, the aim being to excise sufficient muscle to get beyond the limits of the cancer. Having dissected under the cancer, whether this is within the breast tissue or on the pectoral fascia, the cancer and surrounding tissue is grasped between the finger and thumb of the non-dominant hand and excision is completed at the other margins. The specimen is immediately orientated with sutures, Ligaclips or metal markers prior to submission to the pathologist. Metal markers or Ligaclips allow orientated anteroposterior intraoperative specimen radiography to be performed, which helps the surgeon assess whether the target lesion has been excised and also the completeness of excision at radial margins. If the specimen radio-graph shows the cancer or any associated micro-calcification is close to a particular margin, then the surgeon can remove further tissue from the margin of concern, orientate it and send it to pathology.

A number of studies have evaluated the use of cavity shavings and bed biopsies, but only a few of these have compared standard assessment of margins with cavity shavings or bed biopsies. There remain problems with their use. Only a minority of surgeons use cavity shavings and bed biopsies routinely.[23,24] Neither bed biopsies nor cavity shavings have been shown consistently to be reliable indicators of local recurrence. The major concern of using cavity shavings is that significant amounts of breast tissue are removed, particularly if the whole cavity is shaved and this will inevitably have an influence on cosmetic outcome.[24] Most importantly, however, centres who do not use any of these techniques report excellent local control rates. Wide excision with standard examination of margins thus appears to provide sufficient information on margin status. Bed biopsies or cavity shavings are of value where there is concern that one particular margin is involved. Those centres who have established protocols using bed biopsies or cavity shavings and who get good rates of local control and cosmetic outcomes comparable to centres using standard margin assessment can reasonably continue to use these techniques. Nonetheless, removing extra tissue from margins remains unnecessary in the majority of patients undergoing wide local excision. Proponents of their use argue that unsuspected disease is detected by these techniques, but if surgery did remove all foci of disease then radiotherapy would be unnecessary. What clear margins indicate is that any remaining tumour burden is small and can be managed by adjuvant radiotherapy.

Having excised the cancer from the breast, suturing the defect in the breast without mobilisation of the breast tissue frequently results in distortion of the breast contour. Small defects (<5% breast volume) can be left open and produce a good final cosmetic result. Larger defects in the breast should be closed by mobilising surrounding breast tissue from both the overlying skin and subcutaneous tissue and the underlying chest wall. If large defects (>10% breast volume) are not closed they fill with seroma that later absorbs, and as scar tissue forms this contracts, often producing an ugly distorted breast. Following large-volume excisions, having mobilised breast tissue it is usually possible to close the defect in the breast plate with a series of interrupted absorbable sutures. Larger defects can be filled by using a latissimus dorsi miniflap[9,10] (see Chapter 5). Drains are not necessary following wide local excision and should not be used routinely. They do not protect against haematoma formation and increase infection rates. Breast skin wounds should be closed in layers with absorbable sutures, finishing with a subcuticular suture. Staples and interrupted sutures are no longer an acceptable method of wound closure in the breast.

Complications of wide excision include haematoma, infection, incomplete excision and poor cosmetic results. Haematoma requiring evacuation should be rare and occur in less than 2% of patients. Infection requiring treatment affects 2–5% and is more common when combined with an axillary dissection. Incomplete excision rates should be in the range 10–25%. The most common problem following surgery by wide local excision is a poor cosmetic result. Factors influencing cosmetic outcome are considered in detail below.

Excising impalpable cancers

Impalpable lesions can be localised prior to surgery using one of a number of different techniques, including skin marking, injection of blue dye, carbon or radioisotope, insertion of a hooked wire, or intraoperative ultrasound. Excising an impalpable cancer is easier if the skin incision is made directly over the cancer. The location of the lesion can be determined in three ways: (i) the surgeon calculates the position of the breast lesion from the mammogram, (ii) the radiologist marks the skin overlying the lesion or (iii) the surgeon uses a gamma probe to localise the area of maximum radioactivity. An appropriately sized skin incision is made and deepened. If a wire is in place, then dissection continues towards the wire so that it can be located above where it enters the lesion. For instance, if a mammographic abnormality has been localised in the craniocaudal position, then dissection proceeds superiorly. Marked localisation wires, which change diameter or have a guide that can be placed over the wire, help the surgeon to determine exactly how far along the wire the lesion is situated.

The direction of the wire on the preoperative mammogram is only a guide to the actual path of the wire through the breast. Once the wire is in place, the breast is often placed in a different position from standard mammographic views; thus a lesion may be lateral to the entry point of the wire, but on the craniocaudal completion film the wire may appear to be traversing medially. The aim is to remove the mammographic lesion with a 1-cm clear radiological margin.

As for palpable lesions, all specimens should be orientated with Ligaclips or metal markers or secured to an orientated grid so that specimen radiography can be performed. Radiography is performed following compression in a mammogram machine or non-compressed in a Faxitron. There have been conflicting reports about whether compressing the specimen affects the incidence of subsequent positive margins as reported by the pathologist. Orientated specimen radiography improves the rate of complete excision of impalpable cancers.[25] Cooperation between surgeon and pathologist is required to clarify the area of concern and assess the adequacy of excision.

The majority of wide excisions of palpable and impalpable cancers are performed under general anaesthesia, although it is possible to perform wide excision under local anaesthesia. Patients who are unfit for general anaesthesia can usually have surgery safely under local anaesthesia.

FACTORS AFFECTING BREAST-CONSERVING SURGERY AFTER BREAST CONSERVATION

Different centres have reported large variations in recurrence rates following breast-conserving surgery combined with radiotherapy for invasive breast carcinoma. The majority of these recurrences (approximately 80%) occur adjacent to the site of initial excision. The most important treatment-related factor is the use of appropriate doses of radiotherapy. Megavoltage radiation therapy to the whole breast in a dose of 4500–5000 cGy given over 3–5 weeks is routinely used. Radiotherapy significantly reduces the rate of local recurrence and data from the latest overview indicate that addition of radiotherapy improves overall survival.[8] Ongoing studies are evaluating whether localised radiotherapy delivered either during or within a few days of surgery is as effective as whole-breast radiotherapy. As yet it has not been possible to identify groups of patients who do not require radiotherapy. However, there may be a group of older patients with low-risk cancers (completely excised, node negative, and hormone receptor positive on hormone treatment) and women of any age whose cancers have an extremely good outcome (very well differentiated grade 1 or special type cancers that are completely excised, node negative and hormone receptor positive) whose rates of local recurrence without radiotherapy are acceptable. Ongoing studies evaluating the role of radiotherapy in these two groups are underway or have been completed but not yet published. Following whole-breast radiotherapy, it is possible to increase the local dose of radiotherapy by boosting the tumour bed. This reduces local recurrence rates, particularly in younger women.[26]

Patient-related factors

Local recurrence following breast-conserving therapy is significantly more common in younger patients.[27] In contrast, local recurrence is much less of a problem in older patients (>65 years). Ongoing randomised studies are examining whether older patients with hormone-sensitive tumours with limited factors for local recurrence can safely avoid radiotherapy.

Studies have indicated that recurrence is less frequent in women with large breasts but whether this relates to the larger excisions that can be performed in these patients or to alterations in steroid metabolism (fat is known to be an important site of conversion of androgens to estrogens) is uncertain.[28] A family history of breast cancer, particularly carriage of a mutation in one of the breast cancer genes, predisposes a patient to an increased rate of local recurrence unless these women undergo a prophylactic oophorectomy, when local recurrence rates fall to that of the general population.[29]

Tumour-related factors

Tumour location, tumour size, the presence of skin or nipple retraction, and the presence or absence of axillary node involvement have not been consistently shown to be factors predictive of recurrence after breast-conserving surgery.[30–33] The hormone receptor status of a breast cancer does not seem to exert any influence on local control rates.

TUMOUR SIZE

There has been confusion with regard to tumour size. Only 3 of 28 series that have examined the relationship of tumour size and occurrence have shown a significant association.[34] A large study from Boston[35] demonstrated that cancers over 4 cm in size that were treated by breast conservation surgery had the lowest rate of recurrence (**Table 4.1**).

TUMOUR GRADE

A number of reports have analysed the relationship between tumour grade and local recurrence. The lowest rates of local recurrence are reported in grade 1 tumours. Although some series report a higher recurrence rate in grade 3 compared with grade 2 cancers, this is by no means universal.[36–38] The relative risk of local recurrence between grade 1 and grade 2/3 cancer is approximately 1.5. The British Association of Surgical Oncology has undertaken a trial that randomised patients with node-negative grade 1 or special type cancers to no further treatment, tamoxifen alone, radiotherapy alone or both radiotherapy and tamoxifen. No final results have been published. Interim results indicate that there have been very few recurrences in the group receiving both radiotherapy and tamoxifen. There were most recurrences in patients who received no further treatment and small numbers of recurrences

Table 4.1 • Size of tumour related to local recurrence

Size (cm)	Local recurrence
0–1	21%
1.1–2	8%
2.1–3	13%
3.1–4	17%
4.1–5	4%

Data from Eberlein TG, Connolly JN, Schnitt JS et al. Predictors of local recurrence following conservative breast surgery and radiation therapy. The influence of tumour size. Arch Surg 1990; 125:771–9.

in patients receiving radiotherapy or tamoxifen alone. The acceptable annual rate of local recurrence in this very good prognostic group has not yet been defined. It is likely that some of these patients can safely avoid tamoxifen or radiotherapy, but at present in this group of women radiotherapy followed by a discussion of the risks and advantages of adjuvant endocrine therapy remain the standard of care.

HISTOLOGICAL TYPE

There are few data relating histological tumour type and recurrence. There are data indicating that invasive lobular cancer is not associated with a higher recurrence rate than so-called invasive 'ductal' carcinoma.[39–44] One study did suggest that patients with invasive lobular carcinoma who developed local recurrence were more likely to develop multifocal recurrence but this has not been confirmed by others. Patients with invasive lobular cancer are more likely than patients with no special type tumours to have incomplete excision. Patients with invasive lobular cancer on core biopsy should be warned of this.

LYMPHATIC/VASCULAR INVASION

Increased local failure rates have been reported in most, but not all, series in patients with histological evidence of lymphatic/vascular invasion (LVI).[27,30,35–38] Of concern, the percentage of tumours reported to have LVI varies widely between different series by up to a factor of four. Carcinomas with LVI have approximately double the rate of local recurrence compared with tumours with no evidence of this feature. LVI is more common in tumours of younger women (<35 years) than in those of older women (>50 years).

EXTENSIVE IN SITU COMPONENT

The histological factor that has been most frequently shown to be associated with an increased rate of local recurrence is the presence of an extensive in situ component (EIC) within and surrounding an invasive cancer. A tumour is defined as having EIC if 25% or more of the tumour mass is non-invasive *and* non-invasive carcinoma is also present in the breast tissue surrounding the invasive cancer.[45] EIC is a predictor of not only local recurrence but also of residual disease within the breast.[18] Early reports indicated that local recurrence rates were three to four times higher in cancers with EIC.[27,38,40,43,46] The majority of these studies did not take account of margins and the authors did not perform multivariate analysis. More recent studies have clarified the issues surrounding EIC and margins and have shown that in patients who have both EIC and involved margins local recurrence rates are unacceptable, but providing clear margins are obtained, there is no increased rate of local recurrence in patients with EIC.[47,48] There is an interaction between age and EIC, with younger women being more likely to have EIC. It has been suggested that the higher frequency of EIC in younger women might explain some of the increased rate of local recurrence seen in younger women.[38]

MULTIPLE TUMOURS

A patient with macroscopic multiple cancers is more likely to develop local recurrence than a patient with a unifocal cancer. If multifocality is identified only by the pathologist or there are two cancers that are adjacent, then acceptable local recurrence rates can be obtained in these patients providing that all margins of excision are clear of disease.[40]

Treatment-related factors

 The most important surgical-related factor is completeness of excision. Current practice is to aim for at least microscopically disease-free margins. Ideally, there should be a clear rim of normal tissue (>1 mm) around the carcinoma in all directions.[48]

Controversy has surrounded how much extra tissue should be removed and what constitutes an involved or positive margin. Some studies have defined a positive or involved margin as disease at the margin, others as disease within 1 mm or even disease within 2 mm of the margins. Conversely, negative margins or uninvolved margins have been variably defined as no tumour at the margin, 1 mm of normal tissue or greater than 1 mm of normal tissue from the edge of the invasive or in situ cancer. Whatever definition has been used, almost all studies have reported an increased rate of local recurrence in patients with positive, non-negative or involved margins. When comparing patients with involved margins to those with uninvolved or negative margins, the relative risk of local recurrence varies between 1.4 and 9 fold.[30,32,33,38–43,46–53] This is despite the fact that patients with involved or close margins received higher doses of radiotherapy than patients with clear margins in almost half these series. In the few studies which have found that margins were not important predictors of local recurrence, the dose of radiotherapy delivered to the tumour bed ranged from 65 to 72 cGy, i.e. in the dose range that is effective without surgery.[41,48–50,54] In one study of 119 patients with non-negative margins, patients who had re-excision to a negative margin had a zero local recurrence rate compared with a 22% local recurrence rate in patients who had re-excision and non-negative margins (P = 0.001).[48] A recent survey in the UK demonstrated that approximately 50% of surgeons aimed for a margin of more than 2 mm, whereas 50% of surgeons were happy with a margin of 2 mm or less.[23] Few studies have investigated whether wider margins are associated with significantly better rates of local control. One study of 509 patients demonstrated that at 6 years patients with positive margins had a relative rate of local recurrence 3.83 times that of patients with a margin of normal tissue of greater than 5 mm.[52] Within the range of clear margins from 0 to 5 mm there was no suggestion that patients with narrow margins (<2 mm) had a significantly worse rate of local recurrence than those with wider margins (2–5 mm). This study concludes that clear margins are essential but the width of the clear margin is not important.[52] In a separate study from Boston, patients with extensive positive margins had an unacceptable rate of local recurrence at 8 years of 27%.[47] Patients who had only focally positive margins had a rate of local recurrence of 14%. The remaining patients who had either a close margin (clear margins but disease within 1 mm) or a clear margin (>1 mm) had an identical rate of local recurrence of 7% over 8 years. This study confirms that providing margins are microscopically free of both invasive carcinoma and ductal carcinoma in situ, local recurrence rates after breast-conserving therapy will be satisfactory. Studies have looked at the presence of lobular carcinoma in situ[55] and atypical ductal hyperplasia[56] at the margins of excision. Neither of these features significantly increases local recurrence rates and so there is no need for the surgeon to re-excise the margins if the pathologist reports these features alone at any of the margins of excision.

Age interacts with margins. Clear margins are imperative in younger women and if wider margins are important then it is likely to be in women under 45 years of age.[52]

There is also a direct interaction between EIC and margins (**Table 4.2**). Patients with EIC and positive margins had a 37% local recurrence rate in a series from Boston[47] and a 21% recurrence rate in a Stanford series.[48] In contrast, patients with EIC and negative margins had a zero local recurrence rate. These two studies demonstrate that patients with EIC do not have an increased rate of local recurrence if the margins of excision are clear of invasive and in situ cancer and so should not be denied breast-conserving surgery.

Of concern to surgeons is that patients undergoing re-excision for close or involved margins have only a 30% incidence of residual cancer in the re-excised tissue.[57] Patients with more than two foci of microscopic margin involvement had an incidence of residual cancer of 65% in one series, whereas patients with less than two foci had a much lower rate of margin involvement. This study showed that no residual disease at re-excision was associated with a 4% local failure rate at 4.7 years compared with patients who had residual disease at re-excision who had a 13% failure rate. Patients younger than age 50 were more likely to have disease in the re-excision specimen. The conclusion from this study was that the majority of patients who undergo re-excision do not benefit from the procedure. Patients with lucent breasts and a well-defined lesion appeared particularly unlikely to benefit from re-excision if margins were close or focally positive, whereas younger women with dense breasts were much more likely to benefit from further surgery to obtain clear final margins.[57] Further studies in

Table 4.2 ● Local recurrence rates (%) at 5 years in patients from Boston[47] and Stanford[48] subdivided by margin status and the presence (EIC+) or absence (EIC–) of an extensive in situ component

Margins	Boston		Stanford	
	EIC+	EIC–	EIC+	EIC–
Positive/non-negative	37	7	21	11
Close	0	5		
Negative	0	2	0	1

this area are required. If it were possible to identify a group of women who did not benefit from re-excision, this would have great clinical utility.

Adjuvant systemic therapy

Tamoxifen and chemotherapy, in the presence of radiotherapy, reduce local recurrence after breast-conserving surgery.[58-61] In the absence of radiotherapy, tamoxifen or chemotherapy alone do not produce satisfactory rates of local control.[61,62] The interval between surgery and radiotherapy may be important and there are suggestions that the rates of local recurrence increase if radiotherapy is delayed. The sequencing of radiotherapy and chemotherapy are the subject of ongoing trials.

FACTORS INFLUENCING COSMETIC OUTCOME AFTER BREAST-CONSERVING SURGERY

There appears to be great variation in different series in the number of patients with good to excellent cosmetic results after breast-conserving surgery (**Fig. 4.2**).

The importance of good cosmetic results is demonstrated in a study from Nottingham,[2] which showed that there was a significant correlation between cosmetic outcome and levels of anxiety, depression, body image, sexuality and self-esteem.

Patient factors

There is conflicting evidence about whether age influences cosmetic outcome, with some studies claiming that older women have worse cosmetic results than younger women.[1]

There is a trend towards increased fibrosis in large breasts, which leads to poor cosmetic results.[63] The best cosmetic results are obtained in medium- and moderate-sized breasts; cosmetic outcome can be a problem in small breasts.[1]

Tumour factors

Increasing tumour size means that increasingly large amounts of tissue have to be removed. As volume of

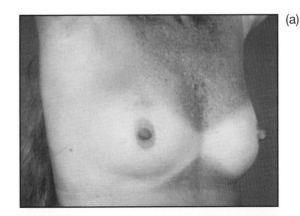

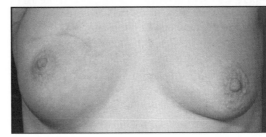

Figure 4.2 • Examples of **(a)** excellent and **(b)** poor cosmetic results from breast-conserving surgery and radiotherapy.

tissue excised is the most important factor relating to cosmetic outcome, not surprisingly patients with larger tumours tend to have worse cosmetic results.[58,64] There are some data that have indicated that when tumours are small and impalpable, a disproportionately large amount of breast tissue is removed to ensure that all the affected tissue is excised. It is likely therefore that not all patients with very small impalpable cancers have a better cosmetic outcome than some patients with small palpable cancers.[1]

LOCATION OF TUMOUR

Cosmetic outcomes tend to be better if the tumour is localised in the upper outer quadrant.[65] Studies have shown that major nipple displacement occurs when surgery is performed on tumours located in the inferior half of the breast.[66] If the tumour is central and the nipple–areola complex needs to be removed, then this can have a major effect on cosmetic outcomes.[1] This is why central tumours have been considered a relative contraindication to breast-conserving surgery. However, studies have suggested that these cancers are not associated with

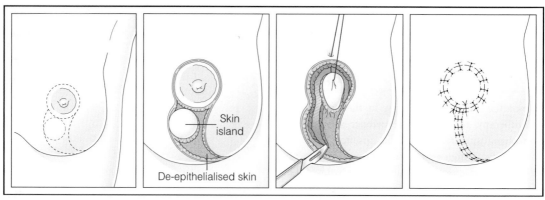

Figure 4.3 • How to excise a central cancer under the nipple and produce a satisfactory cosmetic outcome without major breast distortion. This procedure has also been called central quadrantectomy. The nipple–areola complex is excised and a portion of skin inferior is marked out. An incision around the circular skin island is made and the remaining skin around the island is de-epithelialised. A full-thickness incision is the made in the breast and the skin island is rotated to fill the central defect. Staples are useful to position the flap. When the flap is deemed to be in an optimal position, the staples are removed and the wound closed in two layers with absorbable sutures.

a significantly increased rate of local recurrence compared with more peripherally situated cancers[67] and and good cosmetic outcomes are possible.[64] Cancers directly underneath the nipple–areola complex can be excised by rotating a local flap from the lower part of the breast to fill the defect (**Fig. 4.3**). This so-called central quadrantectomy produces satisfactory long-term results.

Surgical factors

The extent of surgical excision (weight of excision) or the volume of resected breast tissue is the most important factor affecting cosmesis.[1,64] The inferior cosmetic results obtained with quadrantectomy, even in the most experienced hands, compared with wide excision is well documented.[18,66,68]

One option to overcome this problem is to perform a contralateral quadrantectomy.[69] Although techniques have been described using local flaps, small silicone implants and muscular flaps, the volume or the weight of tissue excised has been shown in almost all studies to correlate with cosmetic outcome.[1] Even more critical is the percentage of the breast excised. There is a highly statistical correlation between cosmetic outcome and percentage of the breast excised (**Fig. 4.4**), with excisions of less than 10% of breast volume generally being

associated with a good cosmetic outcome whereas excisions over 10% usually produce a poor cosmetic result (**Fig. 4.5**). Where it is clear that more than 10% of breast volume needs to be excised in order to remove the cancer, then consideration should be given to volume replacement with a latissimus dorsi miniflap,[9,10] an oncoplastic reduction

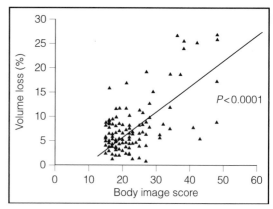

Figure 4.4 • Percentage of breast excised compared with body image score. Percentage of breast excised calculated by measuring total weight of excision and estimating breast volume (from initial diagnostic craniocaudal mammogram). Body image score based on patient-administered questionnaire of 15 questions (score runs from 15, the best possible score, to 60, the worst and highest possible score). Data from a series of 120 patients treated in the Edinburgh Breast Unit.

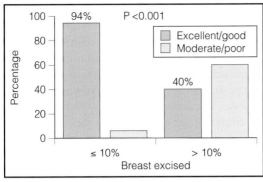

Figure 4.5 • Percentage of good/excellent results in patients subdivided according to whether 10% or less or more than 10% of breast volume was excised by breast-conserving surgery.

procedure, neoadjuvant drug therapy or a mastectomy with or without immediate reconstruction.

RE-EXCISION AND NUMBER OF PROCEDURES

Re-excision of the tumour bed has a negative impact on cosmesis.[1,64] This is mainly as a consequence of the increased total volume of tissue excised from the breast.

SCAR LENGTH

Although some reports have failed to show any correlation between scar length and patient cosmetic self-assessment,[70] others have reported significant association in relation to both cosmesis[71] and patient satisfaction.[72]

AXILLARY SURGERY

Axillary clearance seems to be associated with a worse cosmetic outcome than axillary sampling procedures, primarily because of an increasing risk of breast oedema.[1]

POSTOPERATIVE COMPLICATIONS

Development of a seroma, haematoma or postperative infection is associated with a worse cosmetic result.[1]

Radiotherapy

Increasing doses of radiotherapy, particularly with the use of boost, have a detrimental effect on cosmetic outcomes.[38,70-74] Long-term follow-up is necessary to assess cosmetic outcome; importantly, 3 years after treatment, radiotherapy effects tend to stabilise. Fibrosis is a late effect of radiotherapy and produces breast retraction and contour distortion. Over time a treated breast loses tissue faster than the opposite breast and some patients develop increasing asymmetry over many years. The treated breast will not increase in size to the same extent as the opposite untreated breast, so patients who put on weight develop asymmetry even when the initial cosmetic result was excellent. Boost has a negative impact on cosmesis by producing intense fibrosis and unsightly skin changes.[38,64,71-74]

Other treatment effects

Studies have suggested that tamoxifen has little if any effect on cosmetic outcome, whereas a few studies have shown that chemotherapy has a negative impact on cosmesis.[1]

Treatment of poor cosmetic results after breast-conserving surgery

Options include augmentation of one or both breasts. Swelling after implant insertion in a radiotherapy-treated breast is often marked and takes many months to settle. The opposite breast can be reduced. The whole or part of the treated breast can also be reconstructed. Pedicled myocutaneous latissimus dorsi flaps offer one opportunity to excise unsightly skin and areas of breast distortion and scarring, and provide one option to regain symmetry (**Fig. 4.6**).

SIGNIFICANCE AND TREATMENT OF LOCAL RECURRENCE

Local recurrence rates have varied widely in the literature but rates of 1% or less per year after breast-conserving treatment are achievable. If local recurrence rates for any surgeon or any unit are consistently higher than this, then a thorough audit of the practice of the surgeon or the unit is indicated.

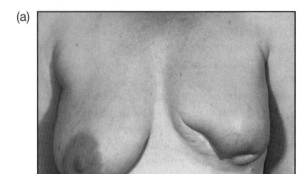

(a)

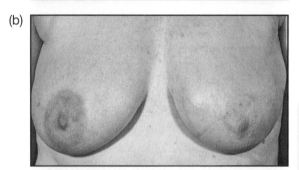

(b)

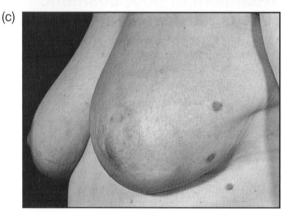

(c)

Figure 4.6 • Patient with a poor cosmetic result after breast-conserving surgery **(a)** before and **(b, c)** after partial breast reconstruction with a pedicled latissimus dorsi myocutaneous flap.

While an isolated local breast recurrence does not appear to be a threat to survival, breast recurrence is a predictor of distant disease;[6,7] the aim of primary treatment is to avoid local recurrence.

Isolated recurrences of the breast can be treated by re-excision or mastectomy.[75] Re-excision is asso-

ciated with a high rate of subsequent local recurrence if the initial recurrence occurs within the first 5 years of treatment.[76] Approximately 80% of local recurrences in the conserved breast occur at the site of the original breast cancer; 90% of local recurrences following breast-conserving surgery are invasive. The majority of disease which develops in the treated breast after 5 years represents a second primary cancer rather than recurrence. Local recurrence within the first 5 years is associated with a much worse long-term outlook than recurrence thereafter.[6,7] The role of systemic therapy following mastectomy for an apparently localised breast recurrence is not clear.[75] Uncontrollable local recurrence is uncommon after breast conservation, but when it does occur it is difficult to treat.

A recent study that extended hormonal treatment with letrozole after 5 years of tamoxifen demonstrated a reduction by almost two-thirds in the number of 'local recurrences' (**Table 4.3**) and reduced the rate of contralateral breast cancer development.[77] Prolonging adjuvant hormonal therapy beyond 5 years may thus have an impact on the rate of subsequent local relapse.

Table 4.3 • Recurrences in 5187 women enrolled into the MA17 study*

	Letrozole (N = 2575)	Placebo (N = 2582)
Total	61 (2.4%)	106 (4.1%)
Breast only	6	19
Local chest wall	2	7
Regional lymph nodes	6	4
Distant site or sites	47	76
Contralateral breast cancer only	14 (0.5%)	26 (1.0%)
Total	75	132

*5187 women were enrolled (median follow-up 2.4 years) into the MA17 study, in which patients who were disease-free after approximately 5 years of tamoxifen were randomised to receive placebo or letrozole. The estimated 4-year disease-free survival rates were 93% with letrozole and 87% with placebo ($P \leq 0.001$ for the comparison of disease-free survival). Modified from ref. 77.

Key points

- For patients with single small breast cancers, survival outcomes from breast-conserving treatment are equivalent to that of mastectomy.
- Radiotherapy reduces the rate of local recurrence after breast-conserving surgery and appears to improve overall survival. No subgroup of patients has yet been identified that can avoid radiotherapy.
- The major surgical factor influencing local recurrence is completeness of excision, and clear margins must be obtained when performing breast-conserving surgery.
- Younger patients have an increased rate of local recurrence after breast-conserving surgery and, conversely, older patients have a lower rate of local recurrence.
- Tumour grade, EIC and LVI have a small influence on the rate of local recurrence. Patients with these factors should not be denied breast-conserving surgery, providing the cancer can be excised with clear margins.
- There is a direct correlation between cosmetic outcome after breast-conserving surgery and psychological morbidity, with better cosmetic outcomes being associated with less anxiety and depression and better body image and self-esteem.
- The most important factor influencing cosmetic outcome after breast-conserving surgery is the percentage volume of breast excised. Removing more than 10% of breast volume results in the majority of women having a poor cosmetic outcome.
- Patients who develop local recurrence after breast-conserving surgery, particularly in the first 5 years, are at increased risk of having systemic relapse.
- Isolated local recurrences after breast-conserving surgery are usually best treated by mastectomy, although re-excision is possible if the recurrence develops more than 5 years after treatment or the patient has not received radiotherapy to the breast.
- Prolonged hormonal therapy beyond 5 years reduces the rate of subsequent local recurrence and the rate of contralateral breast cancer.

REFERENCES

1. Sharif K, Al-Ghazal SK, Blamey RW. Cosmetic assessment of breast-conserving surgery for primary breast cancer. Breast 1999; 8:162–8.

    A comprehensive review of factors that influence cosmetic outcome after breast-conserving surgery. A review of level 2 evidence.

2. Al-Ghazal SK, Fallowfield L, Blamey, RW. Comparison of psychological aspects and patient satisfaction following breast conserving surgery, simple mastectomy and breast reconstruction. Eur J Cancer 2000; 36:1938–43.

3. Shain WS, d'Angelo TM, Dunn ME et al. Mastectomy versus conservative surgery and radiation therapy: psychological consequences. Cancer 1994; 73:1221–8.

4. Early Breast Cancer Trialists' Collaborative Group. Effects of radiotherapy and surgery in early breast cancer: an overview of the randomised trials. N Engl J Med 1995; 333:1444–55.

    This review analyses data on 10-year survival from six randomised controlled trials comparing breast conservation with mastectomy. Meta-analysis of data from five of the randomised trials (3006 women) found no difference in the risk of death at 10 years. Where more than half of node-positive patients in both the mastectomy and breast-conserving groups received adjuvant nodal radiotherapy, both groups had similar survival rates. In contrast, where less than half of node-positive women in both groups received adjuvant nodal radiotherapy, survival was better for the breast-conserving surgery group. Overall risk vs. mastectomy 0.69, 95% CO 0.5, 90%, 0.57. Level 1 evidence.

5. Morris AD, Morris RD, Wilson JF et al. Breast conserving therapy versus mastectomy in early stage breast cancer: a meta-analysis of 10 year survival. Cancer J Sci Am 1997; 3:6–12.

    In this review nine randomised controlled trials involving 4981 women potentially suitable for breast-conserving surgery were analysed. Meta-analysis found no significant difference in the risk of death over 10 years for patients treated by mastectomy or breast-conserving surgery. The authors also found no significant difference in the rates of local recurrence in the six trials where data were available. Level 1 evidence.

6. Fortin A, Larochelle M, Laverdière J. et al. Local failure is responsible for the decrease in survival for patients with breast cancer treated with conservative surgery and postoperative radiotherapy. J Clin Oncol 1999; 17:101–9.

   This study analysed data from 2030 patients. The results showed that local failure was associated with an increase in mortality. The authors conclude that local failure should be considered not only as a marker of occult circulating distant metastases but also as a source of new distant metastases and subsequent mortality. Level 2 evidence.

7. Fisher B, Anderson S, Fisher E et al. Significance of ipsilateral breast tumour recurrence after lumpectomy. Lancet 1991; 338:327–31.

8. Dixon JM, Gregory K, Johnston S et al. Breast cancer: non-metastatic. Clin Evid Concise 2002; 8:355–9.

   This a comprehensive review of all randomised trials in this area. A review of level 1 and 2 evidence.

9. Dixon JM, Venizelos B, Chan P. Latissimus dorsi mini-flap: a technique for extending breast conservation. Breast 2002; 11:58–65.

10. Raja MAK, Straker VF, Rainsbury RM. Extending the role of breast-conserving surgery by immediate volume replacement. Br J Surg 1997; 84:101–5.

11. Fisher ER, Sass R, Fisher B et al. Pathologic findings from the national surgical adjuvant breast project (protocol 6): relation of local breast recurrence to multicentricity. Cancer 1986; 57:1717–24.

12. Kurtz JM, Jacquemier G, Amalaric R et al. Breast-conserving therapy for macroscopically multiple cancers. Ann Surg 1990; 212:38–44.

13. NIH Consensus Conference. Treatment of early-stage breast cancer. JAMA 1991; 265:391–5.

14. Holland DR, Connolly JL, Gelman R et al. The presence of an extensive intraductal component (EIC) following a limited excision predicts for prominent residual disease in the remainder of the breast. J Clin Oncol 1990; 8:113–18.

15. Veronesi U, Banfi A, Salvadore B et al. Breast conservation is the treatment of choice in small breast cancer: long term results of a randomised trial. Eur J Cancer 1990; 26:668–70.

   Results of the first randomised trial performed between 1985 and 1987 involving over 700 patients. This was the first study to compare breast-conserving surgery in the form of quadrantectomy and mastectomy. Importantly, this study showed no difference in outcome. Level 1 evidence.

16. Ghossein NA, Alpert S, Barba J et al. Importance of adequate surgical excision prior to radiotherapy in the local control of breast cancer in patients treated conservatively. Arch Surg 1992; 127:411–15.

17. Veronesi U, Volterrani F, Luini A et al. Quadrantectomy versus lumpectomy for small size breast cancer. Eur J Cancer 1990; 16:671–3.

18. Sacchini V, Luini A, Tana S et al. Quantitive and qualitative cosmetic evaluation after conservation treatment for breast cancer. Eur J Cancer 1991; 27:1395–400.

19. Fisher B, Wolmark N, Fisher ER. Lumpectomy and axillary dissection for breast cancer: surgical, pathological and radiation considerations. World J Surg 1985; 96:692–8.

   The National Surgical Adjuvant Breast and Bowel Project randomised 1850 women for lumpectomy alone, lumpectomy and radiotherapy or mastectomy. The short- and long-term results have shown that lumpectomy followed by breast irradiation is an appropriate therapy for women with breast cancer providing that lumpectomy can be achieved with negative surgical margins and acceptable cosmesis. Level 1 evidence.

20. Langer K. Zur anatomie and physiologie der Haut. Huber Die Spaltbarkiet Der Cutis. S-b-Akad Wiss Wein 1861; 44:19–46.

21. Kraissl CJ. The selection of appropriate lines for elective surgical incisions. Plast Reconstr Surg 1951; 8:1–28.

22. Osteen RT. Partial mastectomy, lumpectomy, quandrantectomy. In: Daly JM, Cady B (eds) Atlas of surgical oncology. St Louis: Mosby-Year Book, 1993; pp. 113–21.

23. Vallasiadou K, Young OE, Dixon JM. Current practices in breast conservation surgery: results of a questionnaire. Br J Surg 2003; 90:44.

24. Beck NE, Bradburn MJ, Vincenti AC et al. Detection of residual disease following breast-conserving surgery. Br J Surg 1998; 85:1273–6.

25. Nedelman R, Dixon JM. Marking of specimens in patients undergoing stereotactic wide local excision for breast cancer. Br J Surg 1992; 79:55.

26. Bartelink H, Horiot JC, Poortmans P et al. Recurrence rates after treatment of breast cancer with standard radiotherapy with or without additional radiation. N Engl J Med 2001; 345:1378–87.

27. Kurtz JM. Factors influencing the risk of local recurrence in the breast. Eur J Cancer 1992; 28:660–6.

28. Chauvet B, Simon JM, Reynaud-Bougnoux A et al. Récidives mammares après traitment conservateur des cancers du sein: facteurs prédictifs et signification pornostique. Bull Cancer 1990; 77:1193–205.

29. Pierce L, Levin A, Rebbeck T et al. Ten-year outcome of breast-conserving surgery (BCS) and radiotherapy (RT) in women with breast cancer

(BC) and germline BRCA 1/2 mutations: results from an international collaboration. Breast Cancer Res Treat 2003; 82:S7.

30. Calle R, Vilcoq JR, Zafrani B. Local control and survival of breast cancer treated by limited surgery followed by irradiation. Int J Radiat Oncol Biol Phys 1986; 12:873–8.

31. Fisher B, Anderson S, Bryant J et al. Twenty-year follow-up of a randomised trial comparing total mastectomy, lumpectomy, and lumpectomy plus irradiation for the treatment of invasive breast cancer. N Engl J Med 2002; 347:1233–41.

Long-term follow-up of one of the two original trials of breast-conserving surgery and mastectomy. After 20 years, this study showed equivalent overall survival rates for patients randomised to receive wide excision alone, wide excision followed by radiotherapy and mastectomy. There were significantly more local recurrences in the group of patients treated by wide excision who did not receive radiotherapy. Level 1 evidence.

32. Fowble BL, Solin LJ, Schultz DJ et al. 10 year results of conservative surgery and irradiation for stage I and II breast cancer. Int J Radiat Oncol Biol Phys 1991; 21:269–77.

33. Haffty BG, Fischer D, Rose M et al. Prognostic factors for local recurrence in the conservatively treated breast cancer patient: a cautious interpretation of the data. J Clin Oncol 1991; 6:997–1003.

34. Asgiersson KS, McCulley SJ, Pinder SE et al. Size of invasive breast cancer and risk of local recurrence after breast-conservation therapy. Eur J Cancer 2003; 39:2462–9

A large recent review bringing together all the evidence relating tumour size and local recurrence. The conclusion of the review is that local recurrence is not influenced by tumour size. Review of level 2 evidence.

35. Eberlein TG, Connolly JN, Schnitt JS et al. Predictors of local recurrence following conservative breast surgery and radiation therapy. The influence of tumour size. Arch Surg 1990; 125:771–9.

36. Clarke DH, Le MG, Sarrazin D et al. Analysis of local–regional relapse in patients with early breast cancers treated by excision and radiotherapy. Experience of the Institut Gustave-Roussy. Int J Radiat Oncol Biol Phys 1985; 11:137–45.

37. Locker AP, Ellis IO, Morgan DAL et al. Factors influencing local recurrence after excision and radiotherapy for primary breast cancer. Br J Surg 1989; 76:890–4.

38. Kurtz JM, Jacquemier G, Amalric R et al. Risk factors for breast recurrence in premenopausal and postmenopausal patients with ductal cancers treated by conservation therapy. Cancer 1990; 65:1867–78.

39. Mate TP, Carter D, Fischer DB et al. A clinical and histopathological analysis of the results of conservation surgery and radiation therapy in stage I and stage II breast carcinoma. Cancer 1986; 58:1995–2002.

40. Zafrani B, Viehl P, Fourqhet A et al. Conservative treatment of early breast cancer: prognostic value of the ductal in situ component and other pathological variables on local control and survival. Long term results. Eur J Cancer Clin Oncol 1989; 25:1645–50.

41. Ryoo MC, Kagan AR, Wollin M. Prognostic factors for recurrence and cosmesis in 393 patients after radiation therapy for early mammary carcinoma. Radiology 1989; 172:555–9.

42. Jacquemier RG, Kurtz JM, Amalric R et al. An assessment of extensive intraductal component as a risk factor for local recurrence after breast-conserving surgery. Br J Cancer 1990; 61:873–6.

43. Fourquet A, Campan F, Zafrani B et al. Prognostic factors of breast recurrence in the conservative management of early breast cancer: a 25 year follow up. Int J Radiat Oncol Biol Phys 1989; 17:719–25.

44. du Toit RS, Locker AP, Ellis IO et al. An evaluation of differences in prognosis, recurrence patterns and receptor status between invasive lobular and other invasive carcinomas of the breast. Eur J Surg Oncol 1991; 17:251–7.

45. Schnitt SJ, Connolly JL, Kettry U. Pathologic findings on re-excision of the primary site in breast cancer patients considered for treatment by primary radiation therapy. Cancer 1987; 59:675–81.

46. Recht A, Danoff BS, Solin LJ et al. Intraductal carcinoma of the breast: results of treatment with excisional biopsy and irradiation. J Clin Oncol 1985; 313:39–43.

47. Gage I, Schnitt SJ, Nixon AJ et al. Pathologic margin involvement and the risk of recurrence in patients treated with breast-conserving therapy. Cancer 1996; 78:1921–8.

48. Smitt MC, Nowels KW, Zdeblick MJ et al. The importance of the lumpectomy surgical margin status in long term results of breast conservation. Cancer 1995; 76:259–67.

Demonstrates that involved margins are the most important risk factor for local recurrence after breast-conserving surgery. Level 2 evidence.

49. Solin LJ, Fowble BL, Schultz DJ et al. The significance of the pathology margins of the tumour excision on the outcome of patients treated with definitive irradiation for early stage breast cancer. Int J Radiat Oncol Biol Phys 1991; 21:279–87.

50. Spivack B, Khanna MM, Tafra L et al. Margin status and local recurrence after breast-conserving surgery. Arch Surg 1994; 129:952–7.

51. Clark RM, McCulloch PB, Levine MN et al. Randomised clinical trials to assess the effectiveness of breast irradiation following lumpectomy and axillary dissection for node-negative breast cancer. J Natl Cancer Inst 1992; 84:683–9.

52. Wazer DE, Jabro G, Ruthazer R et al. Extent of margin positivity as a predictor for local recurrence after breast conserving irradiation. Radiat Oncol Invest 1999; 7:111–17.

53. Borger J, Kemperman, H, Hart A et al. Risk factors in breast-conservation therapy. J Clin Oncol 1994; 12:653–60.

54. Schmidt-Ullrich R, Wazer DE, DiPetrillo T et al. Breast conservation therapy for early stage breast carcinoma with outstanding ten year locoregional control rates: a case for aggressive therapy to the tumour bearing quadrant. Int J Radiat Oncol Biol Phys 1993; 27:545–52.

55. Abner AL, Connolly JL, Recht A et al. The relation between the presence and extent of lobular carcinoma in situ and the risk of local recurrence for patients with infiltrating carcinoma of the breast treated with conservative surgery and radiation therapy. Cancer 2000; 88:1072–1077.

56. Fowble B, Hanlon AL, Patchefsky A et al. The presence of proliferative breast disease with atypia does significantly influence outcome in early-stage invasive breast cancer treated with conservative surgery and radiation. Int J Radiat Oncol Biol Phys 1998; 42:105–15.

57. Swanson GP, Rynearson K, Symmonds R. Significance of margins of excision on breast cancer recurrence. Am J Clin Oncol 2002; 25:438–41.

58. Wazer DE, DiPetrillo T, Schmidt-Ullrich R et al. Factors influencing cosmetic outcome and complication risk after conservative surgery and radiotherapy for early-stage breast carcinoma. J Clin Oncol 1992; 10:356–63.

59. Fisher B, Redmond C, Poisson R et al. Eight year results of a randomised clinical trial comparing total mastectomy and lumpectomy with or without irradiation in the treatment of breast cancer. N Engl J Med 1989; 320:822–8.

60. Rose MA, Henderson IC, Gellman R et al. Premenopausal breast cancer patients treated with conservative surgery, radiotherapy and adjuvant chemotherapy have a low risk of local failure. Int J Radiat Oncol Biol Phys 1989; 17:717–21.

61. Haffty BG, Fischer D, Beinfield M et al. Prognosis following local recurrence in the conservatively treated breast cancer patient. Int J Radiat Oncol Biol Phys 1991; 21:293–8.

62. Forrest P, Stewart HJ, Everington D et al. Randomised controlled trial of conservative therapy for breast cancer: 6-year analysis of the Scottish trial. Lancet 1996; 348:708–13.

Demonstrates that following breast-conserving surgery, giving adjuvant systemic therapy selected on oestrogen receptor status does not protect patients who do not receive radiotherapy from an excess of local recurrences. Conclusion is that radiotherapy is needed even if optimal adjuvant systemic therapy is prescribed. Level 1 evidence.

63. Prosnitz LR, Goldenberg IS, Packard RA et al. Radiation therapy as initial treatment for early stage cancer of the breast without mastectomy. Cancer 1977; 39:917–23.

64. Dewar JA, Benhamou S, Benhamou E et al. Cosmetic results following lumpectomy, axillary dissection and radiotherapy for small breast cancers. Radiother Oncol 1988; 12:273–80.

65. Liljegren G, Holmberg L, Westman G et al. The cosmetic outcome in early breast cancer treated with sector resection with or without radiotherapy. Eur J Cancer 1993; 29A:2083–9.

66. Greco M, Sacchiai V, Agresti R et al. Quadrantectomy is not a disfiguring operation for small breast cancer. Breast 1994; 3:3–7.

67. Haffty BG, Wilson LD, Smith R et al. Subareolar breast cancer: long-term results with conservative surgery and radiation therapy. Int J Radiat Oncol Biol Phys 1995; 33:53–7.

68. Amichetti M, Busana L, Caffo O. Long-term cosmetic outcome and toxicity in patients treated with quandrantectomy and radiation therapy for early-stage breast cancer. Oncology 1995; 52:177–81.

69. Garofalo R, Borioni R, Garofalo RLL et al. Radical tumour excision and cosmetic balance in the surgical treatment of breast carcinoma: biquandrantectomy. Biomed Pharmacother 1992; 46:401–4.

70. Sneeuw KA, Aaronson N, Yarnould J et al. Cosmetic and functional outcomes of breast conserving treatment for early stage breast cancer. 1. Comparison of patients' ratings, observers' ratings and objective assessments. Radiother Oncol 1992; 25:153–9.

71. Christie DRH, O'Brien MY, Christie JA et al. A comparison of methods of cosmetic assessment in breast conservation treatment. Breast 1996; 5:358–67.

72. Patterson M, Pezner R, Hill R et al. Patient self-evaluation of cosmetic outcome of breast-preserving cancer treatment. Int J Radiat Oncol Biol Phys 1985; 11:1849–52.

73. Hamilton CS, Nield JM, Alder GF et al. Breast appearance and function after breast conserving surgery and radiotherapy. Acta Oncol 1990; 29:291–5.

74. Kurtz JM. Impact of radiotherapy on breast cosmesis. Breast 1995; 4:163–9.

75. Anderson EDC. Treatment of breast recurrence after breast conservation. In: Dixon JM (ed.) Breast cancer: diagnosis and management. London: Elsevier, 2000; pp. 1–5.

Review of treatment of local recurrence after breast-conserving surgery. Level 2 evidence.

76. Kurtz JM, Jacquemier G, Amalric R. Is breast conservation after local recurrence feasible. Eur J Cancer 1991; 27:240–4.

77. Goss PE, Ingle JN, Martino S et al. A randomized trial of letrozole in postmenopausal women after five years of tamoxifen therapy for early-stage breast cancer. N Engl J Med 2003; 349:1793–802.

A total of 5187 women were enrolled (median follow-up 2.4 years). At the first interim analysis, there were 207 local or metastatic recurrences of breast cancer or new primary cancers in the contralateral breast (75 in the letrozole group and 132 in the placebo group), with estimated 4-year disease-free survival rates of 93% and 87% respectively in the two groups (P ≤ 0.001 for the comparison of disease-free survival). A total of 42 women in the placebo group and 31 women in the letrozole group died (P = 0.25 for the comparison of overall survival). Low-grade hot flashes, arthritis, arthralgia and myalgia were more frequent in the letrozole group, but vaginal bleeding was less frequent. There were new diagnoses of osteoporosis in 5.8% of the women in the letrozole group and 4.5% of the women in the placebo group (P = 0.07); the rates of fracture were similar. Level 1 evidence.

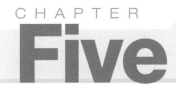

CHAPTER

Five

Partial breast reconstruction

Richard M. Rainsbury and
Krishna Clough

INTRODUCTION

Breast-conserving surgery (BCS) combined with radiotherapy has become the treatment of choice for the majority of women presenting with primary breast cancer over the last 20 years.

A number of prospective randomised trials have compared BCS with mastectomy, showing a survival rate that is unrelated to the type of surgery performed,[1-3] although local recurrence (LR) rates may be higher when the breast is conserved.[1,4]

The risk of LR is related to a number of factors, including positive margins, tumour grade, extensive in situ component, lymphovascular invasion and age. Whole-breast section analysis techniques have been used to show the likelihood of complete excision of unicentric carcinomas using different margins of excision.

Holland et al.[5] showed that a margin of 2 cm would eradicate all microscopic disease in about 60% of cases compared with a margin of 4 cm, which increases this figure to about 90%.

LOCAL RECURRENCE AND COSMETIC OUTCOME

The margins of clearance and to a lesser degree the extent of local excision during BCS are strong predictors of subsequent LR.[6]

The Milan II Trial, which compared tumorectomy and radiotherapy (TART) with quadrantectomy and radiotherapy (QUART),[7] investigated the effect of radical local excision on LR. There was a highly significant reduction in margin involvement and therefore in LR in patients randomised to tumour excision with a 2–3 cm margin (QUART group) compared with those treated by tumorectomy in which the tumour was excised with a minimal margin (TART group).

The extent of local excision remains a controversial issue in BCS. The wider the margin of clearance, the less the risk of incomplete excision and thus of LR (**Table 5.1**), but the greater the amount of tissue removed, the higher the risk of visible deformity leading to an unacceptable cosmetic result. This clash of interests[8] is most evident when attempting

Table 5.1 • Technique-related outcomes of breast-conserving surgery

	Quadrantectomy	Wide local excision
Margin	2–4 cm	1–2 cm
Clearance*	<90%	<58%
Recurrence[†]	2%	7%
Cosmesis	Fair	Good

*Holland et al.[5]
[†]Veronesi et al.[7]

BCS in patients with smaller breast–tumour ratios, for example when planning BCS for a 10-mm tumour in a 200-g breast or a 5-cm tumour in a 700-g breast.

The chances of a poor cosmetic outcome are increased still further when the tumour is in a central, medial or inferior location.[9,10] Cosmetic failure is more common than generally appreciated, occurring in up to 50% of patients after BCS.[11–15] A number of factors are responsible, including volume loss of more than 10–20% leading to retraction and asymmetry, nipple–areola displacement or distortion, ugly and inappropriate incisions, and the local effects of radiotherapy. Volume loss underlies many of the most visible and distressing examples of poor cosmetic outcome and the effects may be compounded by associated displacement of the nipple–areola complex (NAC). Poor surgical technique leading to postoperative haematoma, infection or necrosis will increase the amount of scarring and retraction, and will add to the risks of deformity. Moreover, the use of suction drains, inappropriate incisions and en bloc resections can worsen the cosmetic result still further.

ROLE OF ONCOPLASTIC SURGERY

The interrelationship between breast–tumour ratio, volume loss, cosmetic outcome and margins of clearance is complex, and the widespread popularity of BCS has focused attention on new oncoplastic techniques that can avoid unacceptable cosmetic results. Until now, surgical options have been limited to BCS or mastectomy, the choice depending on fairly well-defined indications and factors. Oncoplastic techniques provide a 'third option' that avoids the need for mastectomy in selected patients and can influence the outcome of BCS in three respects.

1. Oncoplastic techniques allow very wide excision of breast tissue without risking major local deformity.
2. The use of oncoplastic techniques to prevent deformity can extend the scope of BCS to include patients with 3–5 cm tumours, without compromising the adequacy of resection or the cosmetic outcome.
3. Volume replacement can be used after previous BCS and radiotherapy to correct unacceptable deformity[16] and may prevent the need for mastectomy in some cases of LR when further local excision will result in considerable volume loss.

CHOICE OF ONCOPLASTIC TECHNIQUE

The choice of technique depends on a number of factors, including the extent of resection, position of the tumour, timing of surgery, experience of the surgeon and expectations of the patient. Reconstruction at the same time as resection (breast-sparing reconstruction) is gaining in popularity. As a general rule, it is much easier to prevent than to correct a deformity, as the sequelae of previous surgery do not have to be addressed. Immediate reconstruction at the time of mastectomy is associated with clear surgical,[17] financial[18,19] and psychological[20] benefits, and similar benefits are seen in patients undergoing immediate breast-sparing reconstruction after partial mastectomy.

Resection defects can be reconstructed in one of two ways: (i) by volume replacement, importing volume from elsewhere to replace the amount of tissue resected, or (ii) by volume displacement, recruiting and transposing local dermoglandular flaps into the resection site. Volume replacement techniques can restore the shape and size of the breast, achieving symmetry and excellent cosmetic results without the need for contralateral surgery.

67

Volume replacement techniques

Table 5.2 • Comparison of techniques for breast-conserving reconstruction

	Volume replacement	Volume displacement
Symmetry	Good	Variable
Scars	Breast Back	Periareolar Inverted-T
Problems	Donor scar Seroma Flap loss	Parenchymal necrosis Nipple necrosis Volume loss
Theatre time	2–3 hours	1–2 hours (per side)
Convalescence	4–6 weeks	1–2 weeks
Timing	Immediate or delayed	Immediate > delayed
Mammographic surveillance	Possibly enhanced	Unaffected

However, these techniques require additional theatre time and may be complicated by donor-site morbidity, flap loss and an extended convalescence. In contrast, volume displacement techniques require less extensive surgery, limiting scars to the breast and avoiding donor-site problems. These procedures may be complicated by necrosis of the dermoglandular flaps and contralateral surgery is usually required to restore symmetry as volume loss is inevitable (**Table 5.2**).

A number of factors need to be considered when making the choice between volume replacement and volume displacement. Volume replacement is particularly suitable for patients who wish to avoid volume loss and contralateral surgery after extensive local resections. They must be prepared to accept a donor-site scar and be made aware of the possibility of major complications that may result in prolonged convalescence. Volume replacement is equally well suited to immediate and delayed reconstruction and is the method of choice for correcting severe deformity after previous breast irradiation.

Volume displacement techniques are particularly useful for patients with large ptotic breasts who gain benefit from a 'therapeutic' reduction mammoplasty that incorporates wide removal of the tumour. Volume displacement is less reliable in irradiated breasts, and patients need to be warned about the risk of asymmetry that may require simultaneous or subsequent contralateral surgery.

VOLUME REPLACEMENT TECHNIQUES

Several different approaches to volume replacement have been developed over the last 10 years, including myocutaneous, myosubcutaneous and adipose flaps, and implants. Autologous latissimus dorsi (LD) flaps are the most popular option because of their versatility and reliability.

The myocutaneous LD flap carries a skin paddle that can be used to replace skin which has been resected at the time of BCS or as a result of contracture and scarring following previous resection and radiotherapy[16] (**Fig. 5.1**). Although the skin paddle adds to the replacement volume, it can lead to an ugly 'patch' effect because of the difference in colour between the donor skin and the skin of the native breast.

 A myosubcutaneous LD miniflap[21] circumvents this problem by harvesting the flap in a plane deep to Scarpa's fascia. This produces a bulky flap without a skin island and carrying a layer of fat on its superficial surface that is used to reconstruct defects following wide excision with preservation of the overlying skin (**Fig. 5.2**).

Transverse rectus abdominis myocutaneous (TRAM) flaps provide a third alternative, but the bulk of these flaps render them a less attractive choice than LD flaps in this particular situation. Moreover, fat necrosis is a more common complication of TRAM flaps, creating the potential for diagnostic confusion on follow-up. Other flaps, such as the lateral thoracic adipose tissue flap, have been described[22] but their clinical utility is unclear.

Non-autologous volume replacement with saline or silicone implants has been tried with very mixed success.[23,24] Implants can be placed directly into the resection defect or under pectoralis major. They cannot be moulded to fit the resection defect and they form localised capsules, particularly in irradiated tissues. This interferes with not only clinical examination but also mammographic surveillance. Autologous tissue transfer circumvents

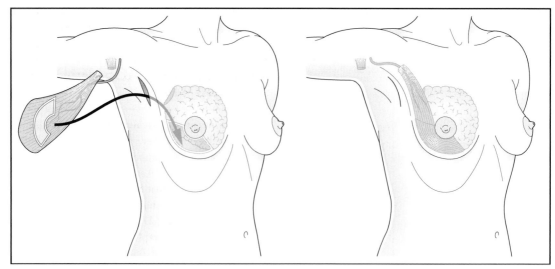

Figure 5.1 • Latissimus dorsi myocutaneous miniflap.

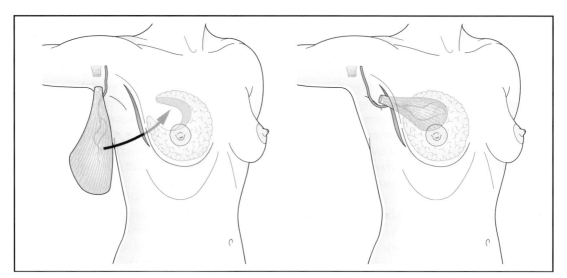

Figure 5.2 • Latissimus dorsi myosubcutaneous miniflap.

these problems, and results in a life-like breast of normal shape and size.

A number of innovative surgical procedures have evolved that facilitate volume replacement at the time of BCS or at a later date.

1. Resection through a radial incision and LD harvest through an axillary incision.[25]
2. Conventional LD myocutaneous flap harvest for correction of major resection defects.[16]

3. Resection through a circumferential incision and endoscopic LD flap harvest and reconstruction through an axillary incision.[26]
4. Resection, LD harvest and reconstruction through a single lateral incision.[22]

Indications for volume replacement

Volume replacement should always be considered when adequate local tumour excision leads to an

Box 5.1 • Selection of patients for volume replacement

Indications

Breast of any size

Resection of 10–50% breast volume

Specimen weight typically150–350 g

Correcting deformity after breast-conserving surgery

When mastectomy declined

When full reconstruction declined

When contralateral surgery declined

When radiotherapy planned after mastectomy

Contraindications

Multicentric tumours

T_4 tumours

Diffuse malignant microcalcification

Comorbidity

Previous division of vascular pedicle

Previous ipsilateral thoracotomy

unacceptable degree of local deformity in those patients who wish to avoid mastectomy or contralateral surgery. Typically, this will occur after loss of 10–20% or more of the breast volume, particularly when this is resected from the central zone, lower pole or medial quadrants of the breast.

Breast conservation with or without reconstruction should be reserved for patients with unicentric tumours and is inappropriate in those with more widespread disease or T4 tumours. Likewise, LD volume replacement is hazardous in patients with a history suggesting damage to the thoracodorsal pedicle or to the LD muscle, and alternative methods should be considered (**Box 5.1**). Patients should be informed that using LD for breast conservation precludes its subsequent use for full breast reconstruction. If a mastectomy is required to treat recurrent disease, the options are limited to TRAM flap or subpectoral reconstruction.

Timing of procedures

Ideally, reconstruction of the partial mastectomy defect should be performed alongside tumour resection in order to prevent deformity rather than to correct deformity months or years later. The emergence of the multiskilled 'oncoplastic' breast surgeon will in future help to circumvent the current problems encountered when organising a 'two-team' approach involving breast and plastic surgeons. Moreover, immediate reconstruction is associated with fewer technical problems and complications than delayed procedures. Delayed reconstruction may be compromised by previous radiotherapy, leading to reduced tissue viability and an increased risk of fat necrosis, infection and delayed wound healing.

Immediate reconstruction can be carried out as a one-stage procedure,[22,27] which involves simultaneous resection and correction of the resulting defect. This requires peroperative confirmation of complete tumour excision using frozen-section techniques. As an alternative, the procedure can be split into two steps.[28] The first step involves the partial mastectomy and the second step includes axillary dissection, flap harvest and reconstruction, and is carried out a few days later after confirmation of clear tumour resection margins. Patients prefer a one-stage procedure, but must be informed that a mastectomy with or without reconstruction may be required if subsequent histopathological analysis confirms incomplete tumour excision.

Volume replacement with latissimus dorsi miniflaps

There are many similarities between the different surgical approaches used in breast-conserving reconstruction and these can be best illustrated by summarising the main steps involved in LD miniflap reconstruction, which has been described in detail elsewhere.[29] This procedure involves the use of a myosubcutaneous flap of LD for immediate reconstruction of a partial mastectomy defect, most commonly in the central zone but also in the upper outer and upper inner quadrants of the breast. The term 'miniflap' is somewhat misleading, as the flap needs to be of sufficient volume to replace resection defects resulting from the excision of 150–350 g of breast tissue. Moreover, the miniflap needs to be bulky enough to allow for a small degree of postoperative flap atrophy.

When planning immediate volume replacement, the patient needs to be fully informed about the nature of the procedure and the possibility that a subsequent total mastectomy may be required if partial mastectomy results in incomplete excision. Careful preoperative mark-up of the tumour, the margins of resection and the line of incision are essential. The operation allows simultaneous partial mastectomy, axillary dissection, mobilisation of part of LD (the miniflap) and reconstruction of the resection defect through a single lateral incision. The procedure is greatly simplified by high-quality equipment, which is essential when developing the narrow optical spaces behind the breast and on the superficial and deep surfaces of the miniflap.

The operation involves tumour resection, axillary dissection, flap harvest and reconstruction. First, the tumour is resected in a subcutaneous plane by separating the skin envelope overlying the tumour-bearing quadrant from the underlying breast disc by sharp dissection, using the preoperative skin marks to determine the exact extent of dissection. By developing a mirror-image retromammary space deep to pectoralis fascia, the mobilised tumour-bearing quadrant is gripped firmly between fingers and thumb and resected with a generous margin of normal breast tissue. Four biopsies taken from opposite poles of the resection defect are sent for frozen-section analysis to allow intraoperative assessment of completeness of excision. The cavity wall is inked in situ with methylene blue to identify the inner surface, and then can be re-excised in its entirety if considered necessary. Further bed biopsies can also be examined after re-excising the cavity wall if frozen-section examination of the initial biopsies shows incomplete excision. A mastectomy is performed if these further bed biopsies fail to confirm complete excision. Next, an appropriate axillary dissection is carried out and the vascular pedicle is prepared.

The third step involves mobilisation of the LD miniflap by developing superficial and deep perimuscular spaces that mirror each other. The myosubcutaneous flap carries a layer of fat on its superficial surface to increase its volume and this is achieved by developing the superficial pocket just deep to Scarpa's fascia. Division of the miniflap around the perimeter of the dissection pocket and division of the tendon of LD near its insertion

ensures unrestricted transposition of the miniflap into the resection defect. Finally, reconstruction of the resection defect is completed by careful use of sutures to model the flap, before fixing it to the cavity walls.

Perioperative outcomes

The time required for breast-conserving immediate reconstruction with a miniflap lies somewhere between BCS alone and total mastectomy combined with immediate LD reconstruction. Early post-operative complications include infection, flap necrosis, haematoma formation and transient brachial plexopathy,[27] although postoperative stay and disability is similar to other types of BCS. Breast oedema is common, particularly after extensive segmental resection and usually settles within 6–8 weeks. It may be caused by division of multiple afferent lymphatic pathways during retromammary dissection. Donor-site seroma formation occurs in almost all patients, and can be reduced by quilting or delaying drain removal. Flap necrosis is rare, and can be avoided by gentle resection and handling of the pedicle and by taking care to prevent traction and twisting injuries during transposition and fixation of the flap after tendon division.

Late sequelae of volume replacement include lateral retraction of the flap, leading to distortion and hollowing of the resection site, and flap atrophy. Flap retraction can be avoided by division and fixation of the tendon and careful suture of the flap into the resection defect. Detectable flap atrophy occurs in a minority of patients followed for up to 10 years.[30] It can be counteracted by over-replacement of the resected volume with a fully innervated flap that has been harvested with a generous layer of subcutaneous fat, or by using a myocutaneous flap.[16]

Frozen-section analysis of bed biopsies has been found to correlate closely with the adequacy of excision determined by formal histopathology (unpublished data). Moreover, the use of LD miniflap reconstruction leads to a significant fall in the number of incomplete excisions compared with BCS alone[22] without compromising the cosmetic outcome. Sensory loss following miniflap reconstruction is minimal compared with the loss following total mastectomy.[31] The sensory innervation of

(a) 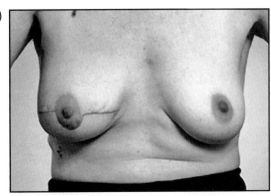 (b)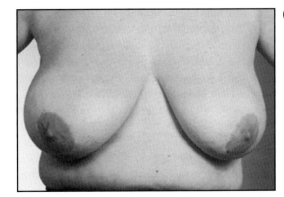

Figure 5.3 • **(a)** Latissimus dorsi myocutaneous miniflap; **(b)** latissimus dorsi myosubcutaneous miniflap.

the breast and NAC is largely intact, except over the resected quadrant. Finally, volume replacement preserves symmetry, avoiding the need for alterations to the contralateral breast in almost all patients (**Fig. 5.3**).

Mammographic surveillance

The mammographic appearance of the partially reconstructed breast compares favourably with the appearances after routine BCS. Symmetry is preserved and the fibres of the isodense flap may be detectable, often associated with a variable zone of radiolucency that corresponds to the layer of surface fat. Flaps may be indistinguishable from the surrounding breast tissue, and important radiological characteristics such as skin thickening, stellate lesions and microcalcifications are easily visualised after flap transfer. Volume replacement does not compromise the early detection of LR,[32] which typically develops at the junctional zone between muscle and breast parenchyma. The appearance of miniflap on mammograms contrasts with the radiodense distorting stellate scars that are a common source of diagnostic confusion following conventional BCS. Lastly, very few patients develop clinically detectable flap atrophy, with the majority of flaps remaining bulky and functional throughout the period of follow-up.

Future prospects

The role of breast-conserving volume replacement is set to increase as more precise, image-guided

resection of specific zones of breast tissue becomes possible. Increasingly sophisticated imaging techniques, such as high-frequency ultrasound and contrast-enhanced dynamic magnetic resonance imaging,[33] may in future enable exact delineation and excision of all malignant and premalignant changes. Endoscopically assisted techniques[34] may increase the ability to harvest more bulky myosubcutaneous flaps, allowing the reconstruction of more extensive resection defects. This will require the further development of novel techniques for endoscopic dissection,[26] including the use of balloon-assisted techniques[34,35] and carbon dioxide insufflation to maintain the epimuscular optical cavities. Current progress is hampered by the use of non-flexible straight endoscopes to carry out dissection over the rigid convex surface of the chest wall.

VOLUME DISPLACEMENT TECHNIQUES

Until recently, little attention has been paid to the cosmetic sequelae of BCS, as most patients are relieved not to lose their breast and many surgeons are unfamiliar with the plastic surgery techniques that can eliminate postoperative deformities. Moreover, there has been a tendency to recommend delayed reconstructive surgery some time after completion of radiotherapy. Although this is possible, partial reconstruction of the breast after surgery and radiotherapy is technically challenging and requires sophisticated techniques, with cosmetic results that are often disappointing.

In order to better assess the surgical approach for these patients, a classification of the cosmetic sequelae after BCS has been published.[36] This defined three groups of patients based on clinical examination (**Fig. 5.4**). The advantage of this classification is that it is a valuable guide for choosing the optimal reconstructive technique, but it is also a good predictor of the final cosmetic result after surgery.

- Type I deformities: patients have a treated breast with a normal appearance but there is asymmetry between the two breasts.
- Type II deformities: patients have a deformity of the treated breast. This deformity can be corrected by partial breast reconstruction and breast conservation, with the irradiated breast tissue being spared in the reconstruction.
- Type III deformities: patients have a major distortion of the treated breast, or diffuse painful fibrosis. These sequelae are so severe that only a mastectomy can be considered.

For type I deformities, a contralateral mammoplasty is performed to restore symmetry, avoiding any surgery on the irradiated breast. This is a simple and reliable approach, the irradiated breast serving as the model for a contralateral breast lift or breast reduction. Type II sequelae are almost always postoperative and are the most difficult to treat. A wide range of techniques can be used to repair these defects, from recentralisation of the nipple to the insetting of a flap to reconstruct a missing quadrant. Type III sequelae require treatment by mastectomy and immediate reconstruction with a myocutaneous flap.

Poor remodelling is one of the reasons for an ugly deformity after lumpectomy or quadrantectomy.[37,38] Some surgeons perform no remodelling at all, leaving an empty defect and relying on a postoperative haematoma to fill the dead space. This may produce acceptable results in the short term but breast retraction of larger defects invariably occurs with longer follow-up, leading to major deformities that are increased by postoperative radiotherapy.[10,36,39,40]

Reshaping of the breast is required after any tumour excision in order to recreate a normal breast shape in one operative procedure. In most cases this can be

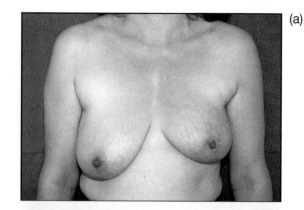
(a)

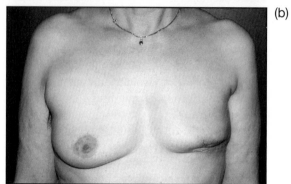
(b)

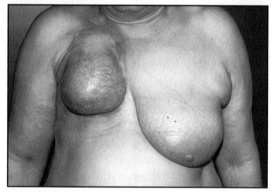
(c)

Figure 5.4 • Deformities after conservative treatment of breast cancer: **(a)** Type I: a symmetrical breast with no deformity of the treated breast. **(b)** Type II: deformity of the treated breast, compatible with partial reconstruction and breast conservation. **(c)** Type III: major deformity of the breast requiring mastectomy. From Klough KB, Claude N, Fitoussi A et al. Oncoplastic conservative surgery for breast cancer. In: Operative techniques in plastic and reconstructive surgery. Philadelphia: WB Saunders, 1999; pp. 50–60, with permission.

achieved with a simple unilateral approach, mobilising glandular flaps to close the defect or by recentralising the NAC. In other cases, a bilateral approach incorporating a bilateral mammoplasty will be the only way to perform a wide excision with no deformity.[41] This graded approach to breast reshaping is discussed below.

Unilateral approach

GLANDULAR FLAPS

Most breast cancers occur in the upper outer quadrant of the breast. In such cases, the glandular defect is easily approximated by mobilising glandular flaps. The skin is undermined extensively, liberating the whole quadrant from its skin attachment. In many cases the central portion of the breast needs to be undermined, separating the NAC from the underlying breast. This allows transfer of some of the central volume of the breast towards the defect, making closure easier and preventing deviation of the NAC towards the tumour bed. This is a safe approach, with no risk of NAC necrosis as long as the subareolar tissue is kept thick enough (0.5–1 cm). The next step is to undermine the posterior part of the breast from the chest wall muscles. This undermining can also be very extensive, leaving only the medial perforating vessels intact, which are branches of the internal mammary vessels. This anterior and posterior undermining allows easy mobilisation of two glandular flaps that are approximated and sutured into the defect (**Fig. 5.5**; see Plate 6, facing p. 116). This approach can be used for most breast cancers in almost any location, except for some lower-pole tumours which require a mammoplasty technique. No drains are used, and these procedures can be performed as an outpatient.

NAC REPOSITIONING

In some cases, wide local excision will cause deviation of the NAC, even when care is taken in reshaping the breast. In such cases, the NAC is always displaced towards the reference quadrant and secondary repair of this deformity is difficult.[10] The solution is to prevent this deformity by transferring the NAC onto the centre of the new breast dome at the time of primary surgery. Recentralisation of the NAC is performed by de-epithelialising a periareolar crescent of skin opposite the lumpectomy.

Bilateral approach

In some cases, the resection is so large that it cannot be closed by simple glandular flap mobilisation. More sophisticated techniques are necessary in order to allow a good cosmetic result. These patients require preoperative planning and patient counselling, and it should not be decided in the operating room that the patient is a candidate for such an approach. One approach is to reconstruct the resection defect with an LD miniflap as described above.[22,28–30] Another approach, when breast volume allows it (B cup or larger), is to perform a remodelling mammoplasty, displacing breast tissue to repair the defect.

The early use of mammoplasty techniques for BCS involved patients with large tumours located in the lower pole of the breast. Lower-pole resections cause more deformity than resections in the upper quadrants[42] and these are impossible to prevent with the simple unilateral techniques just described. Some patients develop a major deformity that presents with a characteristic 'bird's beak' appearance, caused by skin retraction on an underfilled lower pole, and downpointing of the nipple (**Fig. 5.6**). Immediate remodelling should be performed at the time of initial lumpectomy, as the results of delayed procedures based on irradiated tissues are often disappointing.

Conventional breast reduction techniques allow massive excision of tissue from the lower pole of the breast and other sites, without cosmetic penalties. These mammoplasty techniques can be used alongside BCS in order to allow wider resections and prevent postoperative sequelae. There are many advantages to this approach, but the main disadvantage is the need to achieve contralateral symmetry, which can be performed simultaneously in order to avoid secondary procedures. These 'oncoplastic' procedures can be performed as a 'two-team' approach or by a single surgeon qualified in both oncologic and plastic surgery.

SUPERIOR PEDICLE MAMMOPLASTY

Because most post-lumpectomy deformities occur following resection of tumours located in the lower

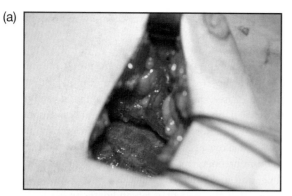

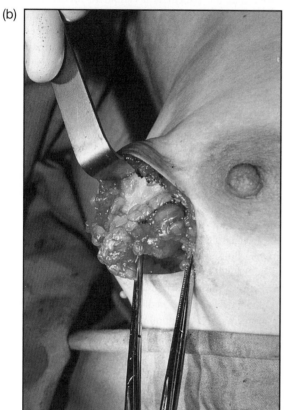

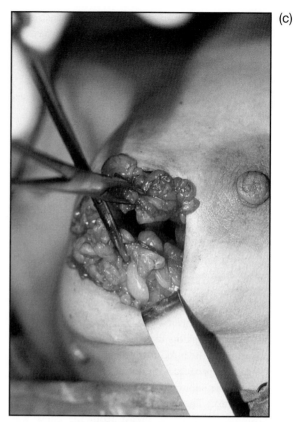

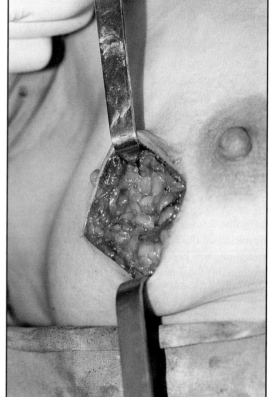

Figure 5.5 • Remodelling with glandular flaps after mastectomy. **(a)** Posterior aspect of breast disc separated from muscle. **(b)** Anterior aspect of breast disc separated from subcutaneous tissue. This may be extended underneath the nipple–areola complex as required. **(c)** Adequacy of mobilisation checked. **(d)** Flaps approximated without distortion.

(a)
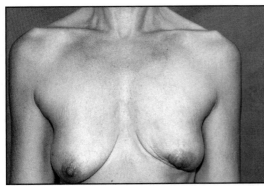

(b)
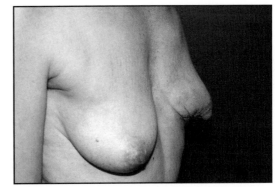

Figure 5.6 • (a, b) Bird's beak deformity following lumpectomy and radiotherapy for lower-pole breast cancer. From Klough KB, Claude N, Fitoussi A et al. Oncoplastic conservative surgery for breast cancer. In: Operative techniques in plastic and reconstructive surgery. Philadelphia: WB Saunders, 1999; pp. 50–60, with permission.

pole of the breast, the technique used most often is a superior pedicle mammoplasty, which allows extensive resection of the breast tissue in the inferior quadrants. Depending on the technique used and the position of the tumour, the final scar is periareolar, with an inverted T as in Pitanguy's technique,[43] vertical as in Lejour's,[44] or a J.[45] Indeed all mammoplasty techniques can be used, the choice between the different procedures depending on each surgeon's expertise, the location of the tumour and the necessity to remove skin en bloc with the lesion.

Inverted-T technique

This is the most versatile technique, as it can be used in most cases. As for all mammoplasty techniques, marking is performed prior to the operation with the patient in a standing position. The principle of the operation is to perform a wide excision of the tumour and surrounding breast tissue, en bloc with the skin of the lower pole of the breast, to reshape the breast and to recentralise the NAC on a de-epithelialised superior pedicle. Both breasts are prepared and draped, as a contralateral symmetrical procedure is needed. The patient is placed on an articulated operating table, as for all breast reconstructions, in order to allow assessment intra-operatively in the sitting position when needed.

The operation begins by de-epithelialisation of the nipple-bearing superior pedicle. Wide undermining of the breast is performed via the inframammary incision, allowing complete separation of the gland from underlying chest wall muscles. The tumour

margins are then very easy to palpate, allowing a wide lumpectomy, with a rim of normal breast tissue around the tumour and any overlying skin if required (**Fig. 5.7**; see Plate 7, facing p. 116). Depending on the size of the breast, centro-inferior resection is then completed to the optimal breast volume, leaving a medial and a lateral glandular column apposed in the midline. In selected cases, a de-epithelialised glandular flap is shaped to fill the defect. Reshaping of the breast starts by resuturing the NAC on its predrawn position. Its vascularisation is checked to ensure that the pedicle is not compressed.

The remaining gland is reshaped by stapling together the skin edges of the vertical scar and of the horizontal scar in the inframammary crease. Minor corrections are then performed when necessary in order to obtain an optimal shape. Staples are removed and replaced by running sutures. This leaves a normal-appearing breast, but smaller and rounder than the contralateral breast. The axillary dissection can be performed through a separate incision or via the inframammary scar. A contralateral mammoplasty is performed immediately to obtain good symmetry in a one-step procedure. Analysis of long-term cosmetic results has confirmed that symmetry is maintained, despite one breast receiving postoperative irradiation.

Other superior pedicle techniques

All superior pedicle mammoplasty techniques can be adapted to allow BCS. The difference between techniques lies in the location of the tissue removed, and the position of the tumour will influence the

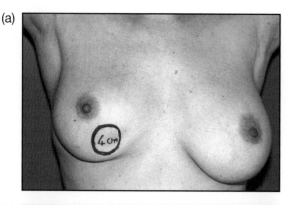

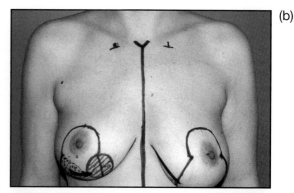

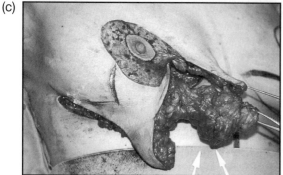

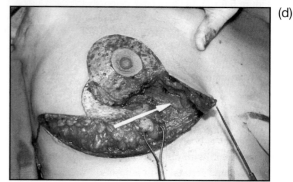

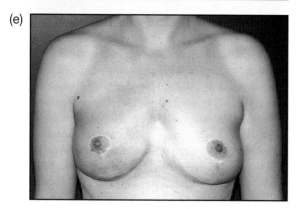

Figure 5.7 • Therapeutic mammoplasty after neoadjuvant chemotherapy. **(a)** Residual 4-cm tumour lower inner quadrant. **(b)** Preoperative markings for superior pedicle mammoplasty and contralateral symmetrisation. **(c)** Excision of the lower inner quadrant. **(d)** De-epithelialisation of the glandular flap, which is advanced into the lower inner quadrant to fill the defect. **(e)** Results 18 months after radiotherapy. From Nos C, Fitoussi A, Bourgeous D et al. Conservative treatment of lower pole breast cancers by mammoplasty and radiotherapy. Eur J Surg Oncol 1998; 24:508–14, with permission.

choice of technique. A vertical mammoplasty[44] can be easily adapted for a tumour located at the junction of the inner and outer quadrants, i.e. at the 6 o'clock position. An oblique technique[45] is more suitable for a patient with a tumour in the lower outer quadrant.

OTHER MAMMOPLASTY TECHNIQUES

Because most postoperative deformities occur for cancers located in the lower pole, superior pedicle techniques are the most commonly used. However, with the increase in indications for conservative treatment and the wish to reduce treatment sequelae, mammoplasty techniques are now frequently used for tumours located in the upper quadrants. In this situation, a superior pedicle technique is not possible, and an inferior or posterior pedicle technique is advocated. These procedures allow wide excision of the upper pole, leaving the NAC vascularised by an inferior pedicle or by the posterior perforators on the deep surface of the breast.

Another option that leaves minimal scarring is the 'round block' or periareolar technique,[46] in which the skin envelope is completely undermined through a periareolar incision. All the breast tissue is then available, allowing wide resection in a radial direction. Reshaping is performed after posterior undermining of the upper pole of the breast, leaving the breast tissue vascularised by the lower perforating branches of the intercostal vessels and by perforating branches of the internal mammary vessels. As for all mammoplasties, the remaining glandular tissue is approximated to fill the defect, and the gland is reshaped in a sitting position. This leaves only a periareolar scar, which is one of the major advantages of this approach. Reshaping of the breast is often more difficult than with a standard technique. The contralateral breast is then made symmetrical using the same approach.

Subareolar breast cancers

One recent additional indication for conservative treatment concerns central subareolar breast cancers. Initially, patients presenting with such a lesion were routinely offered a mastectomy for two reasons: (i) there was fear of a higher risk of multifocality for central cancers, based on previous studies,[47] and (ii) the need for resection of the NAC deterred most surgeons from performing BCS.

These contraindications have been reviewed based on more recent publications. Several studies have demonstrated that conservative treatment is a safe alternative for centrally located breast cancers.[48–50] For any tumour, BCS relies on complete excision followed by radiotherapy. For deep tumours, remote from the nipple, the NAC can be conserved as it is possible to obtain free margins with a standard lumpectomy. For more superficial tumours, NAC resection is necessary because the risk of subclinical NAC involvement is very high. The risk of histological involvement of the NAC is related to the distance between the tumour and the nipple. The more superficial the tumour, the higher the risk, and routine excision of the NAC is indicated when the tumour is less than 1 cm below the nipple. Oncoplastic procedures are then mandatory to reshape a normal breast mound and recreate the NAC. Such procedures can be unilateral, although a bilateral mammoplasty is often necessary. NAC recon-

struction can be performed under local anaesthesia, after completion of radiotherapy.

UNILATERAL APPROACH

The tumour must be removed with free histological margins by performing an en bloc resection of the NAC for any tumour located within 1 cm of the nipple. This can be carried out using a horizontal incision, although different approaches may be preferred depending on the morphology of the breast. In some cases, a vertical or periareolar incision can be used. In the latter case, the final suture is a pursestring suture, producing an almost invisible scar. In all cases, a lumpectomy leaves a large central defect. In most patients, reshaping can be performed by mobilising the remaining breast tissue after detaching the skin extensively from the breast, as in a mastectomy. The breast is then separated from the pectoralis muscle, leaving the external mammary vessels and branches from the internal mammary vessels intact to ensure good vascularisation. This creates two large glandular flaps, one superior, one inferior. These are then slid into the defect and sutured together in order to recreate a central projection. This manoeuvre is essential to prevent flattening of the breast mound and to recreate a normal shape. Reconstruction of the NAC can be performed immediately or, preferably, at a second stage a few weeks after completion of radiotherapy.

BILATERAL APPROACH

In some cases the unilateral approach is not possible, either because the volume of the breast is not large enough to allow mobilisation of two large glandular flaps or because reshaping of the breast cannot be performed easily or this reshaping produces noticeable asymmetry between the two breasts. In such cases, the solution is to use a bilateral mammoplasty technique, which allows an extensive central resection of the treated breast and easy remodelling by redraping the excess skin on the new breast mound. Such an approach allows almost any kind of central lumpectomy, providing the remaining breast volume is sufficient. Because the definitive shape of the breast is then different from its original shape, a contralateral mammoplasty is performed to ensure good symmetry. Any of the mammoplasty techniques described above can be used for a central tumour. As for all oncoplastic techniques, the decision must be made before the operation and discussed with the patient to ensure optimal preoperative planning.

CONCLUSION

Breast-conserving reconstruction extends the role of BCS by enabling complete excision of a greater range of tumours without compromising cosmesis, postoperative surveillance or symmetry. Volume replacement and displacement techniques are likely to become increasingly popular as an alternative to mastectomy in patients with small breast–tumour ratios and localised disease who wish to avoid more major surgery and the use of implants. Further experience of these techniques will lead to a better understanding of their role in the surgical management of primary breast cancer and in the management of local relapse and cosmetic deformity after previous breast-conserving procedures.

Key points

- Local recurrence following BCS can be minimised by extensive local excision.
- Deformity following extensive local excision can be avoided by breast-sparing reconstruction using volume replacement or volume displacement.
- Volume replacement is most suitable for patients with small or medium-sized breasts who wish to avoid contralateral surgery. It can also be used for the correction of deformity following previous BCS.
- Volume displacement is most suitable for patients with medium or large breasts who are willing to undergo bilateral breast reduction, avoiding more major reconstructive surgery.
- Breast-conserving reconstruction should be considered when adequate resection will result in volume loss of more than 20%.
- Breast-conserving reconstruction may be carried out as a one-stage or two-stage procedure.
- Volume displacement allows massive resection of tissue without cosmetic penalty.
- Volume displacement can be designed around modifications of superior pedicle, inferior pedicle and round block techniques.
- The type of breast-sparing reconstruction selected will be determined by the site and extent of resection and by the patient's size, morphology and personal preference.

REFERENCES

1. Fisher B, Redmond C, Posson R et al. Eight-year results of a randomised clinical trial comparing total mastectomy and lumpectomy with or without irradiation in the treatment of breast cancer. N Engl J Med 1989; 320:822–8.

   Seminal trial (NSABP B-06) showing equivalent overall survival in patients with breast cancer treated either by mastectomy or by lumpectomy and radiotherapy.

2. Veronesi U, Banfi A, Del Vecchio M et al. Comparison of Halsted mastectomy with quadrant-ectomy, axillary dissection, and radiotherapy in early breast cancer: long-term results. Eur J Cancer Clin Oncol 1986; 22:1085–9.

   Seminal trial comparing the treatment of patients with breast cancer by radical mastectomy or quadrantectomy, showing equivalent overall survival in each group.

3. Abrams J, Chen T, Giusti R. Survival after breast-sparing surgery versus mastectomy. J Natl Cancer Inst 1994; 86:1672–3.

4. Veronesi U, Saccozzi R, Del Vecchio M et al. Comparing radical mastectomy with quadrantectomy, axillary dissection and radiotherapy in patients with small cancers of the breast. N Engl J Med 1981; 305:6–11.

5. Holland R, Veling SH, Mravunac M, Hendriks JH. Histologic multifocality of T_{IS}, T_{1-2} breast carcinomas: implications for clinical trials of breast-conserving surgery. Cancer 1985; 56:979–90.

   A detailed study using serial whole-breast sections to estasblish the distribution of breast malignancy in relation to the margin of the reference tumour.

6. Dixon J. Histological factors predicting breast recurrence following breast-conserving therapy. Breast 1993; 2:197.

7. Veronesi U, Voltarrani F, Luini A et al. Quadrant-ectomy versus lumpectomy for small size breast cancer. Eur J Cancer 1990; 26:671–3.

A seminal trial comparing very wide local excision (quadrantectomy) with limited excision of breast carcinoma (lumpectomy). Quadrantectomy was associated with significantly lower rates of local recurrence when compared with lumpectomy.

8. Audretsch WP. Reconstruction of the partial mastectomy defect: classification and method. In: Spear SL (ed.) Surgery of the breast: principles and art. Philadelphia: Lippincott-Raven, 1998; pp. 155–95.

9. Pearl RM, Wisnicki J. Breast reconstruction following lumpectomy and irradiation. Plast Reconstr Surg 1985; 76:83–6.

10. Berrino P, Campora E, Sauti P. Postquadrantectomy breast deformities: classification and techniques of surgical correction. Plast Reconstr Surg 1987; 79:567–72.

11. Borger JH, Keijser AH. Conservative breast cancer treatment: analysis of cosmetic role and the role of concomitant adjuvant chemotherapy. Int J Radiat Oncol Biol Phys 1987; 13:1173–7.

12. Van Limbergen E, Rijnders A, van der Schueren E et al. Cosmetic evaluation of conserving treatment for mammary cancer. 2. A quantitative analysis of the influence of radiation dose, fractionation schedules and surgical treatment techniques on cosmetic results. Radiother Oncol 1989; 16:253–67.

13. Van Limbergen E, Van der Schueren E, Van Tongelen K. Cosmetic evaluation of breast conserving treatment for mammary cancer. 1. Proposal of quantitative scoring system. Radiother Oncol 1989; 16:159–67.

14. Olivotto IA, Rose MA, Osteen RJ et al. Late cosmetic outcome after conservative surgery and radiotherapy: analysis of causes of cosmetic failure. Int J Radiat Oncol Biol Phys 1989; 17:747–53.

15. Ray GR, Fish BJ, Marmor JB et al. Impact of adjuvant chemotherapy on cosmesis and complications in stages 1 and 2 carcinoma of the breast treated by biopsy and radiation therapy. Int J Radiat Oncol Biol Phys 1984; 10:837–41.

16. Slavin SA, Love SM, Sadowsky NL. Reconstruction of the irradiated partial mastectomy defect with autogenous tissues. Plast Reconstr Surg 1992; 90:854–65.

17. O'Brien W, Hasselgren P-O, Hummel RP et al. Comparison of postoperative wound complications in early cancer recurrence between patients undergoing mastectomy with or without immediate breast reconstruction. Am J Surg 1993; 116:1–5.

18. Eberlein TJ, Crespo LD, Smith BL et al. Prospective evaluation of immediate reconstruction after mastectomy. Ann Surg 1993; 218:29–36.

19. Elkowitz A, Colen S, Slavin S et al. Various methods of breast reconstruction after mastectomy: an economic comparison. Plast Reconstr Surg 1993; 92:77–83.

20. Dean C, Chetty U, Forrest APM. Effect of immediate breast reconstruction on psychosocial morbidity after mastectomy. Lancet 1983; i:459–62.

 21. Raja MAK, Straker VF, Rainsbury RM. Extending the role of breast-conserving surgery by immediate volume replacement. Br J Surg 1997; 84:101–5.

Original description of latissimus dorsi miniflap reconstruction using myosubcutaneous flaps harvested and transposed through a single lateral incision.

 22. Ohuchi N, Harada Y, Ishida T et al. Breast-conserving surgery for primary breast cancer; immediate volume replacement using lateral tissue flap. Breast Cancer 1997; 4:135–41.

23. Thomas PRS, Ford HT, Gazet JC. Use of silicone implants after wide local excision of the breast. Br J Surg 1993; 80:868–70.

24. Elton C, Jones PA. Initial experience of intramammary prostheses in breast conserving surgery. Eur J Surg Oncol 1999; 25:138–41.

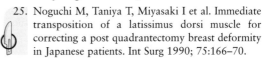 25. Noguchi M, Taniya T, Miyasaki I et al. Immediate transposition of a latissimus dorsi muscle for correcting a post quadrantectomy breast deformity in Japanese patients. Int Surg 1990; 75:166–70.

Original description of latissimus dorsi myocutaneous flaps for immediate reconstruction of resection defects at the time of quadrantectomy.

26. Eaves FF, Bostwick J, Nahai F et al. Endoscopic techniques in aesthetic breast surgery. Clin Plast Surg 1995; 22:683–95.

27. Rainsbury RM, Paramanathan N. Recent progress with breast-conserving volume replacement using latissimus dorsi miniflaps in UK patients. Breast Cancer 1998; 5:139–47.

28. Dixon JM, Venizelos B, Chan P. Latissimus dorsi mini-flap: a technique for extending breast conservation. Breast 2002; 11:58–65.

29. Rainsbury RM. Breast-sparing reconstruction with latissimus dorsi miniflaps. Eur J Surg Oncol 2002; 28:891–5.

30. Laws SAM, Cheetham JE, Rainsbury RM. Temporal changes in breast volume after surgery for breast cancer and the implications for volume replacement with the latissimus dorsi miniflap. Eur J Surg Oncol 2001; 27:790.

31. Gendy RK, Able JA, Rainsbury RM. Impact of skin-sparing mastectomy with immediate reconstruction and breast-sparing reconstruction with miniflaps on the outcomes of oncoplastic breast surgery. Br J Surg 2003; 90:433–9.

32. Monticciolo DL, Ross D, Bostwick J et al. Autogenous breast reconstruction with endoscopic

latissimus dorsi with musculo-subcutaneous flaps in patients choosing breast-conserving therapy: mammographic appearance. Am J Radiol 1996; 167:385–9.

33. Gilles R, Guinebretiere J-M. Magnetic resonance imaging. In: Silverstein MJ (ed.) Ductal carcinoma in situ of the breast. Baltimore: Williams & Wilkins, 1997; pp. 159–66.

34. Bass LS, Karp NS, Benacquista T et al. Endoscopic harvest of the rectus abdominus free flap: balloon dissection in the fascial plain. Ann Plast Surg 1995; 34:274–9.

35. Van Buskark ER, Krehnke RD, Montgomery RL et al. Endoscopic harvest of the latissimus dorsi muscle using balloon dissection technique. Plast Reconstr Surg 1997; 99:899–903.

36. Clough KB, Cuminet J, Fitoussi A et al. Cosmetic sequelae after conservative treatment for breast cancer: classification and results of surgical correction. Ann Plast Surg 1998; 41:471–81.

Original classification of types of deformity following partial mastectomy and the use of therapeutic mammoplasty to avoid rather than correct deformity.

37. Petit J-Y, Rigault L, Zekri A et al. Poor esthetic results after conservative treatment of breast cancer. Techniques of partial breast reconstruction. Ann Chir Plast Esthet 1989; 34:103–8.

38. Rose MA, Olivotto IA, Cady B et al. Conservative surgery and radiation therapy for early breast cancer. Long-term cosmetic results. Arch Surg 1989; 124:153–7.

39. Berrino P, Campora E, Leone S et al. Correction of type II breast deformities following conservative cancer surgery. Plast Reconstr Surg 1992; 90:846–53.

40. Petit J-Y, Rietjens M. Deformities following tumourectomy and partial mastectomy. In: Noone B (ed.) Plastic and reconstruction surgery of the breast. Philadelphia: BC Decker, 1991.

41. Clough KB, Kroll S, Audretsch W. An approach to the repair of partial mastectomy defects. Plast Reconstr Surg 1999; 104:409–20.

Pooled experience of breast-conserving reconstruction from France, USA and Germany using volume replacement and volume displacement techniques.

42. Clough KB, Nos C, Salmon RJ et al. Conservative treatment of breast cancers by mammaplasty and irradiation: a new approach to lower quadrant tumours. Plast Reconstr Surg 1995; 96:363–70.

43. Pitanguy I. Surgical treatment of breast hypertrophy. Br J Plast Surg 1967; 20:78–85.

44. Lejour M. Vertical mammoplasty and liposuction of the breast. Plast Reconstr Surg 1994; 94:100–14.

45. Chairi A. The J short-scar mammoplasty: a new approach. Plast Reconstr Surg 1992; 90:233–46.

46. Goes JC. Periareolar mammoplasty: double skin technique with application of polyglactine or mixed mesh. Plast Reconstr Surg 1996; 97:959–67.

47. Nos C, Fitoussi A, Bourgeois D et al. Conservative treatment of lower pole breast cancer by bilateral mammaplasty and radiotherapy. Eur J Surg Oncol 1998; 24:508–14.

48. Hafty D, Wilson LD, Smith R et al. Subareolar breast cancer: long term results with conservative surgery and radiation therapy. Int J Radiat Oncol Biol Phys 1995; 33:53–7.

49. Bussieres E, Guyon F, Thomas L et al. Conservation treatment in subareolar breast cancers. Eur J Surg Oncol 1996; 22:267–70.

50. Dale PS, Giuliano AE. Nipple–areolar preservation during breast conserving therapy for subareolar breast carcinomas. Arch Surg 1996; 30:430–3.

Six

The axilla: current management including sentinel node

James Kollias and
Melissa A. Bochner

INTRODUCTION

Management of the axilla in early breast cancer has been a subject of great debate and controversy for many decades. The clinical importance of the axilla in the management of early breast cancer lies in the premise that the major group of lymph nodes that receives lymphatic metastases from the breast is the axillary group. As such, management of the axilla may affect survival, provide information regarding staging and prognosis, and have implications for locoregional control of breast cancer. Traditionally, axillary lymph node dissection (ALND) has been the most widely accepted technique for staging the axilla and providing full qualitative and quantitative information. In some centres, radiotherapy is used as an alternative to ALND to treat the involved axilla. Recently, less invasive techniques such as sentinel node biopsy (SNB) have evolved that question the role of routine axillary dissection in early breast cancer.

ROLE OF AXILLARY DISSECTION

Effects on survival

The benefits of ALND on survival are unclear. Studies have reported different effects on survival and most have certain methodological flaws.

The NSABP B-04 trial[1] demonstrated no difference in survival between women who had simple mastectomy and those who underwent mastectomy and ALND. However, 33% of women in the non-dissected group had undergone some form of limited axillary surgery and the power of the study may have been insufficient to demonstrate a clinically significant difference between groups.

Other studies have found benefits in survival when ALND was carried out.[2–4] In a study by Cabanes et al.[2] that evaluated lumpectomy plus breast and axillary irradiation without ALND versus lumpectomy and breast irradiation with ALND, a small but significant improvement in survival at 5 years was demonstrated for women who had axillary surgery (92.6% vs. 96.6%, $P = 0.014$). Interpretation of these results is difficult since a significant proportion of patients in the ALND group received adjuvant systemic therapy based on their nodal status. Two other studies from Guys Hospital[3] and Edinburgh[4] found significantly decreased survival for treatment groups that had a higher rate of locally uncontrolled disease. Both demonstrated long-term benefits in overall survival when ALND was compared with no intervention or radiotherapy to the axilla.

In summary, the data suggest that ALND may have some impact on survival, although the quality of the evidence remains poor.

Effects on axillary recurrence

Control of local disease within the axilla is essential. Uncontrolled axillary recurrence is difficult to treat, causes pain and suffering, and significantly impairs quality of life. There is substantial evidence that ALND reduces the risk of axillary recurrence. The best evidence for this comes from the NSABP B-04 trial,[1] which reported 10-year axillary recurrence rates of only 1% (in node-negative patients) and 3% (in node-positive patients) for women who had undergone ALND at mastectomy, compared with more than 17% in women who had not. Nevertheless, the same trial concluded that despite differences in axillary recurrence between the two study groups, there was no difference in survival. Other studies have shown that axillary recurrence is inversely related to the number of nodes removed from the axilla.[5,6]

Staging the axilla by axillary dissection: advantages

Surgical staging by ALND is currently the usual practice for the majority of women, as it provides prognostic information and data upon which major treatment decisions are made. Although several prognostic indices have been developed, these rely on knowledge of nodal status.[7,8] Axillary lymph node status is the most powerful single variable in the estimation of prognosis for primary breast cancer. The absolute benefit that any individual patient will derive from adjuvant systemic therapy depends on an accurate assessment of her individual risk of relapse. For women considering entry to clinical trials of systemic therapy, some of these trials require a minimum number of lymph nodes to have been examined or require variable numbers of lymph nodes to be involved. Systemic adjuvant therapy can provide a survival benefit[9–13] but these treatments, particularly chemotherapy, are associated with major adverse effects. For women at low risk of systemic relapse, there may be little benefit from systemic adjuvant therapy but potential for considerable morbidity from adverse effects.

Disease-free interval and overall survival are related to the number of axillary nodes that contain metastases.[8,14] As such, ALND provides the most accurate qualitative and quantitative assessment of the axilla. The probability of lymph node involve-ment is related directly to the size of the primary tumour: larger tumours are more likely to have metastasised to axillary lymph nodes than smaller ones. Even in small primary tumours (up to 10 mm), the risk of nodal metastases is in the order of 10%.[15,16] In these patients, identification of involved lymph nodes alters both their prognosis and the adjuvant therapy offered. Screen-detected cancers tend to be small and are associated with an excellent prognosis, and are becoming increasingly common. Adjuvant systemic chemotherapy appears to have little role in many such patients and chemotherapy does not substitute for inadequate local treatment.[17]

Role of micrometastases

Routine histological examination of dissected axillary lymph nodes may be inadequate in identifying the presence of small metastatic tumour deposits. Various approaches have been described in the search for 'micrometastatic disease', including serial sectioning of axillary nodes using haematoxylin/eosin (H&E) or immunohistochemistry and polymerase chain reaction to identify mRNA transcripts from epithelial cells not usually present in lymphoid tissue (**Fig. 6.1**). Previous studies have demonstrated that by using such techniques it is possible to identify micrometastases in up to 50% of lymph node 'negative' cases.[18–20] Although serial sectioning can increase the detection yield of metastases in lymph nodes, the cost and labour involved in processing are disadvantages that make it impractical for many tissue pathology laboratories.

The subject of lymph node micrometastases has recently generated much controversy, particularly with the advent of sentinel node biopsy (SNB; see later). Currently, there is no universal definition for a micrometastasis but the following have been proposed: a single cell or small cluster of cells, cell clusters measuring 0.2–2 mm in diameter, or calculations based on the percentage of the cross-sectional area of the node involved by metastases. The prognostic significance of micrometastases in lymph glands remains in doubt. A number of studies show variability in disease-free and overall survival, although more recent studies with larger patient numbers and longer follow-up suggest that cases initially deemed 'node negative' by routine histological techniques but subsequently shown to

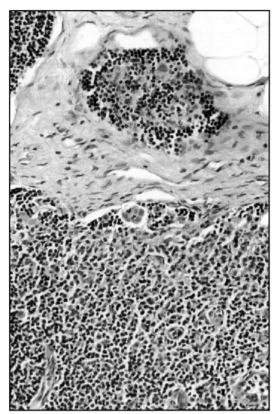

Figure 6.1 • Small cluster of metastatic breast cancer cells located in the subcapsular sinus of a lymph gland demonstrated by immunohistochemistry using cytokeratin stain.

have nodal micrometastases are associated with a worse outcome[19–28] (**Table 6.1**). The prognostic relevance of micrometastatic disease in lymph nodes using immunohistochemistry is unclear. A re-evaluation of the Ludwig V study has confirmed a statistically significant difference in disease-free survival when micrometastases were detected with H&E ($P = 0.001$) but not with immunohistochemistry ($P = 0.09$).[29] Two recent studies of SNB using H&E versus immunohistochemistry failed to demonstrate any survival difference in patients with and without immunohistochemically detected lymph node metastases.[30,31] Longer follow-up of previous retrospective studies or the results of current prospective randomised trials assessing the prognostic role of immunohistochemically detected nodal micrometastases will help determine the need for altering treatment in such cases.

Staging the axilla by axillary dissection: risks and complications

SEROMA

Seromas are common following most types of ALND.[32,33] The management of drain tubes and of seromas is very individualised. Randomised trials have shown little difference in seroma formation,

Table 6.1 • Studies assessing the role of nodal micrometastases in cases of early breast cancer previously deemed 'node negative'

Reference	Year	N	Follow-up (years)	Cases with nodal micrometastases (%)	Outcome	
					DFS	OS
Huvos et al.[21]	1971	208	8	–	NS	NS
Fisher et al.[22]	1978	78	5	24	NS	NS
Rosen et al.[23]	1981	147	10	–	NS	NS
Trojani et al.[19]	1987	150	10	14	$P = 0.0025$	$P = 0.02$
Friedman et al.[24]	1988	456	10	9	–	$P = 0.05$
IBCSG[25]	1990	921	5	9	$P = 0.003$	$P = 0.002$
Hainsworth et al.[20]	1993	343	6	12	$P = 0.05$	NS
Clayton & Hopkins[26]	1993	399	16	–	$P = 0.05$	–
McGuckin et al.[27]	1996	208	5	25	$P = 0.020$	P = 0.007

DFS, disease-free survival; IBCSG, International (Ludwig) Breast Cancer Study Group; OS, overall survival.

regardless of the drainage technique employed. Even with prolonged periods of drainage, some patients still require further aspiration of residual seroma.[33] Recent studies have indicated that not all patients need a drain and that closing the dead space by tacking down the skin flaps reduces the likelihood of seroma development.

WOUND INFECTION

The rate of wound infection in axillary surgery has been reported at approximately 10%.[32] Wound infection is more common in certain groups of patients: the elderly and immunocompromised; those who undergo repeated aspiration of seroma or prolonged wound drainage; and those who have undergone previous recent surgery in the vicinity of the axilla. The prophylactic use of antibiotics has been shown to decrease the rate of wound infection.[34]

REDUCED SHOULDER MOBILITY AND STIFFNESS

Shoulder stiffness is common immediately after ALND.[35] Early mobilisation and exercise is important for retaining normal mobility postoperatively but this increases seroma rates. Patients may be at risk if they have pre-existing arthritis or if the position of the arm during surgery is not carefully monitored. There is little documented evidence on the cause of this problem.

DAMAGE TO MOTOR NERVES

Although the frequency of injury appears to be low, three motor nerves are at risk during axillary lymph node dissection:

- Medial pectoral nerve: when dissecting around pectoralis minor, the medial pectoral nerve, which in up to one-third of patients lies well lateral to the muscle, is at significant risk. In circumstances where there is extensive tumour involvement in the axilla, the nerve and pectoralis minor muscle are often deliberately divided. Damage to the nerve results in minimal morbidity, but leads to wasting of the lower and lateral fibres of pectoralis major. This results in loss of the anterior axillary fold, and an unsatisfactory cosmetic result. Loss of the pectoralis minor and the lateral third of

pectoralis major can cause problems in patients undergoing breast reconstruction using a tissue-expansion technique.
- Long thoracic nerve of Bell or nerve to serratus anterior: this runs along the chest wall in the posterior part of the axilla. Damage to this nerve results in winging of the scapula.
- Thoracodorsal nerve or nerve to latissimus dorsi: this may be divided during dissection of the lateral and posterior aspect of the axilla. Although damage to this nerve results in minimal detectable disability, some reduction in shoulder power may be noticed especially when the arm is raised above the head and in women active in sports.

NUMBNESS AND PARAESTHESIA

Various studies have demonstrated that some numbness can be demonstrated in almost 80% of patients undergoing axillary surgery.[36] The frequency of more significant or disabling pain is in the range of 5%. The alteration to sensory perception is assumed to result from division of the intercostobrachial nerve, although damage to the medial cutaneous nerve of the arm and lower intercostal nerves may also occur. The extent of any deficit is variable but may involve the inner aspect of the upper arm, shoulder, axilla and anterolateral chest wall.

Although many surgeons attempt to preserve the intercostobrachial nerve, this is not necessarily reflected in the preservation of normal sensation. Some units have demonstrated a better outcome at 12 months with intercostobrachial nerve preservation, and randomised studies have shown less sensory loss when the nerve is preserved. Recent studies of sentinel node versus ALND and earlier studies of node sampling versus ALND have shown a much lower rate of sensory change and there is thus a clear relationship between the extent of axillary surgery and the likelihood of having sensory loss.

LYMPHOEDEMA

Lymphoedema is one of the most significant side effects of intervention to the axilla with radiotherapy and/or surgery. Research into lymphoedema is made difficult by the varying definitions used and by the significant differences between the subjective and objective appreciation of this problem. Various studies have reported the incidence of lymphoedema to be between 10 and 25%.[38] The incidence of 'clinically obvious' lymphoedema associated with axillary clearance is approximately 7%. However, the incidence of lymphoedema varies widely depending on when it is assessed after treatment. Some studies suggest that its incidence increases with time following surgery. It remains a difficult treatment problem. Patient size may be the best predictor of lymphoedema risk, with those with a high body mass index (BMI) being at higher risk. Other factors that may contribute to risk are hypertension, disruption of sympathetic nervous input to the limb and anatomical situations where few primary lymphatic channels exist. The risk of lymphoedema or arm swelling appears greater with ALND than with a sampling procedure followed by axillary radiotherapy. The highest incidence of lymphoedema is in patients who have ALND and axillary radiotherapy, and up to 40% of these patients develop symptomatic lymphoedema.

Technical aspects of axillary dissection

There is variation in the extent of ALND in the management of breast cancer. It ranges from no surgical intervention at all, to removal of a few lower nodes, to a complete clearance of soft tissue to the apex of the axilla. This variation has largely been due to a number of differing beliefs about the amount of nodal tissue required for staging, and about the benefits of a clearance procedure.

The axilla is anatomically divided into three levels based around the pectoralis minor muscle. This leads to the definitions of level I, II and III clearance as outlined below.[39]

- *Level I dissection: clearance from the lateral/lower border of pectoralis minor.* This dissection includes all tissue inferior to the axillary vein, lateral to the outer border of the pectoralis minor muscle and extends laterally to the point where the axillary vein crosses the tendon of latissimus dorsi. The rest of the dissection is limited by the axillary fascia and the chest wall.
- *Level II dissection: clearance from the medial/upper border of pectoralis minor.* This

dissection includes all of the level I tissue and fat beneath the pectoralis minor muscle. The pectoralis minor muscle may be either divided or retracted to gain access to this region. No significant difference in morbidity has been demonstrated using either technique, but few surgeons routinely divide pectoralis minor in either level II or III dissections.

- *Level III dissection: clearance from the axillary apex.* This involves the complete removal of all nodal tissue from the axilla. The dissection extends superomedially to the lateral border of the first rib and the costoclavicular (Halsted's) ligament.

There is a wide variation in the number of lymph nodes harvested from any individual nodal basin. In the axilla, complete clearance has been reported as yielding as few as eight nodes and as many as 60 in series from one institution.[40] Average lymph node harvests for the various levels in the axilla have been described: level I alone, nine to thirteen lymph nodes; level II alone, five to nine lymph nodes; level III alone, two to six lymph nodes.[32,41–43] The number of nodes harvested appears to relate as much to the pathologist searching for the nodes as to the surgeon who performs the operation.

ROLE OF AXILLARY IRRADIATION

Effects on survival

The benefits of axillary irradiation on survival from breast cancer remain unclear.

 The results of the Danish Breast Cancer Cooperative Group randomised trial for postoperative radiotherapy[44,45] demonstrated a 9% absolute survival benefit after 10 years for postmastectomy radiotherapy that included the axilla in high-risk patients (T3/T4 and node positive).

Another postmastectomy radiotherapy trial has also demonstrated a trend towards improved survival.[46] In these three trials, postmastectomy radiotherapy included chest wall, axillary, supraclavicular and internal mammary node irradiation. Given that all nodal areas were irradiated in these trials, it is difficult to isolate one area of treatment as being solely responsible for their identified survival improvements. No other trial, overview[47] or meta-analysis, has demonstrated a survival benefit.

Effects on axillary recurrence

In an overview of randomised trials, the Early Breast Cancer Trialists' Collaborative Group[47] demonstrated that radiotherapy reduced the locoregional relapse rate by about two-thirds, from 19.6% to 6.7%. This was independent of the type of axillary surgery or nodal status, and included breast-conserving surgery and mastectomy. There are data reporting no difference in outcome between axillary dissection and radical radiotherapy to the undissected axilla in clinically node-negative axillae.[48,49] Patient factors such as individual preference, performance status and age should be taken into account. Differences in morbidity patterns should also be considered. Axillary irradiation may be added to ALND in some cases where women are identified as being at risk of axillary recurrence, such as where disease remains after ALND. In these situations, axillary irradiation may confer additional benefits over ALND alone in controlling axillary disease and preventing ensuing symptoms, but there is an increased risk of developing lymphoedema (up to 40%).

The benefit of axillary radiotherapy in different subgroups needs to be carefully considered, as the extent of the benefit will differ depending upon the risks and this must be balanced against the known increase in morbidity, of combining extensive axillary dissections and radiotherapy.

AXILLARY IRRADIATION FOLLOWING DISSECTION IN WOMEN WITH LIMITED NODAL INVOLVEMENT

There is little benefit from adding axillary irradiation in women who have had ALND and who have only a small number of involved lymph nodes. The NSABP B-06 trial[17] reported that 90% of patients had less than four positive lymph nodes in a dissected axilla and local axillary relapse in the entire series was low (1–3%). Data from the Mayo Clinic suggest isolated locoregional recurrences (i.e. recurrences on the chest wall or lymphatic areas) of only around 8%, with less than four lymph nodes involved.[50] Similarly, Fowble et al.[51] suggest that

isolated locoregional recurrences occur in 7% of women with limited nodal involvement. Of the 634 patients analysed in this study,[48] only 2.6% recurred in the axilla alone or in multiple sites that included the axilla. Fisher et al.[5] analysed patterns of recurrence in 320 patients who had been treated for stage II or III breast cancer with surgery and chemotherapy without locoregional radiation therapy. Isolated axillary recurrences occurred in only 21 patients (6.6%) at a median follow-up of 77 months. These and other studies[48,52,53] conclude that the addition of radiotherapy after ALND confers little if any benefit where rates of relapse are already very low.

AXILLARY IRRADIATION FOLLOWING DISSECTION IN WOMEN WITH GREATER LYMPH NODE INVOLVEMENT OR REMAINING DISEASE IN THE AXILLA

There may be some benefit from the addition of radiotherapy when it is likely that there is remaining disease in the axilla. This includes cases where the surgeon believes that macroscopic disease has been left behind or transected, or where the pathologist indicates positive margins.

The addition of axillary irradiation after ALND in cases with greater nodal involvement is as controversial as that with limited nodal involvement.[5,6,54,55] Data from the Mayo Clinic[50] suggest isolated locoregional recurrences at 3 years of 14% among women with four to seven positive nodes and 22% for women with eight or more positive nodes. Similar data have been reported by Fowble et al.[51] However, not all relapses are axillary. Most studies have shown at least 50% of recurrences to be on the chest wall. The three randomised trials[44–46] showing an improvement in survival in high-risk disease for patients who had the entire lymphatics and chest wall irradiated reported a reduction in locoregional relapse from 32% to 9% at 10 years. Although the distribution of local relapses was not given, more than half were on the chest wall. Even in patients with heavy nodal involvement, isolated axillary recurrences are uncommon. Not all analyses have demonstrated increased axillary relapse rates with increasing numbers of involved nodes.[5]

It is important to consider the role of axillary irradiation in patients at high risk of local recurrence. Although many cases of axillary recurrence can be managed surgically, not all axillary recurrences can be salvaged. It is particularly difficult to salvage axillary recurrence with radiotherapy where the axilla has been previously selectively excluded from chest wall and supraclavicular fossa fields. The prevention of recurrence in some patients may therefore be preferable, albeit with a significantly increased risk of lymphoedema.

AXILLARY IRRADIATION FOLLOWING DISSECTION IN WOMEN WITH EXTRANODAL SPREAD

The significance of axillary extranodal spread in breast cancer is another controversial issue.[56–63] Retrospective studies have examined the effects of extranodal spread on both survival and local recurrences. Most have demonstrated significant reductions in overall survival in patients with extranodal spread of disease,[58,60–62] and one study[63] showed a non-significant trend.

In examining the risks of locoregional recurrence, two studies have examined the sites of local relapse in patients with axillary extranodal spread.[58,62] Both have demonstrated increased chest wall recurrences but no significant increase in axillary recurrence rates. The axillary recurrence rate in both studies was 7%. Although this figure is higher than reported axillary relapse rates in patients with comparable numbers of involved lymph nodes without extranodal spread, it was not significantly higher than women without extranodal disease in the studies reported. There remains no support for axillary irradiation in patients with breast cancer based solely on reported extranodal spread.

Technical aspects of radiation therapy to the axilla

The axilla is often treated together with the supraclavicular fossa. The depth required to treat the supraclavicular area and the axilla must be determined separately, and the dose should be taken sufficiently posteriorly to include the posterior axillary area fully. Radiation therapy for both areas is generally performed using unmatched anterior and posterior portals. Generally, the supraclavicular portal will be irradiated from the anterior field only, and the axilla from the anterior and posterior fields.

The area of the axillary apex or the coracoid process is generally chosen to determine the medial edge of the posterior field. If the axilla is to be excluded from the treatment volume, the coracoid process forms the most lateral extent of the field. It is desirable to angle the anterior portal away from the spinal cord. If a direct portal is used, it is recommended that the dose to the spinal cord be calculated.

The potential for overlapping fields to produce areas of overdose or underdose at the junctions is now minimised by the following.

1. Isocentric techniques allow the use of asymmetric jaws on all fields so that central axis rays are aligned at the junction. Half-beam blocking may also be used.
2. A calculated gap in the junction area limits the dose to an acceptable threshold.
3. Avoid turning the patient prone to deliver the posterior axillary boost.

Supervoltage equipment (4, 6 or 8 MV or cobalt-60) is preferred because of dose homogeneity and skin sparing. Factors to achieve this in axillary treatment include: (i) choice of beam energy; (ii) using lung correction wherever possible; (iii) giving contours through the nodal areas; and (iv) recording dose as per ICRU 50. The prescribed dose is given in 1.8–2.25 Gy fractions at the rate of nine or ten sessions per fortnight. In general, a dose of 45–52.5 Gy is prescribed. All fields should be treated daily, although the posterior axillary boost is typically given in fewer fractions. Careful attention to the amount of lung included within the treatment volume will decrease the risk of pneumonitis.

Axillary irradiation: risks and complications

LYMPHOEDEMA

The routine addition of radiotherapy to a fully dissected axilla increases the incidence of lymphoedema to at least 30%.[38] Management of the axilla with radiation alone has been reported to induce lymphoedema of the arm in rates similar to that of surgery alone (3–8%).[64,65] However, a randomised study of morbidity comparing ALND and axillary sampling followed by radiotherapy (45 Gy) showed in node-positive patients that there were significantly higher rates of arm swelling with ALND compared with sampling followed by radiotherapy.[66]

Radiation therapy to a conserved breast may include part of level I in the axilla. There is randomised trial evidence that the risk of lymphoedema is not increased in this situation.[65]

SHOULDER AND ARM MOVEMENT RESTRICTION

This is relatively common (approximately 20%), even when the shoulder joint is routinely excluded from the radiation beam.[66] It may be due to the effects of radiation on the pectoral and other muscles associated with shoulder movement.

RIB FRACTURE

This is mostly due to the chest wall or breast fields. The risk of rib fracture in these areas, based on several large reviews, is 1.8%.[67,68] The risk of such fractures in the axillary field areas is much less.

BRACHIAL PLEXUS DAMAGE

This can occur in breast cancer as a result of the effects of radiation or of tumour recurrence in the brachial plexus or supraclavicular fossa. The major factors responsible for radiation-induced plexopathy include a total radiation dose exceeding 50 Gy, high dose per fraction treatment, techniques delivering the dose through a single anterior field, using orthovoltage radiation, and concurrent chemotherapy. The risks range from 0 to 1.8%.[69,70] The use of techniques that lead to field junction overlap increase the risk of this problem.

PNEUMONITIS

This complication occurs in up to 7% of patients.[68] It is seen more commonly where the volume irradiated is large, as when the supraclavicular fossa and axilla are included in the field. The risk is as low as 0.5% for radiation therapy to the breast or chest wall alone. The addition of supraclavicular fossa and axillary radiation fields increases the risk as does the addition of chemotherapy.

SARCOMAS

The development of radiation-induced sarcomas is rare. They occur in bone or soft tissue and most have involved orthovoltage therapy. A review of the evidence in 1995 suggested an incidence of 1–2 per 1000 treated patients alive at 10 years.[71,72]

OMITTING AXILLARY DISSECTION

In certain groups of women, discussed below, the risks associated with ALND outweigh the perceived benefits. In such cases, the decision to omit axillary dissection should be discussed fully with the woman.

Ductal carcinoma in situ

By definition, pure ductal carcinoma in situ (DCIS) has no metastatic potential. A number of studies have demonstrated that the prevalence of axillary nodal metastasis in cases of DCIS is less than 1%.[73] Axillary dissection should be omitted in these patients.

Good-prognosis tumours

In selected cases where the histological features of the breast primary suggest that metastatic disease to the axilla is unlikely, axillary dissection could be omitted. This includes small invasive tumours less than 0.5 cm in diameter or low-grade invasive tumours less than 1 cm in diameter, where the prevalence of axillary lymph node involvement is 3–5%.[74] Furthermore, small well-differentiated invasive tumours of special histological subtype (i.e. tubular, colloid, papillary carcinomas) also have a low prevalence of axillary lymph node involvement. For such tumours, a lesser axillary staging procedure (i.e. SNB) would appear more appropriate.

Elderly women

The management of elderly women with breast cancer and the management of the axilla in such women continues to be an area of debate. Elderly women differ from younger women with regard to anticipated life expectancy, comorbidities and the functional/psychological effects of treatment, and these aspects therefore often influence decisions about how breast cancer should be managed in elderly women. For selected elderly patients in whom ALND is unlikely to influence the decision to use adjuvant systemic therapy, axillary dissection may be omitted. This includes frail elderly women who are deemed unfit for general anaesthesia. The results of the IBCSG Trial 10-93 (which assessed surgical therapy with or without ALND for breast cancer in elderly women receiving adjuvant therapy with tamoxifen) are awaited with interest. In elderly women with small low-grade tumours where knowledge of axillary node status may influence clinical decision-making regarding the use of adjuvant tamoxifen, it seems reasonable to offer a less invasive axillary staging procedure such as axillary lymph node sampling or SNB.

STAGING THE AXILLA: ALTERNATIVES TO AXILLARY LYMPH NODE DISSECTION FOR STAGING

With the advent of population-based mammographic screening programmes, the current trends in breast cancer diagnosis and management have led to a dramatic decrease in tumour size and lymph node involvement.[75,76] As such, a greater proportion of women with early breast cancer undergo ALND only to be ultimately informed that their lymph glands are free of disease and that they have gained nothing from the procedure. In most patients, the surgical staging of breast cancer is a more extensive and expensive procedure than the surgical treatment of the primary cancer. It seems logical that the trend to more conservative surgical management of the breast primary should be combined with reappraisal of the need for routine axillary dissection.

Non-operative approaches

Surgical staging of the axilla has remained the gold standard because no reliable non-operative alternative has yet proven as effective. Clinical examination is unreliable: the sensitivity varies from 30 to 75% and specificity approaches 50%.[77,78] Mammography is a sensitive method of detecting large axillary lymph nodes but its specificity is poor. Careful ultrasound of the axilla supplemented with colour Doppler improves both sensitivity and specificity, but its accuracy relies very much on the experience of the operator and is not routinely used. Other nodal imaging techniques, which have been investigated with limited success, include nuclear scanning and labelled antibody scanning. Magnetic resonance imaging of the axilla has not confirmed its initial promise and cannot be considered at present to be sufficiently sensitive and specific. Fluorodeoxyglucose positron emission tomography (PET) has shown promising early results, with a sensitivity of 75% and specificity of 90%. However, small-volume nodal disease is unlikely to be accurately staged using present PET technology, which is expensive and not widely available. One avenue that offers hope is ultrasound scanning followed by fine-needle aspiration or core biopsy of any abnormal nodes visualised. Up to 40–45% of all patients with involved nodes can be identified using these techniques, which can be performed as part of the initial diagnostic work-up in a multidisciplinary breast diagnostic clinic.

Axillary sampling

Axillary sampling is a non-anatomical dissection and removes significantly less nodal tissue than ALND. It is described as the removal of lymph nodes from principally the lower axilla and aims to provide a qualitative assessment of metastatic disease in the axilla. A formal axillary sample, as described by Steele et al.,[79] removes a minimum of four nodes. The nodes removed are usually from level I but it differs from a formal level I clearance in that the lateral aspect of the axilla and the subcapsular fossa are not dissected and individual nodes are 'cherry picked' from the axilla and only node tissue is removed and sent for pathology. It appears to be effective because involved nodes are harder and larger than non-involved nodes and are thus easier to feel and more likely to be removed by the surgeon. It also works because the low nodes at level I are those most likely to be involved by metastases. The nerves to latissimus dorsi and serratus are not routinely identified. More elaborate descriptions of this procedure sometimes nominate the intercostobrachial nerve as a landmark of the superior extent of an axillary sample.[41,80]

Many argue that axillary sampling is not a reproducible technique. It does not provide total quantitative data in patients with metastatic axillary involvement. The variation in technique explains the variation in the number of lymph nodes harvested from such procedures. Kissin et al.[80] demonstrated a 24% error rate when dissecting to a specific landmark compared with complete axillary clearance. In original reports from the Edinburgh Unit, sampling initially failed to retrieve any lymph nodes in 18% of cases but the success rate improved substantially later.[81]

> The initial results from the Edinburgh Breast Unit of a randomised trial of 417 women undergoing mastectomy comparing ALND versus a four-node lower axillary sample (with axillary irradiation in cases of a positive sample) demonstrated comparable axillary control rates (3.0% vs. 5.4% with median follow-up of 11 years).[79] In a subsequent trial of 466 women undergoing breast conservation, axillary sample alone was associated with the least shoulder and arm morbidity. The lymphoedema rate for radiotherapy following a positive sampling procedure was equivalent to that of a dissected axilla without radiotherapy.[66] Axillary clearance was associated with a higher rate of arm swelling, while axillary sample combined with radiotherapy caused a significant loss of shoulder mobility, which tended to improve with time.

A more recent analysis of these trials at a median follow-up of 10 years has shown a significant increase in regional recurrence in the group undergoing axillary sample, regardless of whether the axilla was positive or negative initially[82] (**Table 6.2**). Despite this, there was no difference in overall survival between the two groups. One reason for this is that patients with a negative axillary sample but who developed isolated axillary recurrences could be salvaged by axillary clearance; 11 of 28 patients in this group were alive at the time of the most recent analysis, whereas all patients who developed axillary recurrence after ALND were dead. Other groups performing axillary sample have not been able to reproduce the Edinburgh data, with the Cardiff local therapy trial showing a higher axillary relapse rate in the group undergoing node sample.[83]

Blue dye-directed axillary sampling is being adopted by increasing numbers of surgeons for

Table 6.2 • Axillary recurrence in women randomised to axillary lymph node dissection (ALND) or axillary node sample (ANS) analysed according to whether the nodes were uninvolved (negative) or involved (positive) by metastases*

Group	Recurrence at 5 years (%)	Recurrence at 10 years (%)	95% CI
ALND negative	2.0	2.0	0.3–3.7
ALND positive	2.9	5.3	1.0–9.6
ANS negative	3.9	7.4	3.9–10.9
ANS positive	6.5	10.9	5.0–16.8

*Axillary recurrence rate was significantly lower in the ALND group than in the ANS group regardless of whether patients were node negative ($P = 0.009$) or node positive ($P = 0.04$).
Adapted from Lambah PA, Dixon JM, Prescott RJ et al. Long-term results of axillary clearance versus nontargeted axillary sampling. Br J Surg 2001; 88(suppl. 1).

patients at low risk of having involved nodes (e.g. small low-grade tumours). Results so far indicate similar false-negative rates to SNB using dye and radioactivity combined. If the sampled lymph nodes contain tumour deposits, further treatment of the axilla (i.e. radiotherapy, further surgery) is indicated.

Sentinel node biopsy

The rationale for SNB was first put forward for penile cancer by Cabanas[84] and then for melanoma by Morton et al.[85] The technique assumes that for any given tumour-bearing site a constant afferent lymphatic channel leads directly to a defined draining lymph node (sentinel node). The sentinel node would be the first site of metastatic disease before progression to higher-echelon nodes. It also relies on the premise that skip metastases do not occur and that the absence of tumour metastases at the sentinel node implies the absence of lymph node metastases in the entire lymphatic basin. Previous detailed pathological studies of axillary nodes have demonstrated a skip metastasis rate of less than 5%.[86,87] The aim of SNB is to provide accurate axillary staging by use of a 'minimally invasive' surgical procedure that potentially has little associated morbidity for lymph node-negative breast cancer patients.

LYMPHATIC MAPPING AND SNB TECHNIQUE

The sentinel node(s) can be identified by the use of lymphatic mapping agents such as radioactive colloid suspensions and/or blue dyes that are selectively taken up by the afferent lymphatic channels draining a tumour-bearing site. A variety of radioactive colloids have been described, including ^{99m}Tc-labelled tin,[88] antimony,[89] albumin or sulphur colloid.[90] Lymphoscintigraphy is often used to identify the location of the sentinel node. Following injection, serial anterior and appropriate lateral images using a large field of view gamma camera are obtained at approximately 15-minute intervals until the initial draining node(s) is visualised (**Fig. 6.2**). While the majority of sentinel nodes are located in the low axilla, other sites include internal mammary, supraclavicular fossa, intramammary and interpectoral nodes.[91] The radioisotope is usually injected on the day of surgery, although injection on the previous day can also be used. Coloured dyes such as Patent Blue V, isosulfan blue and indocyanine green are injected peritumorally, intradermally or in the peri- and subareolar region 5–10 minutes before surgery, and the breast is gently massaged. By using coloured dyes, it is possible to visualise the afferent lymphatic leading to the sentinel node (**Fig. 6.3**; see Plate 8, facing p. 116). Intraoperative identification of the sentinel node is confirmed by a hand-held gamma probe, which detects radioactivity within the node at a much higher level than that of background radioactivity in the nodal basin (**Fig. 6.4**; see Plate 9, facing p. 116). A number of studies have reported an improved rate of sentinel-node identification using both lymphoscintigraphy and dye compared with either technique alone.[91–97]

Similarly, some authors report a better sentinel-node identification rate with an intradermal rather than a peritumoral injection technique.[88] There is a view that peritumoral injection more accurately reflects the physiological drainage of the breast, and that internal mammary drainage may not be evident

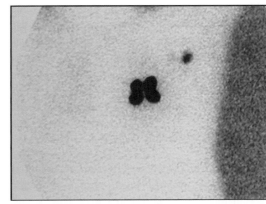

Figure 6.2 • Lymphoscintigram demonstrating transmission image and isotope injection site into left breast with uptake of isotope by single sentinel node in left axilla.

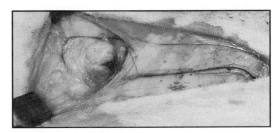

Figure 6.3 • Blue afferent lymphatic leading to blue-coloured sentinel node.

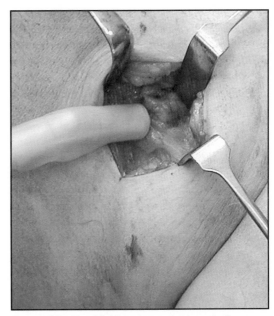

Figure 6.4 • Hand-held gamma probe in protective sterile sheath detecting radioactive blue sentinel node.

with a superficial injection but the rate of node identification is less than other sites.[91,98] Subareolar injection has advantages over both these techniques in that impalpable lesions need no special input to identify the site of injection and reports indicate higher rates of sentinel-node detection and lower rates of false negatives with this technique. On the other hand, superficial injections appear less likely to identify sentinel nodes outside the confines of the axilla.

As with any invasive procedure there are potential risks, the most serious being a low risk of allergic and anaphylactic reactions to Patent Blue V and similar lymphatic mapping dyes.[99] Radiation exposure to surgical, nursing, radiology and pathology per case is negligible but radiation safety standards and requirements for the handling of radioactive pathology specimens should be implemented by centres using radioactive isotopes in order to minimise radiation exposure to staff.[89]

PATHOLOGICAL HANDLING OF THE SENTINEL NODE

Routine pathological assessment of axillary nodes usually involves examining a single section of each node after staining with H&E. Because fewer nodes need to be assessed, SNB has the potential to study each node more comprehensively, leading to a greater detection of micrometastases and consequent upstaging.[97,100] However, protocols vary widely, with some centres continuing to use a single H&E section, while others examine multiple levels with immunohistochemical stains as well as H&E. The optimum pathological evaluation of sentinel nodes has yet to be fully determined.[100,101] A disadvantage of the sentinel node technique is that women with a positive sentinel node usually need a second operation to complete the axillary clearance. Some authors have investigated the use of intraoperative frozen-section or imprint cytology to assess the status of the sentinel node(s) with a view to immediate ALND in cases where the sentinel node contains metastatic tumour deposits.[102–106] Intraoperative assessment must be time efficient, must exhibit high sensitivity, specificity and accuracy, and must not waste nodal tissue needed for definitive analysis. While the false-positive rates for intraoperative frozen-section and imprint cytology assessment are low, false-negative rates are reported in up to 50% of cases, with limited ability to detect micrometastases.[107] Of these two techniques, imprint cytology has the higher sensitivity, is quicker to perform and does not lead to any loss of material for subsequent histological examination. Veronesi et al.[108] have reported specificity and sensitivity comparable to that of definitive histological examination, with intraoperative frozen-section assessment of up to 60 sections per node. However, the intraoperative pathology times in this study exceeded 40 minutes, and would not be feasible for many centres in terms of both time and cost. A summary of recent data is shown in **Table 6.3**. It should be noted that not all authors describe their method of definitive nodal analysis in detail, and it is possible that authors reporting lower sensitivity are performing a more detailed search for micrometastases on definitive analysis.

Table 6.3 • Results of intraoperative imprint cytology (IC) and frozen section (FS)

Reference	No. of patients	Sensitivity (%)	Specificity (%)	Accuracy (%)
Motomura (2003)[88]	101	IC: 91 FS: 52	IC: 99 FS: 100	IC: 96 FS: 88
van Diest et al. (1999)[106]	54	IC: 64 FS: 91	IC: 100 FS: 100	IC: 82 FS: 96
Henry-Tillman et al. (2002)[103]	247	IC: 94 FS: 86	IC: 100 FS: 99	
Llatjos et al. (2002)[102]	76	IC: 68	IC: 100	IC: 87
Bochner et al. (2003)[107]	79	IC: 37	IC: 100	IC: 78

Both Llatjos et al.[102] and Bochner et al.[107] found that almost all false-negative cases occurred with micrometastatic disease only, although the presence of metastatic lobular cancer is also more difficult to detect on imprint cytology. In both these studies over 80% of false-negative metastases in sentinel nodes were micrometastases that would not have been detected had very detailed levels and immuno-histochemistry not been performed. It should also be noted that some centres reporting very high sensitivity also describe false positives, which may lead to unnecessary lymph node clearance. Authors reporting lower sensitivity may be interpreting imprint cytology very conservatively in order to minimise the risk of a false-positive result.

CLINICAL ASPECTS OF SNB

Many groups have now reported extensive experience with SNB in breast cancer, validating the technique by performing an initial series in which SNB is performed in conjunction with axillary clearance. The clinical efficacy of the technique is usually assessed in terms of success at intraoperative identification of the sentinel node, accuracy, false-negative rate and negative predictive value of the sentinel node.

Intraoperative identification of the sentinel node

While increasing experience improves the ability to identify and remove a sentinel node, large series still report rates of 2–11% for non-identification of a sentinel node.[90,93,94,109] The inability to identify a sentinel node at operation may be influenced by non-visualisation of the node at preoperative lymphoscintigraphy,[92,95] surgical inexperience,[95] high BMI[96] and patient age over 60 years.[110] Most authors have not found a correlation between sentinel node identification and tumour size, tumour grade, preoperative open biopsy or tumour position within the breast.[95,96,110]

Accuracy, false-negative rate and negative predictive value of SNB

Most studies from experienced centres report that the status of the sentinel node accurately predicts axillary lymph node status in over 95% of cases.[90,108,111] This is likely to be higher in selected groups of women with a higher probability of being lymph node negative.

A false-negative sentinel node is defined as the absence of histological evidence of tumour deposits in the sentinel node when other axillary nodes contain tumour deposits. The false-negative rate of SNB in a series is determined by the following formula:

$$\text{False-negative rate} = \text{false-negative cases}/(\text{false-negative cases} + \text{true positive cases})$$

This can only be accurately reported when an axillary clearance has been performed in conjunction with SNB. False-negative rates from large series range from 2 to 22%.[92,96,112] While false-negative cases are more common with surgical inexperience,[97] they occur in almost all series and are an inherent flaw of lymphatic mapping and SNB. False-negative sentinel nodes may occur because of incorrect injection of the mapping agent or because the node is replaced by tumour and the obstructed afferent lymphatics do not permit passage of dye and radio-isotope, which are then directed to an uninvolved node.[98] It is likely that such cases may have nodes that are clinically suspicious of tumour involvement at the time of surgery. The surgeon should remove clinically suspicious nodes so that patients are still likely to receive appropriate surgery and adjuvant treatment. Failure of the pathologist to detect small nodal metastases is also a factor determining the false-negative rate. While detailed analysis of sentinel nodes detects more metastatic disease than conventional techniques, much nodal tissue still remains unexamined and metastases, particularly micrometastases, can be missed.[113] False-negative cases may be more common in multifocal cancer, and this should be considered a contraindication to the procedure.

The false-negative rate is principally determined by the prevalence of axillary lymph node involvement in a series. For example, in series where the prevalence of axillary lymph node involvement is high, one or two false-negative cases are likely to lead to a low false-negative rate. Conversely, in series where smaller screen-detected tumours predominate, the prevalence of axillary lymph node involvement is low. As such, one or two false-negative cases are likely to lead to an exaggeratedly high false negative rate. The clinical importance of the predictive value of a negative sentinel node is rarely alluded to in validation studies of SNB. This is defined as the percentage of cases in a series where the sentinel node is free of metastases and the remainder of the axillary nodes is also clear.[112]

Predictive value = cases with overall negative
of negative   axillary nodes/cases with
sentinel node   negative sentinel nodes

In the clinical setting, this is perhaps a more meaningful statistic to an individual woman faced with a result of a tumour-free sentinel node. In most series of SNB, the predictive value of a negative sentinel node is greater than 95%.

Multiple sentinel nodes

In most studies, the number of sentinel nodes identified at surgery ranges from one to eight, with mean values of 1.5–4.0. Extensive dissection of the axilla to remove multiple sentinel nodes is likely to impact on surgical morbidity. The number of sentinel nodes removed may also have an impact on the accuracy of finding a positive sentinel lymph node. The results of recent studies have suggested that in cases of multiple sentinel nodes the removal of more than the first two sentinel nodes is unlikely to significantly impact on the false-negative rate of SNB.[114–117] Nevertheless, these studies demonstrated a small number of cases where the first positive sentinel lymph node was beyond the first two sentinel nodes, suggesting that there is no absolute upper threshold for the number of sentinel nodes that should be removed. Sampling additional sentinel nodes probably adds little morbidity to the procedure, yet may significantly alter the treatment of some individuals. As such, SNB should be continued until all blue and hot nodes are removed.[114]

Internal mammary sentinel lymph nodes

Internal mammary node (IMN) status in breast cancer has previously been shown to have prognostic significance.[118] Patients with IMN metastasis have similar survival prospects to those with axillary lymph node metastasis. In cases of metastasis to both axillary and IMN basins, the prognosis is poor. Nevertheless, historical studies of extended radical mastectomy have not demonstrated improved survival with the routine removal of IMNs in patients treated for breast carcinoma.[118] Although

parasternal recurrence is fortunately rare after modified radical mastectomy or breast-conserving surgery, if left untreated it not infrequently develops as clinically evident disease in patients with histological involvement of IMNs.

The issue of IMN biopsy in breast cancer has recently resurfaced with the advent of lymphatic mapping, where aberrant lymphatic patterns have been demonstrated in up to 56% of cases.[119] In most cases, the aberrant lymphatic drainage is to the IMNs, usually located in the second or third interspace. If lymphatic mapping and SNB is practised with the aim of identifying and removing sentinel nodes, surgeons may need to re-evaluate the role of IMN biopsy dissection for staging purposes, prognosis and treatment.

The technique of IMN biopsy is relatively simple.[120] The procedure can usually be performed through the same incision used to remove the breast cancer for medially placed tumours. For laterally placed tumours, the skin incision can be retracted medially and dissection of the submammary areolar tissue allows satisfactory access to the parasternal area. Using the gamma probe, the position of the sentinel IMN is identified. The pectoral muscle fibres are separated as well as the external and internal intercostal membrane/muscles in order to gain access to the internal mammary paravascular space. With the assistance of careful retraction of the costal cartilages, the sentinel IMN(s) is identified and dissected free of the loose connective tissue using a 'teasing' technique with blunt forceps. The fibres of the pectoralis major muscle are then re-approximated. IMN biopsy is not without risks and potential complications, such as pneumothorax and haemothorax, but with careful attention to surgical technique it can be performed safely and effectively.

Several recent studies have assessed the role of internal mammary SNB in cases of breast cancer. Sentinel IMNs have been identified in 7–56% of cases.[119,121–126] IMN lymphatic mapping is more commonly seen for medial tumours and where the lymphatic mapping agent is injected into the deep aspect of the breast. Periareolar/subareolar or intradermal/subdermal injections of lymphatic mapping agents rarely localise to the IMN basin.[122] The IMN has been successfully biopsied in 60–85% of cases and the prevalence of IMN metastasis ranged from

5 to 27% of cases.[121–126] In these studies, upstaging or change in patient management occurred in 2–8% of all cases, although it is unclear whether this intervention can lead to better survival.

Internal mammary SNB is currently not standard practice but warrants further investigation to determine its safety and efficacy and its effect in improving locoregional recurrence and survival in breast cancer.

MORBIDITY AND RESULTS OF CLINICAL TRIALS

The endpoints of interest for outcome from SNB are early postoperative complications, long-term symptoms in the arm, quality of life, regional recurrence and death from breast cancer. A number of multicentre randomised trials are currently in progress (**Table 6.3**). Results from the ALMANAC trial have reported the expected reduction in arm morbidity with sentinel node biopsy compared to ALND. As the technique of SNB becomes more widely used, surgeons are increasingly performing the technique outside the confines of clinical trials, which has had an effect on the ability of some trials to complete accrual.[127]

 Veronesi et al.[108] reported results of 516 women randomised to either SNB alone or SNB in conjunction with ALND in early breast cancer, with a median follow-up of 46 months. Women were randomised intraoperatively after identification of the sentinel node, and the analysis was performed on a treatment received rather than an intention-to-treat basis. Women undergoing SNB alone experienced less arm swelling, axillary pain and numbness, and better arm mobility. There were no axillary recurrences in either group, and no difference in overall survival.

Chung et al.[128] report a regional recurrence rate, at a median follow-up of 26 months after SNB, of 3 of 208 patients, quoting a clinical false-negative rate of 1.4%. This represents 3.4% of those with positive nodes.

In terms of morbidity, several non-randomised studies with relatively short follow-up periods have demonstrated less arm swelling, numbness and disability in women undergoing SNB compared with those undergoing axillary clearance.[129–132]

SNB IN DCIS

Recently, SNB has been used in DCIS in some centres because of its perceived low morbidity, with reports of 6–9% of patients with DCIS having an involved sentinel node.[96,133] If it has a role in DCIS, then it is probably in patients undergoing mastectomy for a large area of DCIS where the presence of micro-invasion cannot be excluded prior to surgery.

THE FUTURE OF SNB

SNB has great potential to reduce morbidity in patients undergoing lymph node staging procedures for breast cancer. Its impact will be seen in providing improved histological staging of the axilla through greater histological scrutiny of the sentinel node and the avoidance of ALND in lymph node-negative women. Short-term results of current trials should be interpreted with some caution; the message learnt from the Edinburgh trial of sampling versus clearance that a difference in regional recurrence may not be apparent for at least 10 years may also apply in terms of recurrence and survival for SNB. Similar to previous randomised trials of breast-conserving therapy and mastectomy, long-term follow-up of women in current SNB trials is required before the safety of SNB can be determined. The management of women with tumour involvement of the sentinel node has yet to be determined. In a large percentage of women, removal of the sentinel node alone may result not only in accurate staging but also in effective regional control. A number of studies have shown that in 50–70% of cases where metastatic tumour deposits are identified, the sentinel node is the only involved node.[134–137] It is quite possible that after accurate staging with SNB, no residual tumour is left in the remainder of the non-sentinel axillary lymph nodes. However, some women with sentinel node metastases will have micrometastases or macrometastases in non-sentinel nodes that will progress and develop into regional recurrences that may or may not be associated with a diminution of overall survival. On the other hand, it is possible that metastases in non-sentinel nodes could be destroyed or controlled by the adjuvant systemic therapy given to women with involved lymph nodes. In addition, opposing tangential fields of radiation therapy may ablate some metastases. The results of current trials, such as IBCSG 23-01, ACOSOG -Z0011 and others, will

Table 6.4 • Current trials for sentinel node biopsy in breast cancer

Trial	Study population	Study arms	Primary endpoints
NSABP-B32 (USA)	Clinical T1–T3, N0	SNB plus ALND vs. SNB → ALND if positive or SNB → observation if negative	Regional recurrence, DFS, OS, morbidity
ALMANAC (UK)	Any invasive, clinical N0	ALND/ANS vs. SNB → ALND/RT if positive or SNB → observation if negative	Arm morbidity, QOL, resource costs
SNAC (Australia/ New Zealand)	≤30 mm invasive, clinical N0	SNB plus ALND vs. SNB → ALND if positive or SNB → observation if negative	Morbidity, QOL, regional recurrence
ACOSOG Z0010 (USA)	Clinical T1–T2, N0	Non-randomized prospective SNB plus BM → observation if negative or → ANC or Z0011 if positive	OS, DFS, regional recurrence
ACOSOG Z0011 (USA)	T1–T2 invasive with pathological positive sentinel node	ALND vs. observation	Morbidity, OS
IBCSG 23-01	≤30 mm invasive, micrometastasis in sentinel node	ALND vs. observation	Morbidity, DFS, OS
European Institute of Oncology (Italy)	T1	SNB plus ALND vs. SNB → ALND if positive or SNB → observation if negative	Predictive power of positive sentinel node, QOL, regional recurrence

ALND, axillary lymph node dissection; ANS, axillary node sample; BM, bone marrow biopsy; DFS, disease-free survival; OS, overall survival; QOL, quality of life; RT, radiotherapy; SNB, sentinel node biopsy.

therefore be of great clinical importance (**Table 6.4**). SNB requires specialist training, not only for the surgeon but for the whole team, including the nuclear medicine specialist, radiologist, pathologist and ancillary theatre staff in order to obtain results comparable to those achieved in experienced centres.

CONCLUSION

Given that the management of the axilla always involves a balance of the potential risks and benefits of treatment, women undergoing treatment for primary breast cancer must always be fully informed regarding treatment options available and participate in the decision. Advice should be given regarding the value of staging information in determining the best systemic adjuvant treatment if required and about the benefits of axillary surgery and irradiation in reducing the risk of local recurrence and possibly increasing survival. Women should also be informed about the potential side effects of surgery and irradiation, particularly lymphoedema. Patient management is optimal in clinical situations where multidisciplinary communication is greatest. Close communication between the surgeon, radiation oncologist and medical oncologist is required to manage such patients.

Key points

- Lymph node status is the strongest prognostic determinant in early breast cancer.
- ALND may have an impact on survival, although the evidence remains insufficient.
- ALND substantially reduces the risk of axillary recurrence.
- ALND provides the most accurate qualitative and quantitative assessment of the axilla.
- Only cases of axillary nodal micrometastases visible on H & E are associated with a worse outcome.
- ALND is associated with a range of complications including lymphoedema.
- The benefits of axillary irradiation on survival from breast cancer remain unclear.
- ALND should be omitted in cases of DCIS.
- Consideration should be given to replace ALND in elderly women and those with small low-grade screen-detected tumours by SNB.
- Blue dye-directed axillary sampling is practised by some centres familiar with procedure.
- SNB accurately stages the axilla using a minimally invasive approach and reduces axillary morbidity for lymph node-negative cases.
- Randomised trials continue to assess the role of SNB in early breast cancer.

REFERENCES

1. Fisher B, Redmond C, Fisher ER. Ten year results of a randomised clinical trial comparing radical mastectomy and total mastectomy with or without irradiation. N Engl J Med 1985; 312:674–81.

   One of the first large-recruitment randomised studies that demonstrated the importance of ALND but questions its effect on survival.

2. Cabanes PA, Salmon RJ, Vilcoq JR et al. Value of axillary dissection in addition to lumpectomy and radiotherapy in early breast cancer. Lancet 1992; 339:245–8.

   One of few studies that demonstrated a survival benefit in favour of ALND.

3. Hayward J, Caleffi M. The significance of local control in the primary treatment of breast cancer. Arch Surg 1987; 122:1244–7.

4. Langlands A, Prescott R, Hamilton T. A clinical trial in the management of operable cancer of the breast. Br J Surg 1980; 67:170–4.

5. Fisher BJ, Perera FE, Cooke AL et al. Long-term follow-up of axillary node-positive breast cancer patients receiving adjuvant systemic therapy alone: patterns of recurrence. Int J Radiat Oncol Biol Phys 1997; 38:541–50.

6. Vincini F, Horwitz E, Lacerna M et al. The role of regional nodal irradiation in the management of patients with early-stage breast cancer treated with breast-conserving therapy. Int J Radiat Oncol Biol Phys 1997; 39:1069–76.

7. Du Toit RS, Locker AP, Ellis IO et al. Evaluation of the prognostic value of triple node biopsy in early breast cancer. Br J Surg 1990; 77:163–7.

8. Carter CL, Allen C, Henson DE. Relation of tumor size, lymph node status, and survival in 24,740 breast cancer cases. Cancer 1989; 63:181–7.

9. Early Breast Cancer Trialists' Collaborative Group. Systemic treatment of early breast cancer by hormonal, cytotoxic or immune therapy: 133 randomised trials involving 31,000 recurrences and 24,000 deaths among 75,000 women. Lancet 1992; 339:1–15.

10. Early Breast Cancer Trialists' Collaborative Group. Systemic treatment of early breast cancer by hormonal, cytotoxic or immune therapy: 133 randomised trials involving 31,000 recurrences and 24,000 deaths among 75,000 women. Lancet 1992; 339:71–85.

11. Anonymous. Adjuvant systemic therapy for early breast cancer. Lancet 1992; 339:27.

12. Early Breast Cancer Trialists' Collaborative Group. Tamoxifen for early breast cancer: an overview of the randomised trials. Lancet 1998; 351:1451–67.

13. Early Breast Cancer Trialists' Collaborative Group. Polychemotherapy for early breast cancer: an overview of the randomised trials. Lancet 1998; 352:930–42.

14. Fisher ER, Sass R, Fisher B. Pathologic findings from the national surgical adjuvant project (protocol no. 4). X. Discriminants for tenth year treatment failure. Cancer 1984; 53:12–23.

15. Baxter N, McCready DR, Chapman JA et al. Clinical behaviour of untreated axillary nodes after local treatment for primary breast cancer. Ann Surg Oncol 1996; 3:235–40.

16. Kollias J, Murphy CA, Elston CW et al. The prognosis of small primary breast cancers. Eur J Cancer 1999; 35:908–912.

17. Fisher B, Redmond C, Poisson R et al. Eight-year results of a randomised clinical trial comparing total mastectomy and lumpectomy with or without radiation in the treatment of breast cancer. N Engl J Med 1989; 320:822–8.

18. Mann GB, Buchanan M, Collins JP, Lichtenstein M. High incidence of micrometastases in breast cancer sentinel nodes. Aust NZ J Surg 2000; 70:786–90.

19. Trojani M, de Mascarel I, Bonichon F et al. Micro-metastases to axillary lymph nodes from carcinoma of the breast. Br J Cancer 1987; 55:303–6.

20. Hainsworth PJ, Tjandra J, Stillwell RG et al. Detection and significance of occult metastases in node negative breast cancer. Br J Surg 1993; 80:459–63.

21. Huvos AG, Hutter R, Berg JW. Significance of axillary macrometastases and micrometastases in mammary cancer. Ann Surg 1971; 173:44–6.

22. Fisher ER, Swamidoss S, Lee CH et al. Detection and significance of occult axillary node metastases in patients with invasive breast cancer. Cancer 1978; 42:2025–31.

23. Rosen PP, Saigo P, Weathers E et al. Axillary micro- and macrometastases in breast cancer: prognostic significance of tumor size. Ann Surg 1981; 194:585–91.

24. Friedman S, Bertin F, Mouriesse H et al. Importance of tumour cells in axillary node sinus margins (clandestine metastases) discovered by serial sectioning in operable breast cancer. Acta Oncol 1988; 27:483–7.

25. International (Ludwig) Breast Cancer Study Group. Prognostic importance of occult axillary micro-metastases from breast cancer. Lancet 1990; 335:1565–8.

26. Clayton F, Hopkins CL. Pathological correlates of prognosis in lymph node positive breast cancer. Cancer 1993; 71:1780–90.

27. McGuckin MA, Cummings MC, Walsh MD et al. Occult axillary metastases in breast cancer: their detection and prognostic significance. Br J Cancer 1996; 73:88–95.

28. Dowlatashahi K, Fan M, Snider H, Habib L. Lymph node micrometastases from breast carcin-oma. Reviewing the dilemma. Cancer 1997; 80:1188–97.

29. Cote RJ, Peterson HF, Chaiwun B et al. Role of immunohistochemical detection of lymph-node metastases in management of breast cancer. International Breast Cancer Study Group. Lancet 1999; 354:896–900.

30. de Mascarel I, MacGrogan G, Picot V et al. Prognostic significance of immunohistochemically detected breast cancer node metastases in 218 patients. Br J Cancer 2002; 87:70–4.

31. Hansen NM, Grube BJ, Giuliano AE. Clinical significance of axillary micrometastases in breast cancer: how small is too small? Proc Am Soc Clin Oncol 2001; 20:24A.

32. Siegal BM, Mayzel KM, Love SM. Level I and II axillary dissection in the treatment of early stage breast cancer: an analysis of 259 consecutive patients. Arch Surg 1990; 125:1144–7.

33. Shaw JHF, Rumball EM. Complications and local recurrence following lymphadenectomy. Br J Surg 1990; 77:760–4.

34. Platt R, Zucker JR, Zaleznik DF et al. Perioperative antibiotic prophylaxis and wound infection follow-ing breast surgery. J Antimicrob Chemother 1993; 31(suppl. B):43–8.

35. Hladiuk M, Huchcroft S, Temple W et al. Arm function after axillary dissection for breast cancer: a pilot study to provide parameter estimates. J Surg Oncol 1992; 50:47–52.

36. Lin PP, Allison DC, Wainstock J et al. Impact of axillary lymph node dissection on the therapy of breast cancer patients. J Clin Oncol 1993; 11:1536–44.

37. Salmon RJ, Ansquer Y, Asselain B. Preservation versus section of intercosto-brachial nerve in axillary dissection for breast cancer: a prospective randomised trial. Eur J Surg Oncol 1998; 24:158–61.

38. Browning C, Redman S, Pillar C et al. Lymph-oedema: prevalence, risk factors and management: a review of research. Woolloomooloo, NSW, Australia: National Breast Cancer Centre, 1997.

39. Gray H, Bannister L, Berry M et al. (eds) Gray's anatomy: the anatomical basis of medicine and surgery, 38th edn. London: Churchill Livingstone, 1995.

40. Danforth DN Jr, Findlay PA, McDonald HD et al. Complete axillary lymph node dissection for stage I–II carcinoma of the breast. J Clin Oncol 1986; 4:655–62.

41. Davidson T. Why I favour axillary node clearance in the management of breast cancer. Eur J Surg Oncol 1995; 21:5–7.

42. Bundred NJ, Morgan DA, Dixon JM. Management of regional nodes in breast cancer. In: Dixon J (ed.)

ABC of breast diseases. London: BMJ Publishing Group, 1995; pp. 30–40.

43. Veronesi U, Rilke F, Luini A et al. Distribution of axillary node metastases by level of invasion. Cancer 1987; 59:682–7.

44. Overgaard M, Hansen PS, Overgaard J et al. Post operative radiotherapy in high risk premenopausal women with breast cancer who receive adjuvant chemotherapy. N Engl J Med 1997; 337:949–55.

This important randomised trial of 1708 high-risk premenopausal women with breast cancer demonstrated reduced locoregional recurrence and prolongation in survival for women who underwent postoperative radiotherapy.

45. Overgaard M, Hansen PS, Overgaard C et al. Randomized trial evaluating postoperative radio-therapy in high-risk postmenopausal breast cancer patients given adjuvant tamoxifen. Results from the DBCG 82C Trial (abstract). Radiother Oncol 1998; 48(suppl. 1):586.

46. Ragaz J, Stewart M, Jackson NL et al. Adjuvant radiotherapy and chemotherapy in node positive premenopausal women with breast cancer. N Engl J Med 1988; 6:1107–17.

47. Early Breast Cancer Trialists' Collaborative Group. Effects of radiotherapy and surgery in early breast cancer. An overview of the randomized trials. N Engl J Med 1995; 333:1444–55.

48. Baum M, Haybittle JH, Berstock DA et al. The Cancer Research Campaign (King's/Cambridge) Trial for Early Breast Cancer: a detailed update at the tenth year. Lancet 1980; ii:55–60.

49. Recht A, Pierce SM, Abner A et al. Regional nodal failure after conservative surgery and radiotherapy for early-stage breast carcinoma. J Clin Oncol 1991; 9:988–96.

50. Pisansky TM, Ingle JN, Schaid DJ et al. Patterns of tumour relapse following mastectomy and adjuvant systemic therapy in patients with axillary lymph node-positive breast cancer. Cancer 1993; 72:1247–60.

51. Fowble B, Gray R, Gilchrist K et al. Identification of a subgroup of patients with breast cancer and histologically positive axillary nodes receiving adjuvant chemotherapy who may benefit from post operative radiotherapy. J Clin Oncol 1988; 6:1107–17.

52. Veronisi U, Banfi A, Salvadori B et al. Breast conservation is the treatment of choice in small breast cancer: long term results of a randomised trial. Eur J Cancer 1990; 26:668–70.

53. Blichert-Toft M. A Danish randomised trial comparing breast conservation with mastectomy in mammary carcinoma. Br J Cancer 1990; 62(suppl. 12):15.

54. Ung O, Langlands AO, Barraclough B et al. Combined chemotherapy and radiotherapy for patients with breast cancer and extensive nodal involvement. J Clin Oncol 1995; 13:435–43.

55. Diab SG, Hilsenbeck SG, de Moor C et al. Radiation therapy and survival in breast cancer patients with 10 or more positive axillary lymph nodes treated with mastectomy. J Clin Oncol 1998; 16:1655–60.

56. Fisher ER, Gregorio RM, Redmond C et al. Pathologic findings from the National Surgical Adjuvant Breast Project (protocol no. 4). III. The significance of extranodal extension of axillary metastases. Am J Clin Pathol 1976; 65:439–44.

57. Mambo NC, Gallagher HS. Carcinoma of the breast: the prognostic significance of extranodal extension of axillary disease. Cancer 1977; 39:280–5.

58. Fisher BJ, Perera FE, Cooke AL et al. Extracapsular axillary node extension in patients receiving adjuvant systemic therapy: an indication for radiotherapy? Int J Radiat Oncol Biol Phys 1997; 38:551–9.

59. Harviet F. The routine histological investigation of axillary lymph nodes for metastatic breast cancer. J Pathol 1984; 143:87–91.

60. Leonard C, Corkill M, Tompkin J et al. Are axillary recurrence and overall survival affected by axillary extranodal tumor extension in breast cancer? Implications for radiation therapy. J Clin Oncol 1995; 3:47–53.

61. Donegan WL, Stine SB, Samter TG. Implications of extracapsular nodal metastases for treatment and prognosis of breast cancer. Cancer 1993; 72:778–82.

62. Bucci JA, Kennedy CW, Burns J et al. Implications of extranodal spread in node positive breast cancer: a review of survival and local recurrence. In: 49th Annual Scientific Meeting of the Royal Australasian College of Radiologists, October 1998, Brisbane, Queensland.

63. Pierce LJ, Oberman HA, Strawderman MH et al. Microscopic extracapsular extension in the axilla: is this an indication for axillary radiotherapy? Int J Radiat Oncol Biol Phys 1995; 33:253–9.

64. Kissin MW, Querci-della-Rovere G, Easton D et al. Risk of lymphoedema following the treatment of breast cancer. Br J Surg 1986; 73:580–4.

65. Liljegren G, Holmberg L. Arm morbidity after sector resection and axillary dissection with or without postoperative radiotherapy in breast cancer stage I. Results from a randomised trial. Uppsala–Orebro Breast Cancer Study Group. Eur J Cancer 1997; 33:193–9.

66. Chetty U, Jack W, Presett RJ et al. Management of the axilla in patients with operable breast cancer being treated by breast conservation: a randomised trial. Br J Surg 2000; 87:163–9.

A more recent update of the Edinburgh randomised trial of 466 women with breast cancer undergoing breast-conserving treatment having axillary node sample (with radiotherapy to the axilla in node-positive cases) or ALND. There were no differences for local, regional or systemic relapse between groups. Morbidity was least in those who had a node sample alone. Radiotherapy to the axilla in patients who had a node sample resulted in a significant reduction in range of movement of the shoulder. ALND was associated with significant lymphoedema of the upper limb.

67. Steering committee on clinical practice guidelines for the care and treatment of breast cancer. A Canadian consensus document. Can Med Assoc J 1998; 158(3 suppl.).

68. Pierce SM, Recht A, Lingos TI et al. Long-term radiation complications following conservative surgery and radiation therapy in patients with early stage breast cancer. Int J Radiat Oncol Biol Phys 1992; 23:915–23.

69. Pierquin B, Mazeron JJ, Glaubiger D. Conservative treatment of breast cancer in Europe: report of the Groupe Européen de Curietherapie. Radiother Oncol 1990; 18:213–20.

70. Bates T, Evans RGB. Report of the independent review commissioned by the Royal College of Radiologists into brachial plexus neuropathy following radiotherapy for breast carcinoma. London: Royal College of Radiologists, 1995.

71. Pendlebury SC, Bilous M, Langlands AO. Sarcomas following radiation therapy for breast cancer: a report of three cases and a review of the literature. Int J Radiat Oncol Biol Phys 1995; 1:405–10.

72. Doherty MA, Rodger A, Langlands AO et al. Multiple primary tumours in patients treated with radiotherapy for breast cancer. Radiother Oncol 1993; 26:125–31.

73. Silverstein MJ, Gierson ED, Colburn WJ et al. Axillary lymphadenectomy for intraductal carcinoma of the breast. Surg Gynecol Obstet 1991; 172:211–14.

74. Silverstein MJ, Gierson ED, Waisman JR et al. Axillary lymph node dissection for T1a breast carcinoma. Cancer 1994; 73:664–9.

75. Tabar L, Fagerberg G, Duffy SW et al. Update of the Swedish two-county program of mammographic screening for breast cancer. Radiol Clin North Am 1992; 30:187–210.

76. Cady B, Stone MD, Schuler JG et al. The new era in breast cancer: invasion, size and lymph node involvement dramatically decreased as a result of mammographic screening. Arch Surg 1996; 131:301–8.

77. Davies GC, Millis RR, Hayward JL. Assessment of axillary lymph node status. Ann Surg 1980; 192:148–51.

78. Fisher B, Wolmark N, Bauer M et al. The accuracy of clinical nodal staging and of limited axillary dissection as a determinant of histological nodal status in carcinoma of the breast. Surg Gynecol Obstet 1981; 152:765–72.

79. Steele RJC, Forrest APM, Gibson T et al. The efficacy of lower axillary sampling in obtaining lymph node status in breast cancer: a controlled randomised trial. Br J Surg 1985; 72:368–9.

The third trial of axillary sampling versus ALND for women undergoing mastectomy at the Edinburgh Breast Unit. This trial demonstrated a non-significant increase in the rate of axillary relapse favouring the ALND group (3.0% vs. 5.4% with median follow-up of 11 years).

80. Kissin MW, Thompson EM, Price AB et al. The inadequacy of axillary sampling in breast cancer. Lancet 1982; i:1210–12.

81. Forrest AP, Everington D, McDonald CC et al. The Edinburgh randomised trial of axillary sampling or clearance after mastectomy. Br J Surg 1995; 82:1504–8.

82. Lambah PA, Dixon JM, Prescott RJ et al. Long-term results of axillary clearance versus nontargeted axillary sampling. Br J Surg 2001; 88(suppl. 1).

83. Stewart HJ, Everington D, Forrest APM. The Cardiff local therapy trial: results at 20 years. Breast J 1994; 3:40–5.

84. Cabanes RM. An approach for the treatment of penile carcinoma. Cancer 1977; 39:456–66.

85. Morton D, Wen D, Cochran A et al. Management of early stage melanoma by intraoperative lymphatic mapping and selective lymphadenectomy: an alternative to routine elective lymphadenectomy or 'watch and wait'. Surg Oncol Clin North Am 1992; 1:247–59.

86. Veronesi U, Rilke F, Luini A et al. Distribution of axillary node metastases by level of invasion. Cancer 1987; 59:682–7.

87. Berg JW. The significance of axillary node levels in the study of breast cancer. Cancer 1955; 8:776–8.

88. Motomura K. Intradermal radioisotope injection is superior to subdermal injection for the identification of the sentinel node in breast cancer patients. J Clin Oncol 2003; 82:91–6.

89. Kollias J, Gill PG, Chatterton B, Raymond W, Collins PJ. Sentinel node biopsy in breast cancer: recommendations for surgeons, pathologists, nuclear physicians and radiologists in Australia and New Zealand. Aust NZ J Surg 2000; 70:132–6.

90. Krag DN, Harlow S, Weaver D et al. Radiolabeled sentinel node biopsy: collaborative trial with the National Cancer Institute. World J Surg 2001; 25:823–8.

91. Uren RF, Howman-Giles R, Renwick SB et al. Lymphatic mapping of the breast: locating the

sentinel lymph nodes. World J Surg 2001; 25:789–93.

92. Chua B. Outcomes of sentinel node biopsy for breast cancer in British Columbia 1996–2001. Am J Surg 2003; 185:118–26.

93. Cody HS, Hill ADK, Tran KN et al. Credentialing for breast lymphatic mapping: how many cases are enough? Ann Surg 1999; 229:723–8.

94. Cox CE, Pendas S, Cox JM. Guidelines for sentinel node biopsy and lymphatic mapping of patients with breast cancer. Ann Surg 1998; 227:645–53.

95. Kollias J, Gill PG, Coventry BJ et al. Clinical and histological factors associated with sentinel node identification in breast cancer. Aust NZ J Surg 2000; 70:485–9.

96. Cox CE, Bass SS, McCann CR et al. Lymphatic mapping and sentinel lymph node biopsy in patients with breast cancer. Annu Rev Med 2000; 51:525–42.

97. Hill ADK, Tran KN, Akhurst T et al. Lessons learned from 500 cases of lymphatic mapping for breast cancer. Ann Surg 1999; 229:528–35.

98. Nieweg OE, Rutgers EJT, Jansen L et al. Is lymphatic mapping in breast cancer adequate and safe? World J Surg 2001; 25:780–8.

99. Mullan MH, Deacock SJ, Quiney NF et al. Anaphylaxis to patent blue dye during sentinel lymph node biopsy for breast cancer. Eur J Surg Oncol 2001; 27:218–19.

100. Rampaul RS, Miremadi A, Pinder SE et al. Pathological validation and significance of micro-metastases in sentinel nodes in primary breast cancer. Breast Cancer Res 2001; 3:113–16.

101. Treseler PA, Tauchi PS. Pathologic analysis of the sentinel lymph node. Surg Clin North Am 2000; 80:1695–719.

102. Llatjos M, Castella E, Fraile M et al. Intraoperative assessment of sentinel lymph nodes in patients with breast carcinoma: accuracy of rapid imprint cytology compared with definitive histologic workup. Cancer 2002; 96:150–6.

103. Henry-Tillman RS, Korourian S, Rubio IT et al. Intraoperative touch preparation for sentinel lymph node biopsy: a 4-year experience. Ann Surg Oncol 2002; 9:333–9.

104. Anastasiadis PG, Koutlaki NG, Liberis VA et al. Cytologic diagnosis of axillary lymph node metastasis in breast cancer. Acta Cytol 2000; 44:18–21.

105. Ratanawichitrasin A, Biscotti CV, Levy L et al. Touch imprint cytological analysis of sentinel lymph nodes for detecting axillary metastases in patients with breast cancer. Br J Surg 1999; 86:1346–9.

106. van Diest PJ, Torrenga H, Borgstein PJ et al. Reliability of intraoperative frozen section and imprint cytological investigation of sentinel lymph nodes in breast cancer. Histopathology 1999; 35:14–18.

107. Bochner MA, Farshid G, Dodd TJ et al. Intra-operative cytologic assessment of the sentinel node for early breast cancer. World J Surg 2003; 27:430–2.

108. Veronesi U, Paganelli G, Viale G et al. A randomized comparison of sentinel-node biopsy with routine axillary dissection in breast cancer. N Engl J Med 2003; 349:546–53.

    The first report of a randomised trial comparing SNB with ALND. Morbidity was least for lymph node-negative cases that underwent SNB only.

109. Martin RCG, Edwards MJ, Wong SL. Practical guidelines for optimal gamma probe detection of sentinel lymph nodes in breast cancer: results of a multi-institutional study. Surgery 2000; 128:139–44.

110. Motomura K, Komoike Y, Inaji H et al. Patient age affects identification rate of sentinel nodes in breast cancer. Biomed Pharmacother 2002; 56(suppl. 1): 209s–212s.

111. Bergkvist L, Frisell J, Liljegren G et al. Multicentre study of detection and false-negative rates in sentinel node biopsy for breast cancer. Br J Surg 2001; 88:1644–8.

112. Nano MT, Kollias J, Farshid G et al. Clinical impact of false-negative sentinel node biopsy in primary breast cancer. Br J Surg 2002; 89:1430–4.

113. Farshid G, Pradhan M, Kollias J et al. Computer simulations of lymph node metastasis for optimizing the pathologic examination of sentinel lymph nodes in patients with breast carcinoma. Cancer 2000; 89:2527–37.

114. McCarter MD, Yeung H, Fey J et al. The breast cancer patient with multiple sentinel nodes: when to stop? J Am Coll Surg 2001; 192:692–7.

115. Zervos EE, Badgwell BD, Abdessalam SF et al. Selective analysis of the sentinel node in breast cancer. Am J Surg 2001; 182:372–6.

116. Kennedy RJ, Kollias J, Gill PG et al. Removal of two sentinel nodes accurately stages the axilla in breast cancer. Br J Surg 2003; 90:1349–53.

117. Schrenk P, Rehberger W, Shamiyeh A, Wayand W. Sentinel node biopsy for breast cancer: does the number of sentinel nodes removed have an impact on the accuracy of finding a positive node? J Surg Oncol 2002; 80:130–6.

118. Veronesi U, Marubini E, Mariani L et al. The dissection of internal mammary nodes does not improve the survival of breast cancer patients: 30-year results of a randomised trial. Eur J Cancer 1999; 35:1320–5.

119. Uren RF, Howman-Giles R, Renwick SB, Gillett D. Lymphatic mapping of the breast: locating the

sentinel lymph nodes. World J Surg 2001; 25:789–93.

120. Sacchini G, Borgen PI, Galimberti V et al. Surgical approach to internal mammary lymph node biopsy. J Am Coll Surg 2001; 193:709–13.

121. Kollias J, Gill PG, Chatterton B et al. The clinical significance of internal mammary sentinel nodes in primary breast cancer. Aust NZ J Surg 2001; 71:A12.

122. Paganelli G, Galimberti V, Trifiro G et al. Internal mammary node lymphoscintigraphy and biopsy in breast cancer. Q J Nucl Med 2002; 46:138–44.

123. Jansen L, Doting MH, Rutgers EJ et al. Clinical relevance of sentinel lymph nodes outside the axilla in patients with breast cancer. Br J Surg 2000; 87:920–5.

124. van der Ent FW, Kengen RA, van der Pol HA et al. Halsted revisited: internal mammary sentinel lymph node biopsy in breast cancer. Ann Surg 2001; 234:79–84.

125. Tanis PJ, Nieweg OE, Valdes RA et al. Impact of non-axillary sentinel node biopsy on staging and treatment of breast cancer patients. Br J Cancer 2002; 87:705–10.

126. Dupont EL, Salud CJ, Peltz ES et al. Clinical relevance of internal mammary node mapping as a guide to radiation therapy. Am J Surg 2001; 182:321–4.

127. Edge SB, Niland JC, Bookman MA et al. Emergence of sentinel node biopsy in breast cancer as standard-of-care in academic comprehensive cancer centers. J Natl Cancer Inst 2003; 95:1514–21.

128. Chung MA, Steinhoff MM, Cady B. Clinical axillary recurrence in breast cancer patients after a negative sentinel node biopsy. Am J Surg 2002; 184:310–14.

129. Haid A, Koberle-Wuhrer R, Knauer M et al. Morbidity of breast cancer patients following complete axillary dissection or sentinel node biopsy only: a comparative evaluation. Breast Cancer Res Treat 2002; 73:31–6.

130. Schijven MP, Vingerhoets AJ, Rutten HJ et al. Comparison of morbidity between axillary lymph node dissection and sentinel node biopsy. Eur J Surg Oncol 2003; 29:3413–50.

131. Schrenk P, Rieger R, Shamiyeh A et al. Morbidity following sentinel lymph node biopsy versus axillary lymph node dissection for patients with breast carcinoma. Cancer 2000; 88:608–13.

132. Sener SF, Winchester DJ, Martz CH et al. Lymph-oedema after sentinel lymphadenectomy for breast carcinoma. Cancer 2001; 92:748–52.

133. Pendas S, Dauway E, Giuliano R. Sentinel node biopsy in ductal carcinoma in situ patients. Ann Surg Oncol 2000; 7:15–20.

134. Giuliano AE, Kirgan DM, Guenther JM, Morton DL. Lymphatic mapping and sentinel lymphadenectomy in breast cancer. Ann Surg 1994; 220:391–401.

135. Kollias J, Gill PG, Chatterton BA et al. The reliability of sentinel node status in predicting axillary lymph node involvement in breast cancer. Med J Aust 1999; 171:461–5.

136. Albertini JJ, Lyman GH, Cox C et al. Lymphatic mapping and sentinel node biopsy in the patient with breast cancer. JAMA 1996; 276:1818–22.

137. Veronesi U, Paganelli G, Galimberti V et al. Sentinel-node biopsy to avoid axillary dissection in breast cancer with clinically negative lymph nodes. Lancet 1997; 349:1864–7.

Seven

Prevention of breast cancer: the genetics of breast cancer and risk-reducing surgery

D. Gareth R. Evans and
Andrew D. Baildam

INTRODUCTION

The last few years has seen a substantial rise in our knowledge of inherited breast cancer. It is now possible to identify women at very high levels of risk of the disease. While there are promising signs for the reduction in risk from hormonal and other manipulations, the level of risk reduction still falls far short of that provided by surgical removal of breast tissue. Until another reliable risk-reducing measure is developed, risk-reducing surgery will remain a mainstay of management in women at very high risk who want to reduce substantially their chances of developing breast cancer.

GENETIC PREDISPOSITION

The presence of a significant family history is the strongest risk factor for the development of breast cancer. Even at extremes of age, the presence of a BRCA1 mutation will confer significant risks. A 25-year-old woman who carries a mutation in BRCA1 has a greater risk of developing breast cancer in the following decade than a woman aged 70 years in the general population. About 4–5% of breast cancer is thought to be due to inheritance of a high penetrance autosomal dominant cancer-predisposing gene.[1,2]

Inheritance of a germline mutation or deletion in a predisposing gene predisposes to early-onset, and frequently bilateral, breast cancer. Certain mutations also confer an increased susceptibility to other malignancies, such as ovary (BRCA1/2), and sarcomas (TP53)[3–5] (**Table 7.1**).

Multiple primary cancers in one individual or related early-onset cancers in a family pedigree are highly suggestive of a predisposing gene. It is thought that over 25% of breast cancers in women under 30 years of age are due to mutation in a dominant gene, compared with less than 1% in women who develop the disease over 70 years.[2] It has recently been found that at least 20% of breast cancers under 30 years of age are due to mutations in the known high-risk genes BRCA1, BRCA2 and TP53. Nonetheless, this is still largely indicated by family history and the detection rate for mutations in isolated breast cancer cases even at very young ages is considerably less than 10%.[6]

There are few families where it is possible to be certain of a dominantly inherited susceptibility. However, the Breast Cancer Linkage Consortium (BCLC) data suggest that in families with four or more cases of early-onset or bilateral breast cancer, the risk of an unaffected woman inheriting a mutation in a predisposing gene is close to 50%.

Table 7.1 • Hereditary conditions predisposing to breast cancer

Disease	Other tumour susceptibility	Inheritance	BC (%)	Per cent HPHBC	Location
Familial breast cancer *BRCA1*	Ovary/prostate Bowel	AD	1.7	50	17q
Familial breast cancer *BRCA2*	Ovary/prostate Male breast	AD	1.2	35	13q
Li–Fraumeni	Sarcoma, leukaemia, brain, adrenal	AD	0.1	1	17p (*TP53*)
HNPCC	Bowel (proximal) Endometrium, ovary Pancreas, stomach	AD	<1	<1	2p 3p 7q, 3q
Ataxia telangectasia	Homozygous (leukaemia, etc.) Heterozygous (gastric, ?other sites)	AR	0 2	0 4–8	11q
Cowden's	Skin, thyroid, bowel	AD	<l	<l	10q
Reifenstein's	?	?XLR	<l		X
H-ras variant		AD	?8	0	11p
hCHK2	Breast	AD	4	0	22q

AD, autosomal dominant; AR, autosomal recessive; BC, breast cancer; HNPCC, hereditary non-polyposis colorectal cancer; HPHBC, highly penetrant hereditary breast cancer (e.g. more than three affected relatives); XLR, X-linked recessive.

These studies have estimated that the majority of such families harbour mutations in *BRCA1* or *BRCA2*, especially when male breast cancer or ovarian cancer are present. In breast-only families, the frequency of *BRCA1/2* involvement falls to below 50% in four-case families.[7,8] Family and epidemiological studies have demonstrated that approximately 70–85% of *BRCA1* and *BRCA2* mutation carriers develop breast cancer in their lifetime, although the risk is a little lower for *BRCA2*.[7–9] The very low figures published on small numbers of families from population studies have now been addressed by a meta-analysis,[9] which gives risks to 70 years of age of around 70% for *BRCA1* and 55% for *BRCA2*.

The chances that a family with a history of breast and/or ovarian cancer harbours mutations in *BRCA1* or *BRCA2* can be assessed from computer models.[10,11] We have recently validated these models using a dataset of 258 samples tested for *BRCA1/2* mutations. We found that at the lower levels of likelihood for mutations, the computer models substantially overpredict the presence of mutations, particularly for *BRCA1*.[12] Our own manual model was much better at predicting a

mutation in both genes and indeed was better than other manual models (**Table 7.2**). Further indicators for the presence of a *BRCA1* mutation within a family are grade and estrogen receptor status. *BRCA1* tumours are more frequently grade 3 and estrogen receptor negative and often have a medullary-like histology.[13] Ovarian cancers that occur in *BRCA1/2* families are nearly always non-mucinous epithelial cancers.

The likelihood of identifying a *BRCA1/2* mutation should not be confused with the ability to detect a mutation if one is present in the family. No single technique is able to detect all mutations. Even by sequencing the entire gene (exons and intron/exon boundaries), the detection rate only equates to about 85%. If a strategy is added to detect large deletions or duplications in *BRCA1*, this can boost detection to around 95%.[14]

The proportion of breast/ovarian cancers attributable to *BRCA1* or *BRCA2* depends on the ethnic origin of families. Many countries or ethnic groups have particular founder mutations that are not seen in other populations. In countries with a small founder population, very few mutations may account for the vast majority of breast cancer families.

Table 7.2 • Scoring system for identification of a pathogenic *BRCA1/2* mutation

	BRCA1	BRCA2
Female breast cancer <30 years	6	5
Female breast cancer 30–39 years	4	4
Female breast cancer 40–49 years	3	3
Female breast cancer 50–59 years	2	2
Female breast cancer >59 years	1	1
Male breast cancer <60 years	5 (if *BRCA2* tested)	8
Male breast cancer >59 years	5 (if *BRCA2* tested)	5
Ovarian cancer <60 years	8	5 (if *BRCA1* tested)
Ovarian cancer >59 years	5	5 (if *BRCA1* tested)
Pancreatic cancer	0	1
Prostate cancer <60 years	0	2
Prostate cancer >59 years	0	1

Scores for each cancer in a direct lineage are summated. A score of 10 is equivalent to a 10% chance of identifying a mutation in each gene.

The Ashkenazi Jewish population have three founder mutations: 185delAG and 5382insC in *BRCA1*, and 6174delT in *BRCA2*.[15] The three mutations are found in over 2% of the Ashkenazi Jewish population. One study showed that one of the three mutations were present in 59% of high-risk families.[15]

Populations that are more outbred, such as the UK, have larger numbers of mutations, and founder mutations occur at lower frequencies. Nonetheless, many laboratories in the UK have tried to develop a targeted approach to screening, concentrating on the large exons (exon 11 in both genes and exon 10 in *BRCA2*) and the smaller exons commonly reported to be involved, such as exons 2 and 20 in *BRCA1*.

This cuts down the number of polymerase chain reactions using the protein truncation test (PTT) to as little as five for *BRCA1* and four for *BRCA2*. However, this strategy reduces the sensitivity of identifying mutations down to as little as 50%.[14]

GENETIC TESTING

Once a mutation in a predisposing gene like *BRCA1* or *BRCA2* has been identified in a family, definitive genetic testing is possible. This can then more accurately inform women of their risks and give them an informed choice of different options, including risk-reducing surgery. Undertaking mutation analysis on an unaffected individual (without checking an affected relative), particularly in a breast cancer-only family, is problematic. While identifying a pathogenic mutation will confirm a high risk, the absence of a mutation will not exclude the possibility of other genes or even of a mutation refractory to the mutation screening techniques used. Although other genes are being identified (see **Table 7.1**), many more remain to be found and screening for mutations is not clinically useful outside of *BRCA1/2* and in certain circumstances *TP53*.

BREAST CANCER RISK ESTIMATION

Where there is not a dominant family history or it is not possible to identify a mutation in *BRCA1/2*, risk estimation is based on large epidemiological studies, which give 1.5–3 fold relative risks with a family history of a single affected relative.[1,2] Clinicians must be careful to differentiate between lifetime and age-specific risks. Some studies quote ninefold or greater risk associated with bilateral disease in a mother or with severe benign proliferative breast disease. However, these risks are time limited and if these at-risk individuals are followed up for many years, the risk returns to normal levels.[16] Clearly, if one uses these risks and multiplies them on a lifetime incidence of 1 in 10–12, some women will apparently have a greater than 100% chance of having the disease. The risks do not multiply and may not even add. Perhaps the best way to assess risk is to take the strongest risk factor, which in most cases is nearly always the family history. If risk is assessed on this alone, minor adjustments can be made for other factors. It is arguable whether these other factors have a major effect on an 80% penetrant gene other than to speed up or delay the onset of breast cancer. Therefore, we can only really assume an effect on non-hereditary elements of risk. Although studies do point to an increase in risk in family history cases associated with some factors, these may just represent an earlier age expression of the gene. Generally, therefore, we will arrive at risks between 40% and 8–10%, although lower risks are occasionally given. Higher risks are only applicable when a women at 40% genetic risk is shown to have a germline mutation, to have inherited a high-risk allele or to have proliferative breast disease.

Within Europe, risk estimation in the family history setting is based mainly on the Claus dataset.[2,17,18] However, within the USA, the Gail model of risk estimation is widely used.[19]

As well as these datasets allowing estimation of risk, there are specific computer programs available, including Cyrillic and BRCAPRO.[10] These programs take into consideration varying permutations of age of onset of diagnosis, number of affected and unaffected women and hormonal factors; as a consequence, different programs result in different risk estimations. The Gail model does not take into account age of relatives or second-degree relatives. A new model known as Tyrer–Cuzick[20] incorporates all the currently known risk factors.

A major deficiency of the current genetic models is the assumption that all inherited breast cancer is due to a single high-risk dominant gene or two genes (BRCA1 and BRCA2). The problem this causes in a program like BRCAPRO is that in order to obtain an accurate assessment for identifying a BRCA1 or BRCA2 mutation in a family, all other potential genetic factors are overlooked. Therefore while BRCAPRO provides reasonably accurate estimates for the presence of BRCA1/2 mutations in high-risk families,[11] its ability to predict breast cancer incidence is substantially hampered in smaller aggregations of breast cancer. We have recently found that BRCAPRO underestimates the risk of breast cancer in moderate/high-risk families by about 50%.[20] The most accurate computer model was the Tyrer–Cuzick model, although a manual

model incorporating the Claus tables and data from the BCLC and adjustment for hormonal and reproductive factors was similarly accurate. A fuller explanation of the manual model is available elsewhere.[18,21]

MANAGEMENT OPTIONS

Management options available for women at high lifetime risk of breast cancer due to their family history or for those women known to be carrying a mutation in BRCA1/2 are limited. Screening with mammography or magnetic resonance imaging is one option, and this can be combined with a trial of chemoprevention. However, many women are now seriously considering or undergoing risk-reducing mastectomy (RRM) if found to be mutation carriers for BRCA1 or BRCA2. The efficacy of surgical procedures for reducing the risk of breast cancer is controversial,[22,23] although it would appear that the residual risk of breast cancer depends on the amount of residual breast tissue following the surgical procedure. Recent work suggests that more women are considering RRM[24,25] and that protocols should be in place to deal with these requests. It has been suggested that surgery will increase life expectancy in BRCA1 or BRCA2 mutation carriers.[26]

The first study to demonstrate that women with a high risk of breast cancer can significantly reduce their subsequent incidence of the disease with RRM was only published in 1999.[27] This was followed by a Dutch study that confirmed risk reduction in those at highest risk (BRCA1/BRCA2 carriers).[28] Current evidence would suggest that RRM is associated with an approximately 90% reduction in risk.

GENETIC COUNSELLING AND THE FAMILY HISTORY CLINIC

Breast cancer family history clinics started to be established in the UK in 1987,[29,30] and these clinics are now established across Europe and North America. They are generally administered by consultants in medical oncology, clinical genetics and breast surgery, often with a multidisciplinary approach and close involvement of radiologists and a psychiatrist/psychologist. At these clinics unaffected women at increased risk of breast cancer are assessed for their lifetime and shorter-term risks of breast cancer. After assessing risks, women are presented with a number of choices including regular surveillance usually with a combination of mammography and clinical examination that commences between 30 and 40 years depending on the age of cancers in the family and the overall risk. Women are generally divided into three risk groups: average, moderate and high risk. It is only really in the high-risk group that RRM should be considered. This usually equates to a lifetime risk of 1 in 4 (25%) or greater. As a rough guide, this equates to having a heterozygote risk of 1 in 4 with two relatives including one first-degree relative with breast cancer diagnosed below 50 years of age or three affected relatives under 60 years. All affected relatives should be first-degree relatives or related through a male.

In a recent survey of 10 European centres,[31] only three (Manchester, Edinburgh, Heidelberg/Dusseldorf) routinely mention the possibility of RRM to those women with a lifetime risk of 1 in 4 or greater. This information is often only given as a single sentence or a statement of the availability of the procedure as an option for prevention of breast cancer. This then allows women to extend the discussion if they wish to do so, or to state that they are not interested in surgery. Many centres only mention risk-reducing surgery to potential mutation carriers undertaking a genetic test. Indeed, there is a cultural shift across Europe from north to south, with RRM becoming less acceptable to both physician and patient as one moves southward.[32,33] In the USA in centres where mastectomies for severe benign breast disease were commonplace in the 1970s and 1980s,[27] there appears to be less enthusiasm for mastectomy now even among gene mutation carriers.[34] What is absolutely clear is that adequate preparation of a woman contemplating RRM is essential.

THE RRM PROTOCOL

If women wish to discuss the surgical procedure in greater detail, most centres in our European survey offered a further appointment at least 1 month later. This gives women time to consider the procedure more fully and to discuss it with appropriate members of her family. Involvement of partners in the decision-making process is encouraged and they are invited to attend each appointment. At the second appointment, with a geneticist or oncologist, a basic description of the surgery is provided, including the potential residual risk of different procedures. It is emphasised that the residual risk and complication rate may be higher if the surgery preserves the nipple–areola complex (NAC). It is also usually made clear that these procedures, although having proven efficacy in reducing the risk of breast cancer, will still leave some residual risk. The patient is also challenged to consider possible complications, which may result in a potentially poor cosmetic result, as well as considering the impact upon her personal life and family dynamics.

The possibility of genetic testing is also discussed in terms of the availability of a living affected member of the family and the basic underlying structure of the family.[18,35,36] If possible, a time scale for genetic testing is discussed, and the woman is asked to consider the potential impact of proceeding with surgery, particularly if she then undergoes genetic testing which finds that she does not in fact carry the causative mutation. It is also emphasised that the genetic risk of breast cancer decreases with age and that the remaining risk of breast cancer if the woman is older (>40 years) is lower than the lifetime risk.[18] Indeed, a mutation carrier for *BRCA1* may have no more than a 50% risk of breast cancer in her remaining lifetime if she has reached 50 years. If a woman wishes to proceed, a psychological assessment is arranged. At this stage, confirmation of the breast cancers in the family are sought proactively by most centres if this has not already been done. This ensures that the risk assessment is as accurate as possible. We have previously reported the presence of factitious histories within some families where women have fabricated their family history in order to obtain surgery, or are innocently implicated as being at risk by another family member who has promoted an inaccurate family history.[37]

The whole process, from first consultation to the surgical procedure itself, usually takes between 6 and 12 months. This time delay is deliberate; in most centres the greatest delay is at the beginning of the protocol in order to allow women time for the decision-making process. If the protocol is run concurrently with a decision for predictive genetic testing, then the wait will generally be shorter. The full protocol of two sessions at the family history clinic, a session with a psychiatrist and sessions with the surgeon was established in 1993 in Manchester. While only two other centres have a similar written protocol, most clinics adhere to the basic principles. The major difference is that several centres are mainly reactive. Thus prophylactic surgery would usually only be formally discussed in women proven to be *BRCA1/2* mutation carriers. No centre recommends the procedure even in the latter category.

There is also no clear pattern in terms of the surgical procedure recommended in women who decide on surgery. While some units are cautious about offering skin/nipple-preserving mastectomies, these options are generally available in every case in some centres.

THE SURGICAL CONSULTATIONS

After a psychological assessment, at least two detailed surgical consultations are needed to discuss the types of mastectomy and breast reconstruction procedures available and their techniques, limitations, outcomes and potential complications. These should take place unhurriedly with the specialist surgeon, with time for careful communication, evaluation and reflection. Many women may have little understanding of the extent and nature of risk-reducing surgery, with or without breast reconstruction. They may initially regard RRM as a relatively minor cosmetic procedure.

While high-risk women carry their genotype in all cells and the bilateral incidence of cancer is proven, such women seldom develop multifocal cancers in one breast. The objective of surgery is to reduce the incidence of breast cancer, relieve anxiety and diminish breast cancer mortality, and do so in a way that balances risk reduction with aesthetic outcome and quality-of-life concerns. It is impossible to remove completely all breast tissue at risk, with the most complete resection being achieved by a total traditional mastectomy. Some will choose this as the simplest option but for most women the option of simple total bilateral mastectomy without breast reconstruction does not balance risk reduction and

cosmetic outcome. Mastectomy with breast reconstruction can be offered to almost all women, with careful evaluation of the breast and body shape to advise on the most appropriate reconstruction options for each individual. The surgical procedure should aim to reduce as substantially as possible the at-risk glandular breast tissue, including the upper outer quadrants, the area with the highest local incidence of cancer. At all stages of preoperative planning women must be fully involved in the decision-making, and must be aware of the reality that no operation completely removes all risk. Conservation of the natural NAC is controversial, as its preservation confers a small but unknown increase in residual risk. If preserved, loss of NAC sensation or even NAC ischaemia may result; nevertheless, a high proportion of women do opt for NAC preservation.

Risk-reducing surgery should not be undertaken in the following circumstances:

- individual risk cannot be substantiated;
- fictitious family history;
- Munchausen's syndrome;
- gene test result imminent;
- surgery is not the woman's own choice;
- psychiatric disorder, clinical depression, cancer phobia, dysmorphic syndrome;
- comorbidity outweighs potential clinical benefit;
- immovable unrealistic expectation of outcome.

RISK-REDUCING SURGERY AND BREAST RECONSTRUCTION

Innovations in breast surgery over the last few years have resulted in a wide range of mastectomy approaches and incisions, and a full repertoire of reconstruction techniques. These should be presented and discussed in detail at the surgical consultation. Reconstruction often comprises a series of staged procedures extending over a number of months, and it is crucial that realistic outcomes are advised and appreciated. An album of preoperative and postoperative photographs is essential, together with pictures where things have not gone quite so well or complications have occurred. The specialist breast care nurse has an important role during this time of discussion, providing information and facilitating patient–clinician liaison.

Women who opt for RRM with reconstruction have the choice of skin-sparing mastectomy techniques together with immediate reconstruction using expander/implants or myocutaneous flaps, chiefly the latissimus dorsi (LD) flap or the lower abdominal transverse rectus abdominis (TRAM) flap. This myocutaneous flap may be pedicled or a free microvascular transfer, but this escalates substantially the operating time and recovery, and increases risk of major complications.

For a majority the relative 'simplicity' of an implant-based reconstruction makes these the first choice, and many women opt for an immediate sub-muscular tissue expander placement. The cosmetic key is the match of the skin envelope surface area to that achievable by the expanded muscle pocket that constitutes the neo-breast mound. The concept of a single operation to include mastectomy and reconstruction with an immediate fixed-volume permanent implant is an attractive ideal but only rarely gives good cosmesis, and the aesthetic result of the two-stage process for most women is a signifi-cant improvement over a one-stage operation.

Careful preoperative breast evaluation and assess-ment with accurate skin measuring and marking are essential to define which skin areas will be resected in association with the breast parenchyma. Skin surface measures of nipple position relative to the midclavicular point and inframammary fold are recorded, together with full breast morphology (**Fig. 7.1**). Photographs are taken preoperatively and there is agreement between the woman and surgeon as to the proposed postoperative breast size. RRM is a careful time-consuming operation and should not be approached hurriedly. Incisions are planned to optimise glandular access but at the same time placed with appreciation for the need for minimal scarring and long-term aesthetic accept-ability. In the Manchester unit there are two main surgical approaches used: horizontal/oblique and Wise pattern incisions. Inframammary incisions are not used for the mastectomy because of two potential failures: firstly, effective access to remove the whole breast parenchyma including the upper outer quadrant and axillary tail and, secondly, the danger of ischaemia of the breast lower pole skin

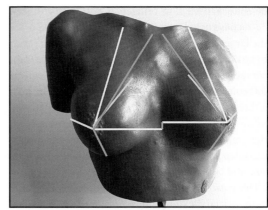

Figure 7.1 • Detailed assessment of breast size, shape, ptosis and nipple position by surface measurements.

between the inframammary incision and the nipple. After early experience in Manchester, when the majority of women having RRM opted to conserve their natural nipples, fewer now do so though some still wish nipple preservation. The main reasons for this are that personal risk reduction is maximised if the nipple is removed and its conservation can result in preservation of some parenchymal and ductal tissue; nipple reconstruction is also usually easy and cosmetically very satisfactory. The majority of women who undergo expander/implant breast reconstruction opt for either the horizontal/oblique approach or the Wise pattern RRM, based on a classical reduction mammoplasty-type incision. In both operations the nipples can be conserved if desired, or removed and subsequently reconstructed using a small local flap and tattooing. The small number of women who choose immediate recon-struction with bilateral LD flaps or bilateral TRAM flaps have a range of skin-sparing mastectomy options open to them and often choose circumareolar incisions to inset the flap skin. The circumareolar approach does not work well with expander/implant breast reconstructions.

RRM using horizontal/oblique approach

The horizontal/oblique mastopexy incision works best for the breast with little ptosis and a weight of no more than 400–450 g. If the NAC is to be preserved, it can be elevated and maintained on de-epithelialised skin bridges; if not, the NAC can be reconstructed across the scar. If undertaken for the larger breast, the horizontal approach can result in a skin envelope/breast mound disparity, and subcutaneous tissue drop-out in the lower pole can be difficult to correct. If the NAC is preserved in such a breast, it may finish too high relative to the inframammary fold. It is a useful guide to maintain the mid-clavicle to NAC distance in the breast meridian at around 19–22 cm, depending on breast size and chest length.

The patient is positioned on the operating table with partial flexion of elbows and hands tucked into the waistband. The incision follows the carefully marked preoperative skin mark-up, which has been accurately measured, planned and discussed with each patient. The width of skin resected between the incisions tightens the skin and subcutaneous tissue onto the expanded muscle pocket lying beneath (**Fig. 7.2**). If the nipple is preserved, de-epithelialised skin bridges are used to maintain its perfusion. Subcutaneous fat is preserved to keep the deep dermal vasculature, and the breast parenchyma removed from this layer by gentle dissection below the layer of Scarpa's fascia. The skin and subcutaneous tissue should not be button-holed but removed in parallel and flaps should be of consistent thickness extending to the pectoralis fascia. The fascia is preserved and the breast tissue removed and weighed.

The subpectoral space is opened by sharp dissection of the lateral border of pectoralis major, and the submuscular pocket developed by sharp and blunt dissection using an illuminated retractor and direct vision. The submuscular pocket is extended under the upper part of rectus abdominis and the external oblique to recreate the breast lower pole fullness. The tissue expander is placed in the pocket with full aseptic precautions, partially inflated and the subcutaneous space closed over closed vacuum drains. The skin is closed with multiple layers of absorbable sutures and wound dressing strips applied. Cosmetic outcome can be excellent (**Fig. 7.3**).

Wise pattern RRM

For the breast with greater ptosis and/or greater weight than that amenable to the horizontal/oblique approach, the Wise pattern RRM technique based on a reduction mammoplasty allows unparalleled

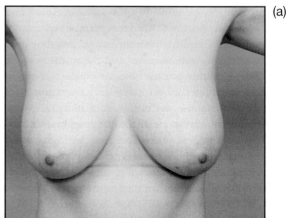
(a)

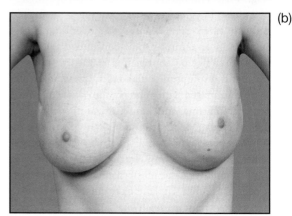
(b)

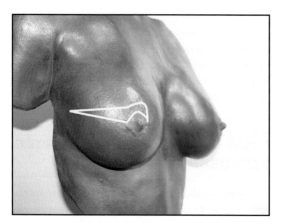

Figure 7.2 • Horizontal/oblique approach for risk-reducing mastectomy with nipple preservation.

Figure 7.3 • Horizontal/oblique risk-reducing mastectomy **(a)** before and **(b)** after operation.

access to all breast quadrants and the axillary tail, and results in cosmetically concealed scarring away from the upper and medial breast poles, as well as providing an opportunity for accurate matching of the residual skin and subcutaneous tissue to the reconstructed breast cone (**Fig. 7.4**). If required, the NAC can be preserved on a superior or supero-medial de-epithelialised pedicle. If the NAC is removed, subsequent bilateral NAC reconstruction can be achieved easily by one of the variety of NAC reconstruction techniques available. This and any tattoo procedure effectively covers the upper half of each of the vertical limbs of the mastectomy scar, reducing further the cosmetic disturbance. These procedures have evolved by attention to detail in order to allow risk reduction and correct possible cosmetic inadequacies of conventional approaches.

In common with the horizontal/oblique RRM, resection of the breast gland is achieved by dissecting along the plane of the subtle Scarpa's fascia that separates the fibro-fatty and glandular tissue of the breast from the subcutaneous fat, which should be preserved deep to the dermis. Removal of the subcutaneous fat results in a high incidence of skin damage or frank necrosis, particularly if the sub-dermal vascular plexus is breached. As always, skin should be closed without undue tension using sutures in layers to create the optimum healing conditions. The mastectomy flaps are retracted gently and handled with great care to minimise trauma from surgical instruments. The plane of dissection is under Scarpa's fascia extending to the pectoralis

fascia, and the subpectoral pocket for the tissue expander is created in an identical way to that described earlier. Special care has to be taken with closure so that the T-junctions are not under tension, as this can lead to wound breakdown. The vertical limb of the wound can be drawn together with multiple layers of absorbable subcuticular sutures in order to shorten its length.

Tissue expanders are chosen to match closely the breast base shape as well as diameter. The chosen volume should be determined by the agreed final breast size rather than the size of the natural breast, as there are opportunities for either increasing or decreasing volume if the woman so wishes and it can be safely and realistically achieved. A full layer of muscle cover for protection and smoothing over the expander requires the elevation of both pectoralis major and the upper part of serratus anterior. This can be vascular and needs careful haemostasis, most easily achieved under direct vision using fibreoptic retractors or headlights and bipolar coagulation. The postoperative result after Wise pattern RRM can be as excellent as that with the horizontal/oblique approach, and has the advantage that there are no scars on the upper or medial breast areas (**Fig. 7.5**). Nipple reconstruction later covers the upper part of each vertical scar, resulting in a highly realistic breast reconstruction (**Fig. 7.6**).

After recovery and healing, the tissue expander is inflated cautiously with injectable saline in the outpatient clinic over several weeks or months, and the woman encouraged to use simple skin creams

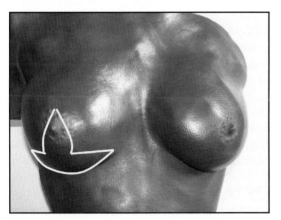

Figure 7.4 • Wise pattern risk-reducing mastectomy planning.

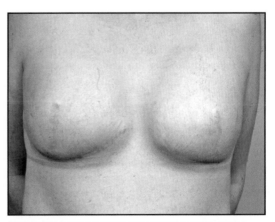

Figure 7.5 • Wise pattern risk-reducing mastectomy

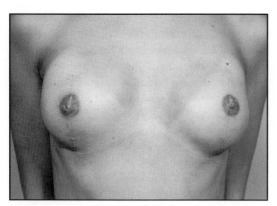

Figure 7.6 • Wise pattern risk-reducing mastectomy after nipple–areola reconstruction.

and massage to promote skin softening and elasticity in the neo-breast mound.

Placement of permanent implants

After full tissue expansion several months later, the tissue expanders are removed and replaced with permanent implants. At full maturation of expansion, permanent implants can be chosen from the extensive ranges now available, with consideration to filler materials, surface textures, size, shape and volume. Permanent implants are specifically ordered for individual women according to breast horizontal width, breast height and projection. For some, round dome-shaped implants are appropriate; for others there is a range of anatomically shaped implants in a wide variety of heights and projections.

This second operation involves accessing the expander pocket either through part of a previous scar or through the inframammary fold, and removing each expander. Shaping of the pocket capsule can be done with bipolar scissors and this helps in forming breast ptosis and filling in and smoothing out areas that may not have expanded fully. Use of implant sizers is helpful prior to permanent implant placement, orientation and closure. Women are sat up on the operating table to judge size, shape and symmetry of the breast reconstructions, and adjustments made accordingly.

For some women the idea of artificially engineered implantable breast prostheses is not acceptable, and they choose instead to undergo breast reconstruction with bilateral LD or TRAM flaps. For this smaller number of women, skin-sparing mastectomy can be achieved through circumareolar incisions in addition to those approaches previously mentioned. Such reconstructions may be very realistic in terms of appearance, shape, movement and warmth (see **Fig. 7.6**). However, the operation and anaesthesia times associated with bilateral RRM and immediate bilateral myocutaneous flaps are substantial, and there is greater opportunity for perioperative and postoperative complications than with implant-based surgery. The extent and nature of donor-site scarring must be appreciated and understood, as well as the operative, inpatient and subsequent recovery periods and needs. Myocutaneous flap complications do occur and should be discussed, including the uncommon but catastrophic scenario of total flap loss.

FOLLOW-UP

Follow-up of women who have undergone surgery is considered an important part of the protocol. In Manchester, women who have undergone prophylactic mastectomy are reviewed annually at a multidisciplinary clinic. As well as discussion of problems/issues with all the relevant clinicians (geneticist, oncologist, psychiatrist, surgeons), each patient is examined. Clinical examination by palpation of the breasts is considered to be adequate, as remaining breast tissue is very superficial in all types of surgical procedure. The mean expected rate of breast cancer for our cohort of women is 1% annually, reflecting a lifetime risk that ranges from 25 to 80%. Even though our own cohort has already a follow-up in excess of 800 woman-years, only eight cancers would have been expected. Follow-up of an extended cohort for more than 5 years will be necessary to address the issue of risk reduction. If this is to be analysed by type of surgery or confined to known *BRCA1/2* mutation carriers, even longer follow-up will be necessary. Published details of the Manchester protocol are available elsewhere.[38]

UPTAKE

Our own data from Manchester show that 8–10% of women at 1 in 4 lifetime risk or above seek further advice about RRM and 6% have undergone surgery; this rises to 11% in those at 40% lifetime risk. Of those proven affected mutation carriers aged under 60 years, 30/65 (45%) have now opted for risk-reducing surgery. Results from the Netherlands show a similarly high uptake (52%).[28] Thus far, three mutation carriers in our series and several in the Dutch series that initially opted not to have surgery have developed breast cancer, whereas none of the operated cases have.

PSYCHOSOCIAL CONSEQUENCES OF RRM

Results from seven studies[39–45] that have evaluated psychosocial outcomes after RRM, two of which had lengthy follow-up periods, show that surgery is associated overall with fairly high levels of satisfaction and reduced anxiety and psychological morbidity among women who undergo this procedure.

A number of studies suggest that provision of pre-surgical multidisciplinary support appears to have had a bearing on outcome. However, a minority of women do express regrets and experience adverse psychosocial events following surgery.

SURGERY FOR HIGH-RISK WOMEN WITH ESTABLISHED BREAST CANCER

Women who are under the care of a high-risk breast cancer team and who are considering RRM may have breast cancer diagnosed at some stage during their clinical assessment or on imaging modalities. Surgery then becomes part of the therapeutic management, and such women can no longer be considered for risk-reducing surgery on the affected breast. The priority is to treat the diagnosed malignancy as effectively as possible, using multimodality treatment within the context of the oncology multidisciplinary team. Therapy will include surgery and any of the adjuvant modalities of radiotherapy, chemotherapy and endocrine manipulation.

Most women will not want breast conservation as primary cancer treatment and will request mastectomy. This is entirely reasonable even if the cancer is small and could be effectively managed under normal circumstances by breast conservation.

These women are often young, and if their family history is attributable to a gene mutation, identified or not, their personal risk of local recurrence or development of a second primary cancer in the same breast is higher than in women with sporadic breast cancer; their risk of contralateral new primary malignancy is also high.[46–48]

Much depends on the stage and grade of the cancer. Nothing is undertaken that might delay or divert necessary adjuvant therapy. Prognosis and life expectancy depend on the recognised prognostic factors of grade, size and lymphovascular invasion. Any reconstructive surgery for the affected breast is considered within the context of total oncology care. It may be that immediate breast reconstruction is not an option, particularly if postoperative radiotherapy is anticipated. Furthermore, any request for contralateral RRM, which is entirely understandable, is considered carefully within the context of the overall stage and prognosis. A woman found to have substantial lymph node involvement will be unlikely to benefit from concurrent RRM for the opposite breast; furthermore, any complications arising from contralateral surgery may delay adjuvant treatment. Each request is discussed in detail with the woman and an agreed treatment strategy is formulated, taking into account all factors. One safe approach is to undertake delayed breast reconstruction for the affected breast and to perform RRM with immediate breast reconstruction for the contralateral side at the same operation, after primary adjuvant therapy has been completed. There are many possible permutations and as individual circumstances vary widely, the decision on how to proceed is individual to each patient.

BILATERAL RISK-REDUCING OOPHORECTOMY

Bilateral risk-reducing oophorectomy (including removal of the fallopian tubes) has been undertaken in women with *BRCA1/2* mutations in order to reduce the risk of ovarian cancer.

In addition to reducing the risk of ovarian cancer, prophylactic oophorectomy has also been shown to decrease the risk of breast cancer in women with a *BRCA1/2* mutation.[49]

This amounts to about a 50% reduction with an oophorectomy at 40 years of age and this risk reduction appears to be unaffected by the subsequent use of hormone replacement therapy (HRT).

However, recent evidence from the Million Women Study would suggest that use of combined estrogen/progesterone HRT doubles the risk of breast cancer after 10 years use.[50]

Using combined HRT in women who retain their uterus may therefore negate the protective effect. Bilateral risk-reducing oophorectomy in high-risk women prior to the menopause is therefore likely to decrease the risk of both breast and ovarian cancer.

Tamoxifen will reduce breast cancer incidence by about 50%, but this is almost exclusively a reduction in estrogen receptor-positive disease.[46–48,51,52]

Key points

- Gene testing can be useful but may not be possible for many women with a strong family history.
- Between 4 and 5% of breast cancer is due to high penetrance cancer-susceptibility genes.
- *BRCA1* and *BRCA2* gene mutations result in breast cancer in young women, often bilateral.
- Familial breast cancer can be associated with ovarian and some other malignancies.
- Gail and Claus data models predict individual breast cancer risk.
- RRM decreases breast cancer incidence by over 90%.
- Common RRM approaches combine breast parenchymal removal with breast reconstruction.
- Breast reconstruction should be appropriate for individual breast morphology.
- RRM can produce profound relief of anxiety, but is major surgery and complications must be avoided wherever possible.
- RRM should be undertaken by multidisciplinary specialised teams working within a protocol.
- Follow-up should ensure that results and outcomes are audited.

REFERENCES

1. Newman B, Austin MA, Lee M et al. Inheritance of human breast cancer: evidence for autosomal dominant transmission in high-risk families. Proc Natl Acad Sci USA 1988; 85:3044–8.

2. Claus EB, Risch N, Thompson WD. Autosomal dominant inheritance of early onset breast cancer: implications for risk prediction. Cancer 1994; 73:643–51.

3. Miki Y, Swensen J, Shattuck-Eidens D et al. A strong candidate for the breast and ovarian cancer gene *BRCA1*. Science 1994; 266:66–71.

4. Wooster R, Bignell G, Lancaster J et al. Identification of the breast cancer susceptibility gene *BRCA2*. Nature 1995; 378:789–92.

5. Malkin D, Li FP, Strong LC et al. Germline TP53 mutations in cancer families. Science 1990; 250:1233–8.

6. Lalloo F, Varley J, Ellis D et al. Family history is predictive of pathogenic mutations in BRCA1, BRCA2 and TP53 with high penetrance in a population based study of very early onset breast cancer. Lancet 2003; 361:1011–12.

7. Ford D, Easton DF, Bishop DT et al. Risk of cancer in BRCA-1 mutation carriers. Lancet 1994; 343:692–5.

8. Ford D, Easton DF, Stratton M et al. The Breast Cancer Linkage Consortium: genetic heterogeneity and penetrance analysis of the BRCA1 and BRCA2 genes in breast cancer families. Am J Hum Genet 1998; 62:676–89.

9. Antoniou A, Pharoah PDP, Narod S et al. Average risks of breast and ovarian cancer associated with mutations in BRCA1 or BRCA2 detected in case series unselected for family history: a combined analysis of 22 studies. Am J Hum Genet 2003; 72:1117–30.

10. Parmigiani G, Berry DA, Aquilar O. Determining carrier probabilities for breast cancer susceptibility genes BRCA1 and BRCA2. Am J Hum Genet 1998; 62:145–8.

11. Berry DA, Iversen ES Jr, Gudbjartsson DF et al. BRCAPRO validation, sensitivity of genetic testing of BRCA1/BRCA2, and prevalence of other breast cancer susceptibility genes. J Clin Oncol 2002; 20:2701–12.

12. Evans DGR, Eccles D, Rahman N et al. A scoring system for prioritising breast/ovarian cancer family genetic testing based on detection rates for BRCA1/2 mutations in families from North West and Southern England. J Med Genet 2004; 41:474–80.

13. Lakhani SR, Van De Vijver MJ, Jacquemier J et al. The pathology of familial breast cancer: predictive value of immunohistochemical markers, estrogen receptor, progesterone receptor, HER-2, and p53

in patients with mutations in BRCA1 and BRCA2. J Clin Oncol 2002; 20:2310–18.

14. Evans DGR, Bulman M, Gokhale D et al. Sensitivity of BRCA1/2 mutation testing in breast/ovarian cancer families from the North West of England. J Med Genet 2003; 40:107.

15. Struewing J, Hartge P, Wacholder S et al. The risk of breast cancer associated with specific mutations of BRCA1 and BRCA2 among Ashkenazi Jews. N Engl J Med 1997; 336:1401–7.

16. Dupont WD, Page DL. Relative risk of breast cancer varies with time since diagnosis of atypical hyperplasia. Hum Pathol 1989; 20:723–5.

17. Vasen HFA, Haites N, Evans DGR et al. Current policies for surveillance and management in women at risk of breast cancer: a survey among 16 European family cancer clinics. Eur J Cancer 1998; 34:1922–6.

18. Evans DGR, Lalloo F. Risk assessment and management of high risk familial breast cancer. J Med Genet 2002; 39:865–71.

19. Gail MH, Brinton LA, Byar DP et al. Projecting individualized probabilities of developing breast cancer for white females who are being examined annually. J Natl Cancer Inst 1989; 81:1879–86.

20. Tyrer JP, Duffy SW, Cuzick J. A breast cancer prediction model incorporating familial and personal risk factors. Stat Med 2004; 23:1111–30.

21. Amir E, Evans DGR, Shenton A et al. Evaluation of breast cancer risk assessment packages in the family history evaluation and screening programme. J Med Genet 2003; 40:807–14.

22. Goodnight JE, Quagliana JM, Morton DL. Failure of subcutaneous mastectomy to prevent the development of breast cancer. J Surg Oncol 1984; 26:198–201.

23. Zeigler LD, Kroll SS. Primary breast cancer after prophylactic mastectomy. Am J Clin Oncol 1991; 14:451–4.

24. Eeles R, Cole T, Taylor R et al. Prophylactic mastectomy for genetic predisposistion to breast cancer: the proband's story. Clin Oncol 1996; 8:222–5.

25. Evans DGR, Lalloo F, Shenton A et al. Uptake of screening and prevention trials in women at very high risk of breast cancer. Lancet 2001; 358:889–90.

26. Schrag D, Kuntz KM, Garbor JE et al. Decision analysis: effects of prophylactic mastectomy and oophorectomy on life expectancy among women with BRCA1 or BRCA2 mutations. N Engl J Med 1997; 336:1465–71.

27. Hartmann LC, Schaid DJ, Woods JE et al. Efficacy of bilateral prophylactic mastectomy in women with a family history of breast cancer. N Engl J Med 1999; 340:77–84.

This retrospective US cohort study examined the incidence of, and risk of death from, breast cancer after a median follow-up of 14 years among 639 women who had a family history of breast cancer and who had undergone bilateral subcutaneous or total prophylactic mastectomy. In the mastectomy group, women were divided into high-risk (N = 214) or moderate-risk (N = 425) subgroups, with most women in each subgroup having undergone subcutaneous mastectomy (89 and 90%, respectively). The study showed a reduction in the risk of breast cancer of 89.5% (P <0.001) in moderate-risk women who had undergone prophylactic mastectomy, and a reduction in risk of 90–94% in the high-risk women.

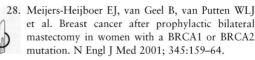

28. Meijers-Heijboer EJ, van Geel B, van Putten WLJ et al. Breast cancer after prophylactic bilateral mastectomy in women with a BRCA1 or BRCA2 mutation. N Engl J Med 2001; 345:159–64.

The incidence of breast cancer after a mean follow-up of 3 years was compared in a Dutch prospective cohort study involving 76 women with BRCA1 or BRCA2 mutations who had undergone bilateral prophylactic mastectomy (total simple, including nipple) and a control group of 63 women with BRCA1 or BRCA2 mutations who underwent surveillance. No cases of invasive breast cancer were observed in the women who had undergone prophylactic bilateral mastectomy whereas in the surveillance group, eight invasive breast cancers were detected. Proportional hazards analysis showed that prophylactic mastectomy significantly (P = 0.003) reduced the incidence of breast cancer.

29. Evans DGR, Fentiman IS, McPherson K et al. Familial breast cancer. Br Med J 1994; 308:183–7.

30. Evans DGR, Cuzick J, Howell A. Cancer genetics clinics. Eur J Cancer 1996; 32:391–2.

31. Evans DGR, Anderson E, Lalloo F et al. Utilisation of preventative mastectomy in 10 European centres. Dis Markers 1999; 15:148–51.

32. Julian-Reynier C, Eisinger F, Moatti J-P, Sobol H. Physician's attitudes towards mammography and prophylactic surgery for hereditary breast/ovarian cancer risk and subsequently published guidelines. Eur J Hum Genet 2000; 8:204–8.

33. Julian-Reynier C, Bouchard L, Evans G et al. Women's attitudes toward preventive strategies for hereditary breast/ovarian cancer risk differ from one country to another: differences between Manchester (UK), Marseilles (F) and Montreal (Ca). Cancer 2001; 92:959–68.

34. Evans DGR, Howell A, Baildam A et al. Risk-reduction mastectomy: clinical issues and research needs. J Natl Cancer Inst 2002; 94:307.

35. Eccles DM, Evans DGR, Mackay J. Guidelines for a genetic risk based approach to advising women with a family history of breast cancer. J Med Genet 2000; 37:203–9.

36. Eeles R. Testing for the breast cancer predisposition gene, BRCA1. Br Med J 1996; 313:572–3.

37. Evans DGR, Kerr B, Cade D et al. Fictitious breast cancer family history. Lancet 1996; 348:1034.

38. Lalloo F, Baildam A, Brain A et al. Preventative mastectomy for women at high risk of breast cancer. Eur J Surg Oncol 2000; 26:711–13.

39. Frost MH, Schaid DJ, Sellers TA et al. Long-term satisfaction and psychological and social function following bilateral prophylactic mastectomy. JAMA 2000; 284:319–24.

40. Hatcher MB, Fallowfield L, A'Hern R. The psychosocial impact of bilateral prophylactic mastectomy: prospective study using questionnaires and semi-structured interviews. Br Med J 2001; 322:76–9.

   The authors compared psychological and sexual morbidity in two cohorts of UK women (total number 154) with a family history of breast cancer who either chose or declined RRM, with psychosocial questionnaires administered at baseline, 6 and 18 months. Results showed that women who underwent RRM showed a reduction in psychological morbidity from baseline to 8 months (P <0.001), whereas in women who declined prophylactic surgery no comparably significant reduction was observed (P = 0.11). Similarly, a reduction in anxiety from baseline to 18 months was observed in women who chose prophylactic mastectomy (P = 0.001) compared with no significant reduction in anxiety over time in women who declined prophylactic surgery (P = 1.00).

41. Hopwood P, Lee A, Shenton A et al. Clinical follow-up after bilateral risk reducing ('prophylactic') mastectomy: mental health and body image outcomes. Psychooncology 2000; 9:462–72.

42. Stefanek ME, Helzlsouer KJ, Wilcox PM et al. Predictors of and satisfaction with bilateral prophylactic mastectomy. Prev Med 1995; 24:412–19.

43. Borgen PI, Hill ADK, Tran KN et al. Patient regrets after bilateral prophylactic mastectomy. Ann Surg Oncol 1998; 5:603–6.

44. Lloyd SM, Watson M, Oaker G et al. Understanding the experience of prophylactic bilateral mastectomy: a qualitative study of ten women. Psychooncology 2000; 9:473–85.

45. Josephson U, Wickman M, Sandelin K. Initial experiences of women from hereditary breast cancer families after bilateral prophylactic mastectomy: a retrospective study. Eur J Surg Oncol 2000; 26:351–6.

46. Eccles D, Simmonds P, Goddard J et al. Familial breast cancer: an investigation into the outcome of treatment for early stage disease. Fam Cancer 2001; 1:65–72.

47. Moller P, Borg A, Evans DG et al. Survival in prospectively ascertained familial breast cancer: analysis of a series stratified by tumour characteristics, BRCA mutations and oophorectomy. Int J Cancer 2002; 101:555–9.

48. Narod SA, Brunet JS, Ghadirian P and the Hereditary Breast Cancer Clinical Study Group. Tamoxifen and risk of contralateral breast cancer in BRCA1 and BRCA2 carriers: a case control study. Lancet 2000; 356:1876–81.

49. Rebbeck TR, Lynch HT, Neuhausen SL et al. Reduction in cancer risk after bilateral prophylactic oophorectomy in BRCA1 and BRCA2 mutation carriers. N Engl J Med 2002; 346:1616–22.

50. Beral V. Breast cancer and hormone-replacement therapy in the Million Women Study. Lancet 2003; 362:419–27.

51. Fisher B, Constantino JP, Wickerham DL et al. Tamoxifen for prevention of breast cancer: report of the National Surgical Adjuvant Breast and Bowel Project PI study. J Natl Cancer Inst 1998; 90:1371–88.

52. IBIS investigators. First results from the International Breast Cancer Intervention Study (IBIS-I): a randomised prevention trial. Lancet 2002; 360:817–24.

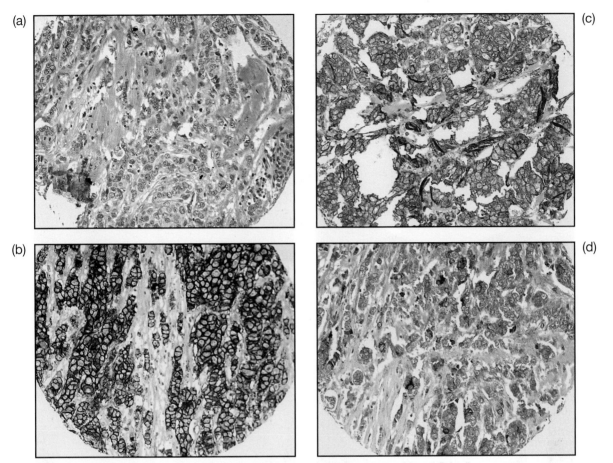

Plate 1 • Photomicrographs of tissue microarray discs: staining is for receptors of the erbB family.

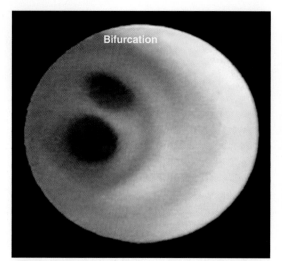

Plate 2 • Bifurcation.

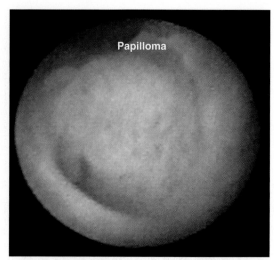

Plate 3 • Papilloma.

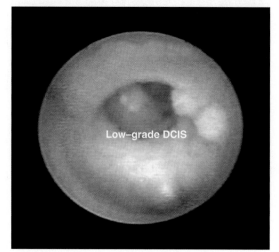

Plate 4 • Low-grade ductal carcinoma in situ.

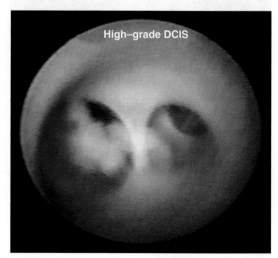

Plate 5 • High-grade ductal carcinoma in situ.

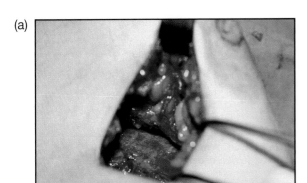

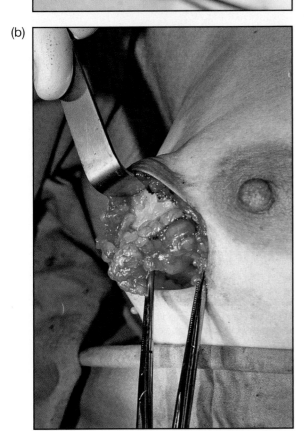

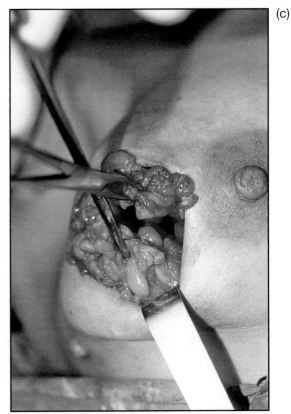

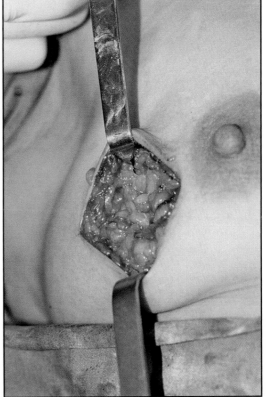

Plate 6 • Remodelling with glandular flaps after
mastectomy. **(a)** Posterior aspect of breast disc
separated from muscle. **(b)** Anterior aspect of breast
disc separated from subcutaneous tissue. This may be
extended underneath the nipple–areola complex as
required. **(c)** Adequacy of mobilisation checked. **(d)** Flaps
approximated without distortion.

(c)

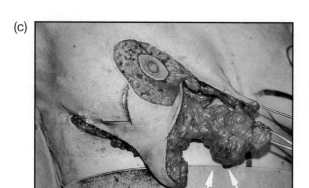

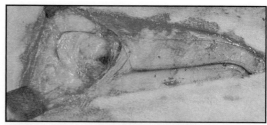

Plate 8 • Blue afferent lymphatic leading to blue-coloured sentinel node.

(d)

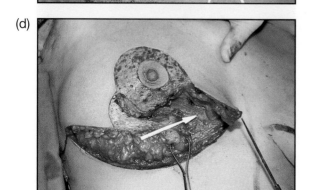

Plate 7 • Therapeutic mammoplasty after neoadjuvant chemotherapy. **(c)** Excision of the lower inner quadrant. **(d)** De-epithelialisation of the glandular flap, which is advanced into the lower inner quadrant to fill the defect.

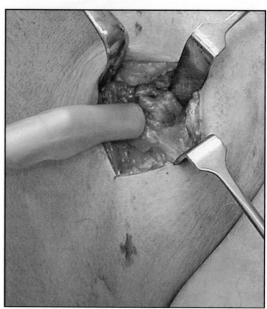

Plate 9 • Hand-held gamma probe in protective sterile sheath detecting radioactive blue sentinel node.

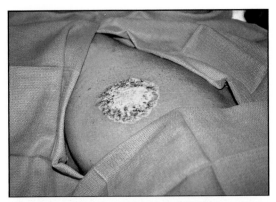

Plate 10 • Advanced changes of Paget's disease with destruction of the nipple and areola and involvement of periareolar skin.

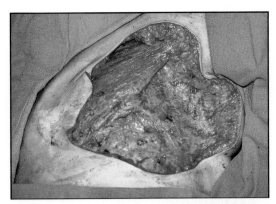

Plate 12 • Extent of resection necessary to obtain negative margins in the patient illustrated in **Fig. 9.4**.

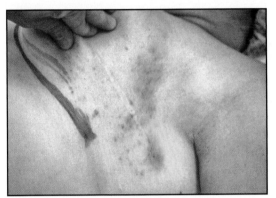

Plate 11 • Appearance of a radiation-induced angiosarcoma on the lateral aspect of a breast treated for adenocarcinoma with lumpectomy and radiotherapy. Multiple reddish-brown cutaneous nodules are visible.

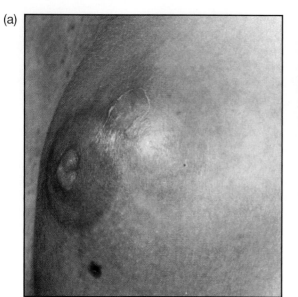 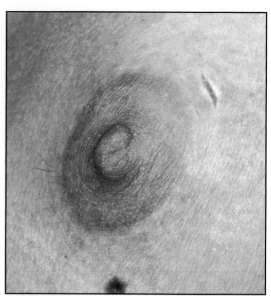

Plate 13 • Abscess of the left breast with thinned overlying skin **(a)** before and **(b)** after incision and drainage through a small stab incision.

Eight
Breast reconstruction

Eva M. Weiler-Mithoff

INTRODUCTION

More breast cancers are now detected at an earlier stage and in younger women. Improved survival means that they will live for much longer with the physical defect and the psychological problems of mastectomy. Mastectomy affects body image and feelings of attractiveness, leading to poor self-esteem, low self-confidence and introversion. A woman subsequently has to cope with the indignity and inconvenience of a breast prosthesis, which serves as a constant reminder of the loss of her breast and resulting deformity. Breast reconstruction can help a woman to feel whole again, re-establish body symmetry, eliminate the external prosthesis, diminish anxiety, increase wardrobe flexibility and the feeling of sexual attractiveness and improve sexual functioning. Breast reconstruction therefore plays a significant role in the woman's physical, emotional and psychological recovery from breast cancer.[1–4]

Even the best reconstruction will not be able to replace the natural breast that has been lost. A totally reconstructed breast will always feel and behave differently and will not have erogenous sensation. Women should be aware of the possibilities of breast reconstruction at the time of planning of the initial surgical treatment even if it may be their personal preference to have a delayed reconstruction or no reconstruction at all.[5–7] A final decision regarding the timing and technique of breast reconstruction should be made by the patient and the oncology team, consisting of ablative surgeon, reconstructive surgeon and oncologist.

Historically, the goals of breast reconstruction were to improve the appearance when clothed and to avoid an external prosthesis. Surgical advances and increased patient expectations have modified these goals. The current aim is to produce symmetry that satisfies the patient's wishes within the limits of technical feasibility, while matching the remaining breast in terms of its contour, dimension and position. This may involve the use of own tissues, breast implants and the use of corrective surgery to the opposite breast.[4]

TIMING

The fundamental aim of breast cancer surgery must be to provide safe and successful oncological treatment. Breast reconstruction can be performed immediately at the time of mastectomy or delayed.

Immediate breast reconstruction

Advantages of immediate breast reconstruction include the potential for a single operation and period of hospitalisation. It allows maximum preservation of breast skin and preservation of the inframammary fold. The reconstructive surgeon can then work with good-quality skin flaps that are unscarred and which do not suffer from the effects of radiotherapy. Skin-sparing mastecotmy in particular facilitates better cosmetic results, with a reduced need for balancing surgery.[8–10]

The disadvantages of immediate reconstruction are the limited time for decision-making by the patient, increased operating time and the difficulties of coordinating two surgical teams in those units where there are no 'oncoplastic' surgeons who can perform both the mastectomy and reconstruction. Concerns that the more complex nature of surgery may have an increased risk of postoperative complications and may therefore compromise adjuvant treatment are not evidence based, although there is a potential in individual patients for complications to result in a delay in starting adjuvant treatment.[11–13] Chemotherapy and radiotherapy can have detrimental effects on some types of breast reconstruction, but these can be reduced by judicious choice of type and timing of reconstructive techniques.[14,15]

Published evidence indicates that immediate breast reconstruction does not adversely affect breast cancer outcome. The reconstruction does not interfere with the delivery of adjuvant treatment and there is no significant difference in the survival rates between immediate and delayed reconstruction.[16–20] Breast reconstruction may be indicated even in disease with poor prognosis in order to improve the overall psychological rehabilitation and quality of remaining life. It is no longer necessary to make a woman mourn the loss of a breast by experiencing its absence.[4,21,22]

Delayed breast reconstruction

Delayed breast reconstruction, on the other hand, allows the patient unlimited time for decision-making, avoids any potential delay of adjuvant treatment and removes the detrimental affects of radiotherapy or chemotherapy on the reconstruction but requires replacement of a larger amount of breast skin. The mastectomy flaps may be thin, scarred, contracted or irradiated and the end result of the breast reconstruction is often not as aesthetically pleasing. A second episode of hospitalisation is required and treatment costs are increased compared with immediate reconstruction (**Box 8.1**).

Box 8.1 • Advantages and disadvantages of immediate and delayed breast reconstruction

Advantages of immediate breast reconstruction
Potential for a single operation and period of hospitalisation
Maximum preservation of breast skin
Preservation of the inframammary fold
Good-quality skin flaps
Better cosmetic results in skin-sparing mastectomy
Reduced need for balancing surgery to the contralateral breast
Lower cost than delayed reconstruction

Disadvantages of immediate reconstruction
Limited time for decision-making by patient
Increased operating time
Difficulties of coordinating two surgical teams when required
Potential in individual patients for complications to result in delay of adjuvant treatment

Advantages of delayed breast reconstruction
Allows unlimited time for decision-making by patient
Avoids any potential delay of adjuvant treatment
Avoids detrimental effects of radiotherapy or chemotherapy on the reconstruction

Disadvantages of delayed breast reconstruction
Requires replacement of a larger amount of breast skin
Mastectomy flaps may be thin, scarred, contracted or irradiated
Mastectomy scar may be poorly positioned
May result in a less aesthetically pleasing outcome
Requires separate episode of hospitalisation
Increased treatment cost compared with immediate breast reconstruction

CONTRAINDICATIONS

Contraindications for breast reconstruction include uncontrolled and non-resectable local chest wall disease, rapidly progressive systemic disease, patients who have serious comorbidity and patients who are psychologically unsuitable.[4]

TECHNIQUES

Breast reconstruction involves replacement of breast skin and breast volume. Surgical options for reconstruction include the use of tissue expanders and breast implants and the use of autologous tissue. The most commonly used surgical techniques are tissue expansion, latissimus dorsi (LD) myocutaneous flap with or without implant, the use of lower abdominal tissue and other free tissue transfers.

Implant-based techniques require limited surgery initially but have limitations and are not always quick and trouble-free. These procedures allow some patient control over breast size, but the quality of the long-term result is directly related to the tolerance of breast implants. Further procedures may be required for complications and maintenance. The aesthetic results from autologous reconstruction are superior to those of implant-based reconstruction due to their versatility, their more natural appearance, consistency and durability. Autologous tissue can also better withstand radiotherapy. The autologous LD flap is highly versatile and has acceptable donor-site morbidity. The skin and fat of the lower abdomen are ideal for autologous breast reconstruction but donor-site morbidity is increasingly being appreciated. Muscle-sparing techniques preserve the abdominal wall function at the cost of a more complex procedure. The effects of adjuvant radiotherapy on breast reconstruction using lower abdominal tissue are still under investigation.[23–27]

The ultimate choice of technique depends on patient fitness, breast size, body habitus, laxity and thickness of remaining breast skin, the condition of the underlying muscles, availability of flap donor sites, stage of disease and the need for adjuvant radiotherapy. The final decision depends on the personal preference of the patient if more than one reconstructive option is feasible. Because of the variable needs of individual patients, the reconstructive surgeon must be able to provide the full range of reconstructive options.[4,28]

Tissue expansion reconstruction

Tissue expansion is the simplest method of immediate breast reconstruction. An inflatable silicone balloon is placed into a submuscular pocket on the anterior chest wall and subsequently expanded by a series of postoperative saline injections. This ingenious method of breast reconstruction is based on the gradual stretching of the skin with a single or double-lumen tissue expander to replace the skin loss after mastectomy. The tissue expander or a breast implant will simultaneously replace the breast volume[29] (**Fig. 8.1**). Patient selection and implant selection are crucial. Several techniques are possible:

- fixed volume implant (single stage);
- variable volume expander implant (single stage);
- issue expansion followed by permanent implant (two stage).

Tissue expansion is a simple and flexible technique that does not involve any additional scarring. The breast is reconstructed with local tissues with similar colour and texture. This short procedure requires 1 hour operating time, a short period of hospitalisation and 2–4 weeks recovery time.

INDICATIONS

This technique is suitable for patients with small non-ptotic breasts, when performing bilateral reconstruction or for women who are happy to accept a mastopexy procedure on the opposite breast. This procedure is ideal for patients who want minimal scarring, are not worried about a silicone implant and are unwilling or unfit to undergo autologous tissue reconstruction.[28]

CONTRAINDICATIONS

Patients are unsuitable for implant reconstruction if the chest wall tissues are thin, damaged, inelastic or irradiated, if a radical mastectomy has been performed, if there is an extensive infraclavicular tissue deformity after resection or atrophy of the pectoralis major muscle, or if there is a vertical mastectomy scar.[28]

SURGICAL TECHNIQUES

Tissue expansion can be used in immediate or delayed breast reconstruction. The expander is only partially inflated at insertion to allow safe closure of overlying muscle and skin. The actual expansion

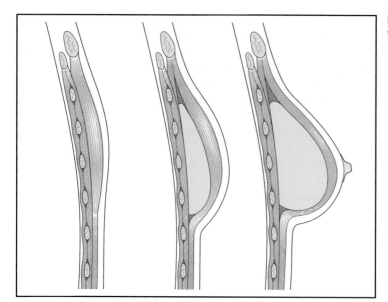

Figure 8.1 • Breast reconstruction with submuscular tissue expander.

starts 2–4 weeks postoperatively and is usually performed at weekly intervals. Numerous visits to the outpatient department may be required and inflation can sometimes be painful. Overexpansion by 50–200% of the breast volume for several months is thought to create a more natural ptosis.[30] Reconstruction of the breast mound can take up to 6 months using tissue expansion. Secondary procedures may be necessary to achieve a more natural appearance of the reconstructed breast. Over one-third of patients require further surgery within the first 5 years after implant-based breast reconstruction.[31] Implant-only breast reconstructions lack ptosis and significant alterations of the contralateral breast to improve symmetry are usually necessary (**Fig. 8.2**). The long-term results of implant-based reconstruction can be disappointing and are characterised by periods of asymmetry due to continuous changes of the contralateral breast as a consequence of the effects of gravity and fluctuations in weight.[32]

COMPLICATIONS

The complications of tissue expansion can be grouped into those related to wound failure such as haematoma, wound infection, breast skin necrosis and wound dehiscence, those due to implant failure, and those of breast implants such as capsular con-

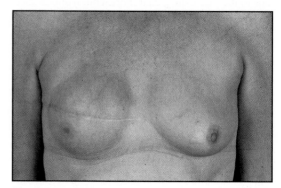

Figure 8.2 • Delayed breast reconstruction by tissue expansion.

tracture, asymmetry, displacement and thinning of overlying skin. The incidence of skin-flap necrosis and implant exposure can be as high as 10% and 30–50% respectively.[18,33,34] The commonest and least predictable complication of implant reconstruction is capsular contracture. Hardening of the scar tissue around the implant leads to firmness on palpation and distortion of the breast as well as discomfort and pain. Further surgical revision is necessary in severe cases. The risk of capsular contracture is significantly increased in the presence of preoperative or postoperative radiotherapy.[35,36] Textured implants reduce capsular contracture rates and their use is now routine.

Latissimus dorsi flap reconstruction

The LD myocutaneous flap, originally described for chest wall reconstruction by Tansini at the turn of the century, was rediscovered and became the standard method of breast reconstruction in the 1970s, allowing the immediate reconstruction of larger, more pendulous breasts[28,37] (**Fig. 8.3**).

The LD muscle is a large triangular back muscle of variable thickness. The cutaneous territory of this flap consists of the skin superficial to the entire muscle and approximately 3 cm beyond. Numerous myocutaneous perforators allow the design of skin islands in various patterns but orientation of the skin paddle in the skin crease allows maximum skin harvest with a good scar, which can be hidden under the bra strap.

LD flap breast reconstruction is a very versatile, safe and reliable technique with a success rate of over 99%, and is even suitable for high-risk patients. Disadvantages include a donor scar on the back, unless endoscopic techniques are used. The colour match of back and breast skin may not be ideal and there is a potential for further impairment of shoulder movement, which may have already been compromised by previous surgery. The functional deficit after transfer of an LD muscle affects only very specific activities like rowing, cross-country skiing or mountain climbing but has little effect on most other activities. Additional physiotherapy may be required to restore full shoulder mobility.[28,38] LD breast reconstruction is a major operation but a lesser procedure than free tissue transfer. Approximately 3–4 hours operating time, a hospital stay of 5–7 days and a recovery time of 4–8 weeks are required.

INDICATIONS

Indications for this technique include the reconstruction of large breasts where an implant alone would not be sufficient for size, if the chest wall tissues are unsuitable for tissue expansion and if there are additional tissue requirements after mastectomy. Additional indications are congenital breast hypoplasia such as Poland's syndrome, chest wall reconstruction, partial breast reconstruction after conservation surgery or partial loss of an abdominal tissue flap.[28]

CONTRAINDICATIONS

Contraindications for LD breast reconstruction are previous surgery that may have compromised the vascular supply to the flap such as thoracotomies or

(a) 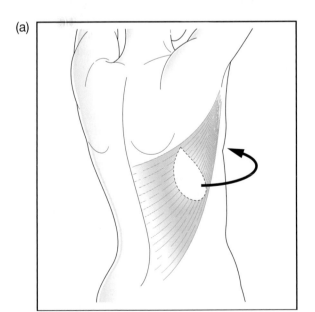 (b)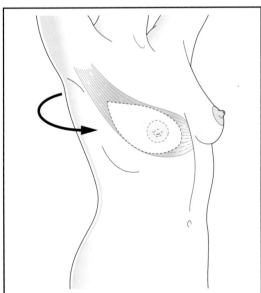

Figure 8.3 • Breast reconstruction using latissimus dorsi myocutaneous flap.

extensive and radical axillary surgery, absence of the LD muscle and serious patient comorbidity.[4]

SURGICAL TECHNIQUES

Several variations of this flap are possible. The LD muscle can be transferred as muscle-only flap without a skin island, avoiding a donor-site scar on the back. A myocutaneous flap can be used with or without a breast implant or tissue expander if muscle cover and skin are required. It is also possible to reconstruct a small to moderate-sized breast with an extended or autologous LD flap. This type of reconstruction includes taking the maximum amount of both skin and subcutaneous fat overlying the muscle and avoids the use of implants or tissue expanders (**Fig. 8.4**). A muscle-sparing or perforator-based technique, the so-called thoracodorsal artery perforator (T-DAP) flap, can be employed if preservation of muscle function is desirable.[39–42] The sections that follow describe the technique of autologous LD flap reconstruction.

Preoperative planning

Preoperative planning takes into account the size and shape of the opposite breast or the planned breast size and, in the case of an immediate breast reconstruction, the area of breast skin excision. In delayed breast reconstruction additional factors such as the thickness and quality of the skin flaps, the condition and function of the pectoralis major muscle, the extent of radiotherapy damage, and the position and quality of the mastectomy scar are assessed and additional soft tissue requirements noted.

The function of the LD muscle must be tested prior to surgery. If necessary, colour Doppler or magnetic resonance imaging may be used to establish the continuity of the thoracodorsal vessels. The amount and distribution of excess skin and soft tissue are assessed. A lean back can yield 300–400 cm³, an average back 600–800 cm³ and a plump back 1200–1500 cm³.

Prior to surgery, breast base, inframammary fold, anterior axillary fold and the take-off point of the breast from the chest wall are marked with the patient in a sitting or standing position. On the back, the limits of the LD muscle and the skin ellipse are marked. This should be centred over the fat roll on the back and positioned in the relaxed skin tension

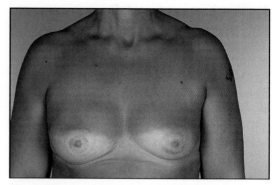

Figure 8.4 • Immediate breast reconstruction by autologous latissimus dorsi flap after skin-sparing mastectomy.

lines. A maximum width of 7–9 cm allows closure without tension. The resulting scar should lie in the middle to lower bra strap area. The additional areas of soft tissue harvest are marked.

Positioning in the operating theatre

The patient is positioned in a lateral decubitus position and secured with well-padded table attachments. The arm is suspended or supported with attachments at 90° to allow easy access to the axilla. The mastectomy and any axillary surgery can be performed in this position as well. Such a combined approach in immediate reconstruction can save up to 1.5 hours operating time. A separate incision may be required for axillary clearance in skin-sparing mastectomy and the different spatial orientation of the axilla has to be taken into account.

Flap harvest

Infiltration of the area of incision and the subcutaneous space overlying the area of soft tissue harvest with a weak solution of local anaesthetic with or without adrenaline (epinephrine) and normal saline helps to plump up this space and facilitates dissection at the level of Scarpa's fascia. The skin island is incised and Scarpa's fascia is identified. Raising the skin flaps at this level protects the blood supply to the overlying skin flaps and ensures maximum soft tissue harvest with the flap. At the border of the previously marked soft tissue harvest the dissection is carried down to the LD muscle, the muscles overlying the scapula and the rhomboid muscles. The superomedial extent of the soft tissue harvest is the anterior border of the trapezius muscle. The adipofascial parascapular flap extension is lifted caudally until the upper edge of the LD flap is exposed at the tip of the scapula. The proximal portion of the muscle is dissected up to the tendinous junction at the level of the muscle fascia to avoid excess bulk in the axilla after flap transfer. The borders of flap harvest are now marked and the muscle can then be raised from cranial, posterior and inferior. All intercostal perforators are divided and haemostasis is secured. A strip of thoracolumbar fascia can be harvested and protects the posterior and inferior flap borders. The anterior border with the additional soft tissue anterior to the muscle is elevated last, taking care to identify the posterior border of serratus anterior and avoid harvest of slips of external oblique or serratus posterior muscle. As the LD is lifted off the serratus anterior, the neurovascular pedicle to serratus and the serratus branch are identified and carefully preserved. The posterior border of the LD muscle is detatched from the teres muscles up to the tendinous insertion. The posterior half of the tendon may be divided if it is very broad in order to provide maximum mobility of the flap. The anterior border of the muscle is freed, carefully avoiding damage to the thoraco-dorsal neurovascular bundle. A high tunnel to the mastectomy defect is fashioned to position the upper part of the muscle parallel to the anterior axillary fold. The muscle is transferred and the tension on the pedicle is assessed. It is generally not necessary to divide the LD tendon (although some do this routinely) or the serratus branch, which can provide additional vascularity particularly in delayed reconstruction when the main thoracodorsal vein may be encased by scar tissue. The thoracodorsal nerve is preserved to maintain muscular bulk. Muscle twitching tends to decrease with time and is rarely a problem. The donor site may be quilted and then closed in three layers with absorbable sutures after insertion of two drains. The flap is secured temporarily on the anterior chest wall to allow repositioning of the patient for the final flap inset.

Flap inset

The patient is repositioned supine and both breasts are prepared and redraped. The flap is then sutured into position after securing the upper part of the LD muscle to the lateral border of the pectoralis major muscle. The flap is then rotated 180° and the scapular adipofascial flap is folded under for extra projection in the lower pole. The edges of the flap are sutured into the borders of the mastectomy defect, and the anterior axillary fold and the infra-mammary fold are recreated. An upper abdominal advancement flap can provide extra skin for the breast envelope in delayed breast reconstruction or chest wall resurfacing. Any excess skin island is de-epithelialised for additional volume. The projection of the neo-breast can be adjusted with plication sutures. The size of the reconstructed breast should be approximately 25% larger than the opposite breast to allow for some postoperative atrophy. Two drains are inserted and the skin is closed.

Postoperative management

The patient is encouraged to wear a well-supporting brassiere for the final moulding of the reconstructed breast. Physiotherapy is started on the first post-operative day with shoulder shrugging and exercises up to 90°. Rehabilitation of the scapular region follows after 4 weeks.

COMPLICATIONS

Potential postoperative complications include wound failure, expander failure and complications of breast implants. Flap-related wound complications include haematoma, infection, partial or total flap necrosis, breast skin flap necrosis and delayed healing. Donor site-related complications include haematoma, seroma, wound infection and wound dehiscence. Seroma formation is common after extended LD harvest and may require repeated aspiration. Several strategies have been suggested in order to reduce the incidence of postoperative seroma, including quilting the skin onto the underlying chest wall and the use of triamcinolone injected into the cavity at first aspiration.[43]

Localised fat necrosis in autologous LD flaps has been reported in up to 14% of cases. Partial flap necrosis occurs in less than 5–7% and total flap necrosis in less than 1%. Implant failure and rates of complications of breast implants are similar to those of implant-only reconstructions (**Table 8.1**).[39,44,45]

There is some evidence that the autologous LD flap may withstand adjuvant radiotherapy better than the LD flap with additional implant.[46,47]

Table 8.1 • Complications of breast reconstruction using latissimus dorsi (LD) flap

	Autologous LD	LD with implant
Flap-related complications		
Total flap loss	0–1%	0.6%
Partial flap loss	1–7%	3%
Fat necrosis	4–14%	19%
Breast skin necrosis	10%	19%
Wound infection	2%	5%
Donor-site complications		
Seroma	20–80%	9–50%
Haematoma	3–6%	0.6%
Wound dehiscence	10–25%	16%
Implant-related complications		
Capsular contracture	NA	20–56%
Displacement	NA	1%
Implant rupture	NA	2%

NA, not appropriate or not relevant.

THE SILICONE ISSUE

All available information on the safety of silicone breast implants has been assessed by the Independent Review Group and the findings published in a very thorough report in 1998.[48] This report shows clearly that there is no histopathological or immunological evidence of an abnormal immune response to silicone and no epidemiological evidence of any link between silicone and an established connective tissue disease such as rheumatoid arthritis or autoimmune diseases. There is lack of evidence for an atypical connective tissue disease or 'silicone poisoning' and no toxic reaction could be found. There is no evidence that children of women with breast implants are at risk of connective tissue disease. However, there is currently not enough information about the actual lifespan of implants and any patient receiving an implant- or tissue expander-based breast reconstruction should be aware that the implant may require replacement.[48] Patients who receive implant-based breast reconstructions should be encouraged to have their details forwarded to the National Breast Implant Registry (Plastic Surgery Department, Salisbury District Hospital, Salisbury SP2 8BJ).

Breast reconstruction with lower abdominal tissue

The lower abdomen is often an abundant source of tissue for autologous breast reconstruction. A sizeable and natural-feeling breast mound can be created without any implant or tissue expander tissue, which is usually discarded during an aesthetic abdominoplasty procedure. The donor defect is acceptable and often a cosmetic improvement. Although this technique can provide excellent long-term results, donor-site morbidity should not be underestimated.[49,50]

INDICATIONS

Lower abdominal tissue can be used for immediate and delayed breast reconstruction. Good candidates are young and healthy with sufficient lower abdominal tissue available. It is also indicated if the contralateral breast is large, in bilateral breast reconstruction, if there have been previous complications with breast implants and if the LD muscle has been divided or is atrophic. Reconstructions using lower abdominal tissue can be associated with significant complications and morbidity.[4]

CONTRAINDICATIONS

Contraindications are obesity, smoking, diabetes, autoimmune disease, vasospastic or cardio-respiratory disorders, psychosocial problems, abdominal scars disrupting the vascular anatomy, inadequate recipient vessels or an inexperienced surgeon. The potentially detrimental effects of adjuvant radiotherapy on the reconstructed breast are currently under investigation.[22,27,51]

SURGICAL TECHNIQUES

Myocutaneous perforators through the rectus abdominis muscle and direct cutaneous vessels provide the blood supply to the lower abdominal apron by three main vascular routes. The deep inferior epigastric artery (DIEA), a branch of the external iliac vessel, is the primary source of circulation to the rectus abdominis muscle. The deep superior epigastric artery (DSEA), the terminal branch of the internal mammary artery and lesser vessel of supply, anastomoses with the DIEA within the substance of the muscle. Additional direct cutaneous supply of the abdominal apron exists through the superficial inferior epigastric artery (SIEA). The triple blood supply to the lower abdominal tissue allows it to be used in a variety of techniques:[52–58]

- pedicled transverse rectus abdominis myocutaneous (TRAM) flap;
- free TRAM flap;
- free deep inferior epigastric perforator (DIEP) flap;
- free superficial inferior epigastric artery (SIEA) flap.

The reason why surgeons have moved from pedicled TRAM flaps to free perforator flaps is to try to reduce the morbidity of the donor site and preserve abdominal wall integrity and function. The complications encountered with techniques using lower abdominal tissue for breast reconstruction are related to the extent of muscle resection, extent of fascia resection and the use of a mesh to repair the abdominal wall. These factors should be borne in mind when selecting the appropriate procedure for an individual patient (**Table 8.2**). All these techniques will interfere with abdominal wall sensation (**Fig. 8.5**).

Pedicled TRAM flap

The pedicled TRAM flap relies on blood flow through the deep superior epigastric vessels within the substance of the rectus abdominis muscle to supply a horizontal ellipse of lower abdominal skin and fat. The flap is transferred onto the chest wall through a large subcutaneous tunnel. It is not an appropriate technique for individuals in whom the distance from nipple to costal margin is greater than the distance from costal margin to the umbilicus (short waisted).[52–54]

The pedicled TRAM flap does not require microvascular skills. However, the perfusion of the flap through microscopic connections only between the DSEA and DIEA results in reduced vascularity and an incidence of fat necrosis of up to 42%. A very large amount of muscle is sacrificed, causing a dramatic reduction in abdominal wall function, a

Table 8.2 • Flap survival and donor-site morbidity after breast reconstruction using abdominal tissue

	Pedicled TRAM flap	Free TRAM flap	Free DIEP flap
Total flap loss	<1%	5–7%	1–5%
Partial flap loss	28–60%	6–8%	6%
Fat necrosis	27–40%	7–13%	6–10%
Abdominal bulge	8–28%	5–8%	0.3–5%
Abdominal hernia	>6%	4–6%	0–1.4%

DIEP, deep inferior epigastric perforator; TRAM, transverse rectus abdominis myocutaneous.
Modified from Weiler-Mithoff E, Hodgson ELB, Malata CM. Perforator flap breast reconstruction. Breast Disease 2002; 16:93–106.

long recovery time, costal nerve compression and complications of mesh, which is usually required to repair the abdominal wall.[50,59–61] The development of reliable free tissue transfer techniques has provided an alternative to the pedicled TRAM flap in an attempt to reduce abdominal wall damage and lower the risk of partial or total flap necrosis. The double pedicled flap should be avoided if possible.[62]

Free TRAM flap

The deep inferior epigastric vessels are the dominant blood supply for a free TRAM flap. The lower abdominal skin is transferred with a segment of rectus abdominis muscle and the deep inferior epigastric vessels, which are longer and of larger diameter compared with other free tissue transfers. These are then anastomosed to the recipient vessels of the subscapular axis or the internal mammary system.[55] The donor site is closed most commonly by insertion of synthetic mesh. This technique provides better tissue perfusion than the pedicled TRAM flap and a larger portion of the abdominal apron can be transferred safely with reduced risks of partial flap necrosis or fat necrosis. This is more appropriate for the reconstruction of a larger breast. A smaller amount of rectus muscle is harvested, causing less interference with abdominal wall function. The free TRAM flap requires a high level of surgical expertise and microsurgical skills.

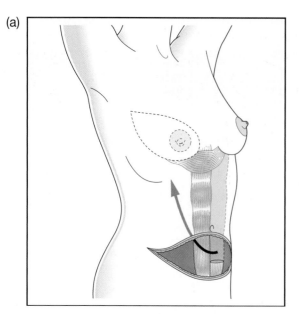

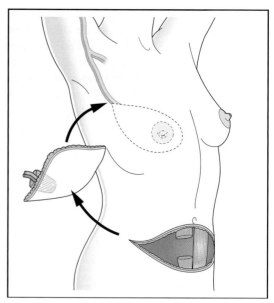

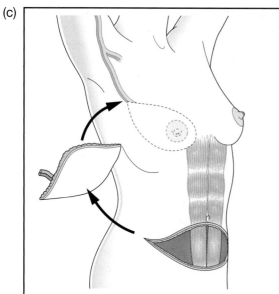

Figure 8.5 • Techniques of breast reconstruction using abdominal tissue: **(a)** pedicled TRAM flap; **(b)** free TRAM flap; **(c)** free DIEP flap. See text for explanation of abbreviations.

necrosis, partial or total flap loss and delayed wound healing. Success rates in many centres are around 98%. Donor-site complications include haematoma, wound infection, problems with mesh closure, asymmetry, bulging, hernia formation and reduced abdominal strength. Although the free flap is preferred to the pedicled variant due to its more reliable blood supply, it still causes some functional impairment of the abdominal wall.[63-68]

Free DIEP flap

The free DIEP flap spares the whole of the rectus abdominis muscle. The flap relies on meticulous dissection of perforating vessels within the rectus abdominis muscle.[56,57,69-71] This technique is particularly indicated for young athletic patients and when performing bilateral breast reconstruction. The DIEP flap still has all the potential flap complications of any free tissue transfer but donor-site complications and morbidity are reduced.

No muscle or fascia is harvested and no mesh is required for donor-site closure. Preservation of the rectus muscle preserves abdominal and back extensor muscle strength and reduces donor-site morbidity, postoperative pain and hospital stay. Preliminary studies have shown that this technique

Free tissue transfer; although routine in many centres, is a major surgical procedure and requires 6–8 hours operating time, hospital stay of 7–10 days and postoperative recovery of 2–3 months. There is an increased risk of general complications, such as deep vein thrombosis, pneumonia or acute respiratory distress syndrome. Specific complications of free TRAM flaps are related to the flap or donor site. Flap-related problems include microsurgical problems with the anastomosis, haematoma, fat

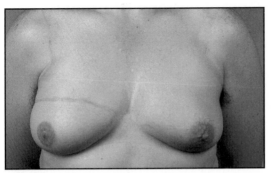

Figure 8.6 • Delayed breast reconstruction with free DIEP flap.

is as safe and reliable as the free TRAM flap. The vascularity of the transferred tissue is not compromised and the incidence of fat necrosis is no different from that of the standard free TRAM flap.[4,69–72] Disadvantages are increased operating time and an even higher level of surgical expertise requiring specialised training in dissection techniques (**Fig. 8.6**).

Free SIEA flap

The free SIEA flap does not disturb the rectus abdominis or the abdominal fascia. It relies on a branch of the femoral artery, the SIEA and its vein, which supply the fat and skin of the lower abdomen.[73]

The advantages of this technique are that there is no damage to the muscular or aponeurotic part of the abdominal wall without any risk of postoperative weakness. This operation is also quicker, with an easier dissection of the vascular pedicle, and the postoperative morbidity is comparable to an abdominoplasty procedure. Unfortunately, this vessel is absent in one-third of patients, while in others the vascular pedicle is short with a very small diameter of 1.5–2 mm and may have been damaged by previous surgery. The smaller vessel diameter may result in decreased flap perfusion, with a higher risk of partial or total flap necrosis.[73–75]

Alternative free flap donor sites for breast reconstruction

There are further types of free flap transfer for breast reconstruction. However, the expertise required for these is extremely demanding and the failure rates are potentially higher. They should be reserved for women in whom conventional techniques are deemed inappropriate.

Alternative options of autologous tissue breast reconstruction include the free superior and inferior gluteal flaps, which can be raised as perforator flaps as well; the lateral transverse thigh flap, using the so-called saddlebag area of the upper thigh; the Rubens peri-iliac fat pad flap; the anterolateral thigh flap; and the free LD flap from the contralateral side. These may be indicated if the lower abdomen or back have insufficient tissue, have already been used, cannot be used due to disruption of the vascular pedicles, or if the patient wants to avoid scars in more obvious parts of the body.[76–80]

FINISHING TOUCHES

Further surgery may be necessary to the reconstructed breast, the opposite breast or the donor site of the breast reconstruction. Complete breast reconstruction including nipple–areola reconstruction requires on average 3.3 separate procedures.[81]

Surgery to the reconstructed breast

The reconstructed breast may require adjustment in size or shape by liposuction, excision, mastopexy or augmentation. Further adjustments of the position of the breast on the chest wall, improvement of projection, adjustment of the inframammary fold, or revisional surgery for capsular contracture are necessary in a significant number of cases. Involuntary muscle contraction of the LD or pectoralis major muscle can be treated by temporary paralysis with botulinum toxin or permanent division of the motor nerve, physiotherapy or change of reconstruction.

Surgery to the contralateral breast

There are two situations in which contralateral surgery needs to be considered. One is where it is necessary to operate in order to achieve symmetry. The other is where a woman, deemed at high risk of contralateral breast cancer after a formal assessment of genetic risk, wishes a risk-reducing mastectomy with reconstruction.

Surgery to the flap donor site

Scar revision, liposuction, treatment of persistent seroma, correction of dog ears or repair of an abdominal bulge or hernia may be necessary. Donor-site morbidity is becoming more and more appreciated. Permanent loss of function at the donor site is considered by many almost as serious as failure of the reconstruction itself.[4]

Nipple–areola reconstruction

The final part of breast reconstruction is restoration of the nipple–areola complex. Some patients are happy with a prosthetic nipple but patients should have the opportunity to proceed to nipple–areola reconstruction. This leads to increased satisfaction with the breast reconstruction, a sense of completeness and an enhanced sense of attractiveness, especially unclothed.[82] The two main options for nipple reconstruction are (i) composite grafts from the opposite breast, toe pulp, ear lobe or dog ears following previous surgery and (ii) local flaps, which have been described in a multitude of variations. Areola reconstruction can be performed by full-thickness skin grafting or by tatooing. Donor sites of skin grafts for areolar reconstruction are selected on the basis of pigmentation. Grafts can be obtained from the contralateral areola, the postauricular area, the upper inner thigh, the labia majora and scarred skin from the mastectomy or old abdominal scars. However, the colour match of these grafts with the contralateral areola may not be acceptable and further tattooing may be necessary. Nowadays skin grafting has been largely abandoned in favour of tattooing, which is a quick and simple technique with minimal morbidity and very few complications apart from colour mismatch. Improved colour match can be achieved by the use of a three-dimensional colour chart.[83,84]

SALVAGE SURGERY

Salvage surgery may be required for complications of the reconstruction or for oncological reasons.

Complications of breast reconstruction

Where there has been breast skin-flap loss, the situation can be redeemed by advancement of breast skin or flap and direct closure, split-thickness skin graft or LD flap salvage. Implant extrusion due to wound dehiscence may require either implant removal and later reinsertion or conversion to an LD flap. Partial flap loss can be treated with débridement and direct closure, split-thickness skin grafting, or a further flap procedure such as an LD flap or a thoraco-epigastric flap. Unexpected loss of volume in the reconstructed breast after radiotherapy or following atropy of the muscle components in myocutaneous flaps can be corrected by augmentation of the reconstructed breast or additional surgery to the opposite breast in order to achieve symmetry. Complete flap loss can be dealt with by débridement of all necrotic tissues and direct closure or split-thickness skin graft without reconstruction. A further flap procedure or the insertion of tissue expander or implant as a space filler are indicated if the patient wishes a further attempt at breast reconstruction.

Local recurrence

Salvage surgery for chest wall recurrence often creates a surgical dilemma. Although the patient has recurrence, they may have significant life expectancy. These reconstructions are often difficult because they rely on poor-quality tissues and are often best dealt with in a multidisciplinary setting. The aims of surgery in this situation include local control of disease, palliation of symptoms and enhancement of the quality of remaining life. Resurfacing the chest wall with non-irradiated flap tissues may facilitate further radiotherapy or adjunctive treatment such as brachytherapy. Reconstruction of the resultant defect requires often extensive surgery in the form of local flaps or abdominal advancement, regional flaps such as LD, pectoralis major and parascapular flaps, omental transposition, pedicled or free abdominal flaps or even a combination of these techniques.[85–90]

SUMMARY

Immediate breast reconstruction after mastectomy for breast cancer has been accepted as safe and has no known oncological disadvantages. The ideal breast reconstruction is a soft natural-feeling breast that maintains its characteristics over time as a natural ptosis or droop and a permanent and natural inframammary fold.

It is important for any woman undergoing mastectomy to make an informed decision about reconstruction and to be provided with information about the techniques, advantages and disadvantages. There is a high degree of patient satisfaction with breast reconstruction but high levels of preoperative information and psychological support are necessary.

Close collaboration between oncological and reconstructive surgeons or management by an oncoplastic surgeon, careful patient selection and counselling, and refinements in surgical techniques can provide a range of safe and predictable techniques for breast reconstruction.

• Key points

- Breast reconstruction plays a significant role in the woman's physical, emotional and psychological recovery from breast cancer.
- Even the best reconstruction will not be able to replace the natural breast that has been lost.
- Surgical options for reconstruction include the use of tissue expanders or breast implants and the use of autologous tissue.
- The most commonly used surgical techniques are tissue expansion, LD myocutaneous flap with or without implant, lower abdominal tissue and other free tissue transfers.
- Implant-based techniques require limited surgery initially but have limitations and are not always quick and trouble-free. The quality of the long-term result is directly related to the tolerance of breast implants.
- Further procedures are often required for complications and maintenance. Asymmetry may reoccur due to the effects of gravity on the contralateral breast and fluctuations in body weight.
- The aesthetic results from autologous reconstruction are superior to those of implant-based reconstruction due to their versatility, their more natural appearance, consistency and durability.
- Autologous tissue can better withstand radiotherapy.
- The autologous LD flap is highly versatile and has acceptable donor-site morbidity.
- The skin and fat of the lower abdomen are ideal for autologous breast reconstruction but donor-site morbidity is being increasingly appreciated. Muscle-sparing techniques preserve abdominal wall function at the cost of a more complex procedure.
- Further surgery may be necessary to the reconstructed breast, the opposite breast or the donor site of the breast reconstruction.
- Nipple–areola reconstruction leads to increased satisfaction with breast reconstruction.
- Salvage surgery may be required for complications of the reconstruction or for oncological reasons.
- It is important for any woman undergoing mastectomy to be able to make an informed decision about reconstruction and information about different techniques, advantages and disadvantages should be freely available.
- Due to the variable needs of individual patients, the reconstructive surgeon must be able to provide the full range of reconstructive options.

REFERENCES

1. Schain WS. Breast reconstruction. Update of psychosocial and pragmatic concerns. Cancer 1991; 68(suppl. 5):1170–5.

2. Stevens LA, McGrath MH, Druss RG et al. The psychological impact of immediate breast reconstruction for women with early breast cancer. Plast Reconstr Surg 1984; 73:619–28.

3. Goin MK, Goin JM. Psychological reactions to prophylactic mastectomy synchronous with contralateral breast reconstruction. Plast Reconstr Surg 1982; 70:355–9.

4. Weiler-Mithoff EM. Breast reconstruction: techniques, timing and patient selection. CML Breast Cancer 2001; 13:1–11.

5. Handel N, Silverstein MJ, Waisman E et al. Reasons why mastectomy patients do not have breast reconstruction. Plast Reconstr Surg 1990; 86:1118–22.

6. Scottish Intercollegiate Guidelines Network, Scottish Cancer Therapy Network. Breast cancer in women. Edinburgh: Royal College of Physicians, 1998.

7. Harcourt DM, Rumsey NJ, Ambler NR et al. The psychological effect of mastectomy with or without breast reconstruction: a prospective, multicenter study. Plast Reconstr Surg 2003; 111:1060–8.

8. Kroll SS, Ames F, Singletary SE et al. The oncologic risks of skin preservation at mastectomy when combined with immediate reconstruction of the breast. Surg Gynecol Obstet 1991; 172:17–20.

9. Toth BA, Lappert P. Modified skin incisions for mastectomy: the need for plastic surgical input in preoperative planning. Plast Reconstr Surg 1991; 87:1048–53.

10. Bensimon RH, Bergmeyer JM. Improved aesthetics in breast reconstruction: modified mastectomy incision and immediate autologous tissue reconstruction. Ann Plast Surg 1995; 34:229–33.

11. Yule GJ, Concannon MJ, Croll G et al. Is there liability with chemotherapy following immediate breast reconstruction? Plast Reconstr Surg 1996; 97:969–73.

12. Furey PC, Macgillivary DC, Gastiglione CL et al. Wound complications in patients receiving adjuvant chemotherapy after mastectomy and immediate breast reconstruction for breast cancer. J Surg Oncol 1994; 55:194–7.

13. Wilson CR, Brown IM, Weiler-Mithoff EM et al. Immediate breast reconstruction is not associated with a delay in the delivery of adjuvant chemotherapy. Eur J Surg Oncol 2004; 30:324–7.

14. Hussien M, Salah B, Malyon A et al. Impact of adjuvant radiotherapy on the choice of immediate breast reconstruction. Eur J Cancer 2000; 36 (suppl. 5):58.

15. Von Smitten K, Sundell B. The impact of adjuvant radiotherapy and cytotoxic chemotherapy on the outcome of immediate breast reconstruction by tissue expansion after mastectomy for breast cancer. Eur J Surg Oncol 1992; 18:119–23.

16. Malata CM, McIntosh SA, Prurushotham AD. Immediate breast reconstruction after mastectomy for cancer. Br J Surg 2000; 87:1455–72.

17. Rosenquist S, Sandelin K, Wickmann M. Patients' psychological and cosmetic experience after immediate breast reconstruction. Eur J Surg Oncol 1996; 22:262–6.

18. Petit JY, Le MG, Mouriesse H et al. Can breast reconstruction with gel-filled silicone implants increase the risk of death and second primary cancer in patients treated by mastectomy for breast cancer? Plast Reconstr Surg 1994; 94:115–19.

19. Noone RB, Frazier TG, Noone GC et al. Recurrence of breast carcinoma following immediate reconstruction: a 13-year review. Plast Reconstr Surg 1994; 93:90–106.

20. Townsend CM Jr, Abston S, Fish JC. Surgical adjuvant treatment of locally advanced breast cancer. Ann Surg 1985; 201:604–10.

21. Godfrey PM, Godfrey NV, Romita MC. Immediate autogenous breast reconstruction in clinically advanced disease. Plast Reconstr Surg 1995; 95:1039–44.

22. Eberlein TJ, Crespo LD, Smith BL et al. Prospective evaluation of immediate reconstruction after mastectomy. Ann Surg 1993; 218:29–36.

23. Hunt KK, Baldwin BJ, Strom EA et al. Feasibility of postmastectomy radiation therapy after TRAM flap breast reconstruction. Ann Surg Oncol 1997; 4:377–84.

24. Williams JK, Carlson GW, Bostwick J III et al. The effects of radiation treatment after TRAM flap breast reconstruction. Plast Reconstr Surg 1997; 100:1153–60.

25. Tran NV, Evans GRD, Kroll SS et al. Postoperative adjuvant irradiation: effects on transverse rectus abdominis muscle flap breast reconstruction. Plast Reconstr Surg 2000; 106:313–20.

26. Tran NV, Chang DW, Gupta A et al. Comparison of immediate and delayed free TRAM flap breast reconstruction in patients receiving postmastectomy radiation therapy. Plast Reconstr Surg 2001; 108:78–82.

27. Rodgers NE, Allen RJ. Radiation effects on breast reconstruction with the deep inferior epigastric perforator flap. Plast Reconstr Surg 2002; 109:1919–24.

28. Bostwick J III. Plastic and reconstructive breast surgery. St Louis: Quality Medical Publishing, 1990.

29. Radovan C. Breast reconstruction after mastectomy using the temporary expander. Plast Reconstr Surg 1982; 69:195–208.

30. Woods JE, Mangan MA. Breast reconstruction with tissue expanders: obtaining an optimal result. Ann Plast Surg 1992; 28:390–96.

31. Gabriel SE, Woods JE, O'Fallon WM et al. Complications leading to surgery after breast implantation. N Engl J Med 1997; 336:677–82.

32. Clough KB, O'Donoghue JM, Fitoussi AD et al. Prospective evaluation of late cosmetic results following breast reconstruction: implant reconstruction. Plast Reconstr Surg 2001; 107:1702–9.

33. Slavin SA, Colen SR. Sixty consecutive breast reconstructions with the inflatable expander: a critical appraisal. Plast Reconstr Surg 1990; 86:910–19.

34. Gruber RP, Kahn RA, Lash H et al. Breast reconstruction following mastectomy: a comparison of submuscular and subcutaneous techniques. Plast Reconstr Surg 1981; 67:312–17.

35. Dickson MG, Sharpe DT. The complications of tissue expansion in breast reconstruction: a review of 75 cases. Br J Plast Surg 1987; 40:629–35.

36. Rosato RM, Dowden RV. Radiation therapy as a cause of capsular contracture. Ann Plast Surg 1994; 32:342–5.

37. McCraw JB, Papp CTh. Latissimus dorsi myocutaneous flap. In: Hartrampf CR (ed.) Breast reconstruction with living tissue. Norfolk, VA: Hampton Press, 1991; pp. 211–48.

38. Clough KB, Louis-Sylvestre C, Fitoussi A et al. Donor site sequelae after autologous breast reconstruction with an extended latissimus dorsi flap. Plast Reconstr Surg 2002; 109:1904–11.

39. Delay E, Gounot N, Bouillot A et al. Autologous latissimus breast reconstruction: a 3 year clinical experience with 100 patients. Plast Reconstr Surg 1998; 102:1461–78.

40. McCraw JB, Papp C, Edwards A et al. The autogenous latissimus breast reconstruction. Clin Plast Surg 1994; 21:279–88.

41. Germann G, Steinau HU. Breast reconstruction with the extended latissimus dorsi flap. Plast Reconstr Surg 1996; 97:519–26.

42. Fatah MFT. Extended latissimus dorsi flap in breast reconstruction. Operative Tech Plast Reconstr Surg 1999; 6:38–49.

43. Titley OG, Spyrou GE, Fatah MFT. Preventing seroma in the latissimus dorsi flap donor site. Br J Plast Surg 1997; 50:106–8.

44. Kroll SS, Baldwin B. A comparison of outcomes using three different methods of breast reconstruction. Plast Reconstr Surg 1992; 90:455–62.

45. Roy MK, Shrotia S, Holcombe C et al. Complications of latissimus dorsi myocutaneous flap breast reconstruction. Eur J Surg Oncol 1998; 24:162–5.

46. Arnold PG, Lovic SF, Pairolero PC. Muscle flaps in irradiated wounds: an account of 100 consecutive cases. Plast Reconstr Surg 1994; 93:324–7.

47. Scott JR, Malyon A, Hussien M et al. Immediate breast reconstruction: the effect of adjuvant radiotherapy on latissimus dorsi flap reconstructions with and without implants. BAPS Summer Meeting, Stirling, 2001.

48. Report of the Independent Review Group. Silicone gel breast implants. London: HMSO, 1998.

49. Clough BC, O'Donoghue JM, Fitoussi AD et al. Prospective evaluation of late cosmetic results following breast reconstruction. II. TRAM flap reconstruction. Plast Reconstr Surg 2001; 107:1710–16.

50. Petit JY, Rietjens M, Ferreire MAR et al. Abdominal sequelae after pedicled TRAM flap breast reconstruction. Plast Reconstr Surg 1997; 99:723–9.

51. Hartrampf CR Jr. The transverse abdominal island flap for breast reconstruction. A 7-year experience. Clin Plast Surg 1988; 15:703.

52. McCraw JB. Clinical definition of independent myocutaneous vascular teritories. Plast Reconstr Surg 1977; 60:341–52.

53. Robbins TH. Rectus abdominis myocutaneous flap for breast reconstruction. Aust NZ J Surg 1979; 49:527–30.

54. Hartrampf CR. Breast reconstruction with a transverse abdominal island flap. Plast Reconstr Surg 1982; 69:216–24.

55. Holmstroem H. The free abdominoplasty flap and its use in breast reconstruction. Scand J Plast Reconstr Surg 1979; 13:423–6.

56. Koshima I, Soeda S. Inferior epigastric artery skin flaps without rectus abdominis muscle. Br J Plast Surg 1989; 42:645–8.

57. Allen RJ, Treece P. Deep inferior epigastric perforator flap for breast reconstruction. Ann Plast Surg 1994; 32:32–8.

58. Antia NH, Buch VI. Transfer of an abdominal dermo-fat graft by direct anastomosis of blood vessels. Br J Plast Surg 1971; 24:15–19.

59. Mitzgala CL, Hartrampf CR, Bennett GK. Abdominal wall function after pedicled TRAM flap surgery. Clin Plast Surg 1994; 21:255–72.

60. Mizgala CL, Hartrampf CR Jr, Bennett GK. Assessment of the abdominal wall after pedicled TRAM flap surgery: 5- to 7-year follow-up of 150 consecutive patients. Plast Reconstr Surg 1994; 93:988–1002.

61. Lejour M, Dome M. Abdominal wall function after pedicled rectus abdominis transfer. Plast Reconstr Surg 1991; 87:1054–68.

62. Jensen JA. Is the double pedicle TRAM flap reconstruction of a single breast within the standard of care? Plast Reconstr Surg 1997; 100:1592–3.

63. Arnez ZM, Bajec J, Bardsley AF et al. Experience with 50 free TRAM flap breast reconstructions. Plast Reconstr Surg 1991; 87:470–8.

64. Schustermann MA, Kroll SS, Weldon ME. Immediate breast reconstruction: why the free TRAM over the conventional TRAM flap? Plast Reconstr Surg 1992; 90:255–61.

65. Grotting JC, Urist MM, Maddox WA et al. Conventional TRAM flap versus free microsurgical TRAM flap for immediate breast reconstruction. Plast Reconstr Surg 1989; 83:828–41.

66. Grotting JC. Immediate breast reconstruction using the free TRAM flap. Clin Plast Surg 1994; 21:207–21.

67. Kroll SS, Schusterman MA, Reece GP et al. Abdominal wall strength, bulging and hernia after TRAM flap breast reconstruction. Plast Reconstr Surg 1995; 96:616–19.

68. Feller AM. Free TRAM: results and abdominal wall function. Clin Plast Surg 1994; 21:223–32.

69. Hamdi M, Weiler-Mithoff EM, Webster MHC. Deep inferior epigastric perforator flap in breast reconstruction: experience with the first 50 flaps. Plast Reconstr Surg 1999; 103:86–95.

70. Futter CM, Webster MHC, Hagen S et al. A retrospective comparison of abdominal muscle strength following breast reconstruction with a free TRAM or DIEP flap. Br J Plast Surg 2000; 53:578–83.

71. Blondeel PN, Vanderstraeten GG, Monstrey SJ et al. The donor site morbidity of free DIEP flaps and free TRAM flaps for breast reconstruction. Br J Plast Surg 1997; 50:322–30.

72. Weiler-Mithoff E, Hodgson ELB, Malata CM. Perforator flap breast reconstruction. Breast Disease 2002; 16:93–106.

73. Stern HS, Nahai F. The versatile superficial inferior epigastric artery free flap. Br J Plast Surg 1992; 95:270–4.

74. Arnez ZM, Khan U, Pogorelec D et al. Breast reconstruction using the free superficial inferior epigastric artery (SIEA) flap. Br J Plast Surg 1999; 52:276–9.

75. Arnez ZM, Khan U, Pogorelec D et al. Rational selection of flaps from the abdomen in breast reconstruction to reduce donor site morbidity. Br J Plast Surg 1999; 52:351–4.

76. Shaw WW. Breast reconstruction by superior gluteal microvascular free flap without silicone implants. Plast Reconstr Surg 1983; 72:490–501.

77. Boustred AM, Nahai F. Inferior gluteal free flap breast reconstruction. Clin Plast Surg 1998; 25:275–82.

78. Allen RJ, Tucker C Jr. Superior gluteal artery perforator free flap for breast reconstruction. Plast Reconstr Surg 1995; 95:1207–12.

79. Elliot LF. The lateral transverse thigh free flap for autogenous tissue breast reconstruction. Perspect Plast Surg 1989; 3:80–4.

80. Hartrampf CR, Elliot LF. Ruben's fat pad for breast reconstruction: a peri-iliac soft-tissue free flap. Plast Reconstr Surg 1994; 93:402–7.

81. Malyon AD, Husein M, Weiler-Mithoff EM. How many procedures to make a breast? Br J Plast Surg 2001; 54:227–31.

82. Wellisch DK, Schain WS, Noone RB et al. The psychological contribution of nipple addition in breast reconstruction. Plast Reconstr Surg 1987; 80:699–704.

83. Little JW. Nipple–areola reconstruction. In: Spear SL (ed.) Surgery of the breast: principles and art. Philadelphia: Lippincott-Raven, 1998; pp. 661–9.

84. Henseler H, Cheong V, Weiler-Mithoff EM et al. The use of Munsell colour charts in nipple areola tattooing. Br J Plast Surg 2001; 54:338–40.

85. Hathaway CL, Rand RP, Moe R, Marchioro T. Salvage surgery for locally advanced and locally recurrent breast cancer. Arch Surg 1994; 129:582–7.

86. Burk RW III, Grotting JC. Conceptual considerations in breast reconstruction. Clin Plast Surg 1995; 22:141–52.

87. Sultan MR, Smith ML, Estabrook A et al. Immediate breast reconstruction in patients with locally advanced disease. Ann Plast Surg 1997; 38:345–9; discussion 350–1.

88. Rivas B, Carrillo JF, Escobar G. Reconstructive management of advanced breast cancer. Ann Plast Surg 2001; 47:234–9.

89. Brower ST, Weinberg H, Tartter PI et al. Chest wall resection for locally recurrent breast cancer: indications, technique, and results. J Surg Oncol 1992; 49:189–95.

90. Hasse J. Reconstruction of chest wall defects. Thorac Cardiovasc Surg 1991; 39(suppl. 3):241–7.

Nine

Breast cancer treatments of uncommon diseases

Swati Kulkarni and
Monica Morrow

PAGET'S DISEASE

In 1874, Sir James Paget described the clinical entity now known as Paget's disease as 'an eczematous change in the skin of the nipple preceding an underlying mammary cancer'.[1] More than 95% of women with Paget's disease of the nipple have an underlying malignancy, although almost half are clinically and mammographically undetectable.[2]

Incidence

Paget's disease accounts for 0.7–4.9% of breast malignancies, and has also been reported in males.[3,4] The time from first symptoms to treatment is 10–12 months. Misdiagnosis as eczema and treatment with topical steroids is the most common reason for delay in diagnosis.[5–8]

Pathology

There are two hypotheses regarding the development of Paget's disease of the nipple. The in-situ-transformation hypothesis suggests that Paget's cells arise from transformed malignant keratinocytes and that it is a type of in-situ carcinoma of the skin.[4,5,9] Consistent with this is that Paget's cells and the underlying cancer are often separated by some distance. The epidermotropic hypothesis of Paget's

disease suggests that ductal cells migrate along the basement membrane of ducts into the nipple epidermis.[10] Support for this comes from immunohistochemical studies that show similar staining patterns of Paget's cells and the underlying carcinoma.[11] Proponents of this hypothesis believe that carcinoma is present in 100% of women with pagetoid changes but that it is not always identified during pathological evaluation.[12]

On histological examination, Paget's cells appear as large, round or ovoid intraepidermal cells with abundant clear pale cytoplasm and enlarged pleomorphic and hyperchromatic nuclei with prominent nucleoli. Reactive changes in the dermis, such as plasma cell infiltration, neovascularisation, serous exudate and hyperaemia, result in the characteristic appearance of the nipple in Paget's.[13] One study suggests that Paget's is found in association more often with high-grade ductal carcinoma in situ (DCIS) and high-grade invasive carcinomas than with lower-grade lesions.[5]

Clinical presentation

Burning, itching and a change in sensation of the nipple and areola are the first symptoms of Paget's disease. This is followed by the development of skin lesions that may be raised and irregular and have a sharp demarcation from the surrounding skin. The

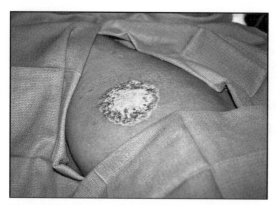

Figure 9.1 • Advanced changes of Paget's disease with destruction of the nipple and areola and involvement of periareolar skin.

nipple may appear erythematous and scaling may be visible. Nipple deformity or retraction may be present if there is tethering from an underlying malignancy, but is not a classic sign. Characteristically, Paget's begins on the nipple and spreads to the areola and subsequently to the surrounding skin. Later stages of Paget's may result in ulceration, bleeding and destruction of the nipple–areola complex. (**Fig. 9.1**; see Plate 10, facing p. 116). Nipple discharge has also been reported in association with Paget's disease but is not common, and bleeding is usually due to ulceration of the nipple epithelium rather than discharge from the underlying ducts.[14]

The differential diagnosis of Paget's disease is chronic eczema, benign papilloma of the nipple, basal cell carcinoma, malignant melanoma and Bowen's disease.[15] Paget's disease can present in association with an underlying mass or calcifications. It can also present as an abnormality of the nipple–areola complex alone or it can be subclinical (reported as a histological finding after a mastectomy for DCIS or invasive cancer). Approximately half of patients with the characteristic nipple changes will have an underlying palpable abnormality at presentation.[16]

Diagnosis

A full-thickness biopsy of the nipple should be performed to confirm diagnosis. This can be done with a punch biopsy.[17] Exfoliative cytology or incisional biopsy may be done if a punch biopsy is

not available.[18] Immunohistochemistry is helpful in differentiating Paget's disease from other nipple pathology. Paget's cells stain positive for CK7, CAM-5.2, AE1/AE3 and S100 but do not express HMB-45 and high-molecular-weight keratins, which helps differentiate them from melanomas.[19–21] As in all patients with breast cancer, bilateral diagnostic mammography is recommended for revealing multicentric disease, suspicious microcalcifications and non-palpable masses, as well as for assessing the contralateral breast. Ultrasound may be useful if mammography is unable to detect an underlying mass. Magnetic resonance imaging (MRI) is a promising method for evaluating patients with Paget's disease due to its high sensitivity in detecting occult malignancy.[22,23] Because of its greater sensitivity, MRI has the potential to play a significant role in planning surgical therapy.

Treatment

Treatment of Paget's disease should always include excision of the nipple–areola complex. If a tumour is evident in the periphery of the breast, either clinically or mammographically, mastectomy is the preferred treatment. Some have advocated mastectomy as the procedure of choice in all cases due to the frequent finding of multicentric disease in association with Paget's disease of the nipple. Kothari et al.[5] reported 67 patients with Paget's disease treated by mastectomy. In addition to disease in the central part of the breast, 75% had a malignancy in another quadrant.

However, multiple small studies of breast-conserving therapy in Paget's disease indicate low rates of local recurrence after treatment with excision and irradiation. These are summarised in **Table 9.1**.[8,24–28] A recent prospective study of 61 patients with Paget's with no clinically identifiable disease and centrally located DCIS treated with excision of the nipple–areola complex to negative margins, removal of a cone of underlying breast tissue and 50 Gy of irradiation reported a local recurrence rate of 5.2% after a median follow-up of 6.4 years.[25]

Attempts to treat Paget's disease with excision without irradiation have been less successful. Dixon et al.[8] and Polgar et al.[29] reported recurrence rates of 40% and 33% after excision alone in patients

Table 9.1 • Conservative management of Paget's disease of the nipple

Reference	Year	N	Median follow-up (months)	Radiation	Recurrence	No. of local recurrences	No. of distant recurrences	No. of deaths
Marshall et al.[24]	2003	36	113	Yes	11%	4	0	0
Bijker et al.[25]	2001	61	77	Yes	5.2%	4	2	1
Fu et al.[26]	2001	12	42	No	25%	3	0	0
Kollemorgen et al.[27]	1998	10	71	No	20%	0	2	2
Dixon et al.[8]	1991	10	56	No	40%	4	0	0
Fourquet et al.[28]	1987	20	90	Yes	6.7%	3	0	0

with or without clinical evidence of malignancy in the underlying breast tissue. Similarly, attempts to preserve clinically uninvolved areas of the nipple–areola complex have also resulted in high rates of local recurrence.[26,30]

In patients with coexisting invasive cancer, axillary staging by sentinel lymph node biopsy (SLNB) or axillary dissection should be undertaken. The prognosis of Paget's disease is determined by the stage of the coexisting carcinoma. Guidelines for systemic therapy are the same as those used in women without Paget's disease of the nipple.

• **Key points**

- Local therapy for Paget's disease consists of mastectomy or breast-conserving therapy that includes excision of the nipple–areola complex followed by radiation therapy.
- Axillary dissection or SLNB is performed when invasive cancer is present.
- Adjuvant therapy is based on the stage of the underlying malignancy.

PREGNANCY-ASSOCIATED BREAST CANCER

The term 'pregnancy-associated breast cancer' (PABC) includes breast cancer diagnosed during pregnancy, up to 1 year after delivery or at any time while the patient is lactating.[31] Breast cancer is the second most common malignancy in pregnant women after cervical cancer.[32] There is often a delay in diagnosis due to anatomical and physiological changes in the breast and a low index of suspicion of malignancy.

Epidemiology

The average age of patients with PABC is 32–38 years.[33] The estimated incidence of PABC is 0.2–3.8% of all breast cancers and PABC is reported to occur in 1 in 10 000 to 1 in 3000 pregnancies.[34,35] PABC is diagnosed at later stages than breast cancer in non-pregnant women of the same age.[36] It is unknown if this is due to a more aggressive biology of PABC or because of a delay in diagnosis.[37]

Aetiology/risk factors

A case–control study in Japan of 383 patients found that those with PABC were three times more likely than age-matched, non-pregnant, non-lactating women with breast cancer to have a family history of breast cancer.[38] In general, young age of first full-term pregnancy and multiparity are associated with a decrease in the risk of breast cancer. The opposite appears to be true for women who carry the *BRCA1/BRCA2* germline mutation. Carriers of the *BRCA1* or *BRCA2* mutation who had a full-term pregnancy were significantly more likely than nulliparous women with the *BRCA1* or *BRCA2* mutation to develop breast cancer before the age of 40.[39] This may be due to an increased sensitivity of the breast epithelium to estrogen and progesterone in gene carriers.[39]

In general, the infrequent occurrence of PABC has prevented a detailed assessment of the risk factors that differentiate it from breast cancer in general.

Clinical presentation

The most common presentation of PABC is a painless mass.[40,41] During pregnancy, levels of estrogen, progesterone, prolactin and chorionic gonadotrophin rise. The breasts undergo marked ductal and lobular proliferation. Mammary blood flow increases by 180% and the weight of the breast can double.[42] Clinical breast examination can be difficult because of the increased nodularity of the breast. Because of these physiological changes and a reluctance to investigate masses discovered during pregnancy, PABC tends to be diagnosed at a more advanced stage and consequently is associated with a worse prognosis. A study of 63 women with PABC indicated that fewer than 20% were diagnosed prior to delivery and the median size of the cancer at diagnosis was 3.5 cm. In the same study, 62% of patients with PABC had lymph node metastasis compared with 39% of matched non-pregnant controls.[31] Additionally, patients with PABC are more likely to have larger tumours, vascular invasion and distant metastasis.[43] It is not known whether these finding are due to a different biology of PABC or because of delay in diagnosis.

Differential diagnoses

Of breast biopsies performed during pregnancy, 70–80% are benign.[37] The differential diagnosis of a breast mass in pregnancy includes lactating adenoma, fibroadenoma, cystic disease, lobular hyperplasia, galactocele, abscess, lipoma and hamartoma. Rarely, other malignancies present in the breast during pregnancy.[44] A mass in a pregnant woman should be investigated by imaging and biopsy if it has the characteristics of a dominant breast mass. If, clinically, a mass cannot be distinguished from the nodularity of pregnancy, ultrasound is useful in excluding the presence of a suspicious lesion. In women felt to have prominent areas of nodularity, a short-interval follow-up examination in 3–4 weeks is appropriate.

Diagnostic techniques

Mammography is not routinely used to screen the pregnant woman. In contrast, diagnostic mammography is useful for evaluating masses during pregnancy and can be performed safely with the use of abdominal shielding. Mammography was able to detect 78–88% of palpable breast cancers in reports of 21 and 22 cases respectively.[45,46] Ultrasound is also a safe imaging tool in pregnancy and can reliably identify cystic lesions and help to characterise solid masses. However, dominant solid masses require histological confirmation that they are benign before the decision is made to observe them.[42] As in the non-pregnant patient, core needle biopsy is the preferred method of diagnosis. A study of 331 pregnant women showed that fine-needle aspiration (FNA) is accurate in pregnancy. The increased proliferation of the breast epithelium in pregnancy may result in false-positive cytological diagnosis of carcinoma or atypia unless the cytopathologist is specifically informed of the patient's pregnancy. In addition, benign lesions such as fibroadenomas increase in size during pregnancy. A specific histological diagnosis by core biopsy will allow continued observation of these lesions, while an increase in size of a lesion diagnosed as 'benign' by FNA is usually an indication for surgical excision.[47] For these reasons, core biopsy is the diagnostic technique of choice in pregnancy. However, there have been case reports of milk fistula formation after core biopsy and this technique should be used with caution for centrally located lesions in lactating women.[48] If FNA and core biopsy are not diagnostic, excisional biopsy should be performed. Breastfeeding should be stopped before biopsy in order to reduce the risk of milk fistula formation. In general, guidelines for the diagnosis of a dominant breast mass in the pregnant woman are the same as those in the non-pregnant woman.

The need for a metastatic work-up should be guided by symptoms and the clinical stage of the cancer, as in non-pregnant patients. Chest radiography can be done safely with abdominal shielding. Bone scans have been performed in pregnant women using lower doses of radioisotope, but their use is generally not recommended during pregnancy.[49] MRI is promising for use in pregnancy in order to evaluate liver and bony metastasis since it does not involve ionising radiation. MRI has also been used for fetal imaging in utero with no untoward effects reported.[50] No studies have examined the use of positron emission tomography (PET) during pregnancy.

Pathology

PABC is histologically similar to carcinoma in non-pregnant patients.[38] PABC tends to be negative for both estrogen receptor and progesterone receptor.[51] Conflicting data exist on overexpression of erbB-2 or HER-2/neu in PABC. Tumours associated with PABC are reported to have a high positivity for Ki67 and p53, although the significance of these findings is uncertain.[52]

Prognosis

Early studies reported a dismal prognosis for PABC.[53,54] Recent studies indicate a similar prognosis for patients with stage I and II PABC compared with non-pregnant matched controls; however, there appears to be trend towards a worse prognosis in stage III and IV PABC.[31,51] In a study by Petrek et al.,[31] patients with PABC who had negative lymph node involvement had the same 5-year survival as non-pregnant controls. However, the survival of those patients with PABC with positive lymph nodes was 47% versus 59% in the non-pregnant controls. This may reflect differences in tumour biology or delays in therapy due to concerns about fetal safety. However, some studies suggest that pregnancy is an independent poor prognostic factor.[51,55] Additionally, there appears to be an increased relative risk of dying from breast cancer if it develops within 4 years after giving birth compared with women, matched for age and stage, who have never been pregnant and who develop breast cancer.[43,56]

Treatment of the primary tumour

LOCAL THERAPY OF CLINICAL STAGE I AND II PABC

Treatment should not be delayed because of pregnancy. The approach should involve a multi-disciplinary team that includes the surgeon, medical oncologist and high-risk obstetrician. Surgery can be safely performed during all trimesters of pregnancy. Duncan et al.[56] found no increase in congenital anomalies in 2565 pregnant women who underwent surgery compared with pregnant controls who did not have surgery. When planning surgery, the surgical team must be aware of the physiological changes associated with pregnancy, including increased cardiac output, increased blood volume, decreased systemic vascular resistance, hyper-coagulable state, delayed gastric emptying and a physiological dilutional anaemia that decreases oxygen-carrying capacity.[57] Additionally, a pillow should be placed on the right side of the patient to relieve pressure on the inferior vena cava. The fetus should be monitored closely during and after surgery.

The type of surgery should be tailored to the gestational age of the fetus and breast cancer stage of the mother. Breast-conserving therapy is generally not recommended in the first trimester of pregnancy because of the need to delay radiotherapy until after delivery, with the potential for increased risk of local recurrence. However, for the patient who receives adjuvant chemotherapy this delay is no longer than that seen in the non-pregnant patient. The effects of increased vascularity of the breast and hormonal changes of pregnancy on local recurrence rates are unknown. The decision to undertake breast-conserving therapy in the pregnant woman is much more complex than in the non-pregnant woman and requires a detailed assessment of the individual tumour characteristics and a frank discussion of the uncertainties associated with this approach. Mastectomy can be safely performed during any trimester of pregnancy, although immediate reconstruction is not usually recommended due to the increased operating time and the difficulty in achieving symmetry with the contralateral breast as it continues to change as pregnancy advances.

SLNB is not recommended in the pregnant or lactating woman. Lymphazurin blue or patent blue V, the dyes most commonly used to localise the sentinel node, have not been studied in pregnant women and therefore their safety has not been established. Technetium-99m, the radioactive tracer commonly used to localise sentinel nodes, results in low doses of radiation (1.85–3.7 MBq) to the breast; fetal exposure would be minimal. Some have advocated its use for SLNB during pregnancy but it is not standard practice and no studies have been conducted to examine the long-term adverse effects on the fetus.[58] Axillary dissection remains the standard approach in pregnant women with invasive breast cancer.

SYSTEMIC THERAPY

Chemotherapy is contraindicated in the first trimester of pregnancy. First-trimester exposure to chemotherapy results in a 14–19% risk of fetal malformation,[59] which falls to 1.3% with exposure in the second trimester. Spontaneous abortion has also been reported after first-trimester exposure.[60]

Berry et al.[61] conducted a prospective cohort study of 24 women who received 5-fluorouracil, doxorubicin and cyclophosphamide during the second and third trimesters of pregnancy and found no congenital malformations or postpartum complications in the infants. Long-term follow-up is needed to monitor the occurrence of late adverse effects in these children, including the risk of cancer development. In general, methotrexate should be avoided during pregnancy due to a high reported risk of associated abnormalities. Because of limited experience with taxanes during pregnancy their use is not recommended, although cases of normal neonates after taxane exposure during pregnancy have been reported.[62,63] Chemotherapy should be stopped 3 weeks before delivery to avoid myelosuppression and septic complications in the mother and the newborn infant.[52]

Endocrine therapy is not recommended during pregnancy. Tamoxifen is known to cause spontaneous abortions, birth defects and fetal demise.[64]

The risk–benefit ratio for chemotherapy is shifted during pregnancy because of the potential for fetal injury. While each woman must make an individual decision about the level of risk that is acceptable to her, some general guidelines can be employed. Women with positive lymph nodes should receive chemotherapy after the first trimester of pregnancy. Since adjuvant studies have suggested that chemotherapy is effective if administered within 6 weeks of surgery, delays of this duration or slightly longer to allow treatment after delivery are appropriate. For the low-risk node-negative woman, where the survival benefit of chemotherapy is 5% or less, treatment during pregnancy is usually avoided. For the node-negative woman with larger high-grade cancer with unfavourable prognostic features, treatment decisions must be made on an individual basis.

LOCALLY ADVANCED BREAST CANCER AND INFLAMMATORY CANCER

In women who present with advanced breast cancer during early pregnancy, the need for prompt treatment must be balanced against the risk to the fetus. Termination of pregnancy should be discussed in this circumstance, although it is not an option all women will choose. It is essential that there is a frank discussion with the patient of not only the potential toxicity of chemotherapy to the fetus but also the risk of death both with and without prompt therapy. After the first trimester, chemotherapy can be administered as discussed above. Surgery as an initial approach to inflammatory cancer should be avoided. **Figure 9.2** is a summary of the management strategy for PABC.

Termination of pregnancy

In the past, the prognosis of PABC was considered so dismal that therapeutic abortion was advocated in all women. Comparisons of survival in women opting to continue pregnancy and those undergoing abortion do not suggest a survival advantage for abortion.[40,65] Currently, there are no formal recommendations for therapeutic abortion in women with PABC. However, therapeutic abortion can simplify treatment in patients with advanced disease. A detailed discussion about treatment options and the potential risks to the fetus should be undertaken with the patient. Additionally, the patient and family should be informed of the risk of recurrence, overall survival and risk of infertility due to therapy when making a decision regarding termination of pregnancy.

Breast cancer after pregnancy

Pregnancy after breast cancer appears to be safe. Retrospective studies indicate an equivalent or better survival in patients treated for breast cancer who subsequently become pregnant, although this

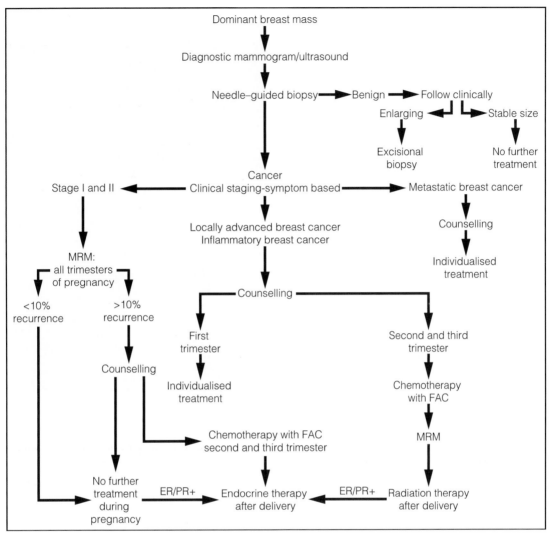

Figure 9.2 • Management algorithm for the pregnant woman presenting with a dominant breast mass. ER/PR+, estrogen and progesterone receptor positive; FAC, fluorouracil, doxorubicin and cyclophosphamide; MRM, magnetic resonance mammography.

may be due to selection bias.[31] There is no absolute time interval that is known to be safe for becoming pregnant after a diagnosis of breast cancer. Some advocate waiting 2 years after treatment of PABC for women with low-risk tumours, with a longer waiting period for those with high-risk tumours.[52]

However, since the rate of relapse is fairly constant for the first 10 years after breast cancer diagnosis, the rationale for these recommendations is unclear. The ability of the breast cancer survivor to delay pregnancy is often limited by older age and concerns about decreased fertility related to treatment.

• Key points

- A multidisciplinary approach is necessary in managing the woman with PABC. Patient and family counselling is also important.
- Mammography, sonography and image-guided biopsy can be performed safely during pregnancy.
- Surgery can be safely performed during any trimester of pregnancy, while radiation is contraindicated during pregnancy.
- Chemotherapy can be given if necessary during the second and third trimesters.
- Recognising PABC and understanding the management issues associated with it is of increasing importance as more women delay childbirth.

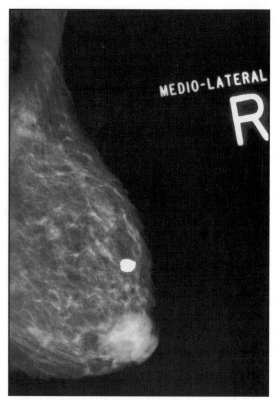

Figure 9.3 • Mammogram of a primary breast lymphoma in the subareolar space. The appearance is indistinguishable from that of a primary adenocarcinoma.

OTHER BREAST MALIGNANCIES

Primary breast lymphomas

Primary breast lymphoma (PBL) arises from lymphoid tissue in the breast and is defined as lymphoma localised to the breast and its draining lymph node basins.[66,67] The incidence of PBL is 0.14% of all breast malignancies and 0.65% of all non-Hodgkin's lymphomas.[66] The most common subtype is diffuse large B-cell lymphoma.[66–68] The mean age of onset is 65 years. PBL most often presents as a painless, enlarging, rubbery mass. Mammographic and ultrasound findings tend to be non-specific (**Fig. 9.3**). PBLs are categorised using the Working Classification and the Ann Arbor Classification of lymphomas.

PBL is usually not suspected in the absence of constitutional symptoms until a core biopsy is obtained. Once the diagnosis is known, a complete history and physical examination should be done, focusing on the presence of constitutional symptoms and evaluation of the lymph node basins. Additionally, computerised tomography (CT) of the chest, abdomen and pelvis and a bone marrow biopsy are needed to adequately stage the patient. Single-institution reports have indicated that surgery alone or surgery with radiation results in a high incidence of local and disseminated recurrence, and surgery is no longer recommended for the treatment of PBL.[66] The only role of surgery is in obtaining tissue for diagnosis if core biopsy is inadequate. Treatment of PBL consists of chemotherapy with agents appropriate for the histological type of lymphoma followed by appropriately targeted radiation.[68,69] The 2-year overall survival is 63%, which is comparable to similar lymphomas elsewhere in the body.[66]

Angiosarcomas of the breast

Although rare, radiation-induced primary angiosarcoma of the breast is an important clinical entity. The first case of angiosarcoma following radiation to the breast was reported in 1981.[70] The incidence of this problem may be increasing due to the increase in the number of women receiving radiation therapy following breast-conserving surgery. Approximately 60 cases have been reported to date.[71] The average time from radiation therapy to diagnosis is 75 months.[71] For an angiosarcoma to be considered radiation induced, it must occur in the radiated field and have a long latency period.[72]

Post-radiation sarcoma usually presents in a multifocal pattern with painless skin nodules. The nodules may be violet, blue, black or red (**Fig. 9.4**; see Plate 11, facing p. 116).[73] The differential diagnosis includes adenocarcinoma of the breast, radiation-related skin changes and melanoma.[74] The diagnosis is made by full-thickness punch biopsy or incisional or excisional biopsy. FNA is not recommended and mammography and ultrasound are generally not helpful. Molecular markers such as factor VIII-related antigen are positive in most angiosarcomas and can help to distinguish angiosarcomas from other sarcomas.[75] Staging of angiosarcoma follows the guidelines for other sarcomas, where staging is based on size, grade and depth of the tumour. As in other sarcomas, grade is the most important determinant of prognosis. Most radiation-induced angiosarcomas are high grade.[73] Treatment consists of mastectomy with wide resection of the skin of the breast. The microscopic extent of cutaneous angiosarcoma is often greater than clinically evident, so efforts should be made to achieve widely negative skin margins (**Fig. 9.5**; see Plate 12, facing p. 116). Axillary staging is not recommended since most sarcomas do not metastasise to regional lymph nodes. The recurrence rate is approximately 40% and the prognosis is poor. In a study of 58 patients, almost half had died at an average follow-up period of 15 months.[71] Adjuvant treatment follows recommendations for other sarcomas, but individual reports do not indicate a clear benefit.

Melanoma of the breast

Primary cutaneous melanoma of the skin of the breast is extremely rare; only 0.28% of all melanomas are reported to occur in this site.[76] Melanoma is more commonly found in the breast as a result of distant metastasis from a primary elsewhere in the body.[77] A history focusing on risk factors for developing melanoma as well as change

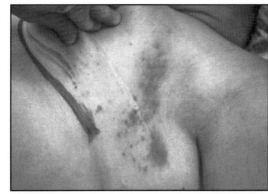

Figure 9.4 • Appearance of a radiation-induced angiosarcoma on the lateral aspect of a breast treated for adenocarcinoma with lumpectomy and radiotherapy. Multiple reddish-brown cutaneous nodules are visible.

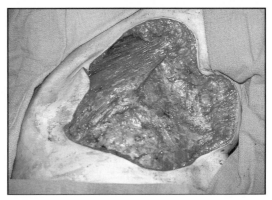

Figure 9.5 • Extent of resection necessary to obtain negative margins in the patient illustrated in **Fig. 9.4**.

in the appearance of the lesion should be obtained. Physical examination for the presence of other melanomas and lymphadenopathy should also be performed.

Mammography and ultrasound are generally not helpful in diagnosis and therapeutic planning. Core biopsy or surgical biopsy at the thickest portion of the melanoma should be performed to determine the depth of invasion of the melanoma. Staging follows the American Joint Committee on Cancer (AJCC) or International Union Against Cancer (UICC) guidelines.[78] Immunohistochemistry for HMB-45 and S100 can help differentiate melanoma from other cutaneous lesions.

All patients should undergo measurement of lactate dehydrogenase, and staging with CT or PET is indicated for patients with thick melanomas. Primary treatment for cutaneous melanoma is surgical excision. In the past, mastectomy was the recommended treatment but this is no longer considered necessary. Wide local excision of the lesion is recommended, with margins depending on the depth of invasion. SLNB for intermediate-thickness melanomas and thin melanomas with poor prognostic characteristics should also be done at the time of excision.[79] Lymphoscintigraphy should be performed prior to SLNB as in all trunk melanomas. Complete axillary dissection should be performed in patients with clinically suspicious adenopathy, those with positive SLNB and patients with melanomas greater than 4 mm.[80] Adjuvant treatment for primary melanoma of the breast follows current guidelines for treatment of melanoma found elsewhere in the body.

Metastasis to the breast

Metastatic disease to the breast is uncommon, with an incidence of 0.5–6.6% of breast malignancies.[81,82] The contralateral breast is the most common site of metastatic malignancy found in the breast.[83] Other common malignancies that metastasise to the breast are lymphoma, melanoma, rhabdomyosarcoma and small cell lung cancer.[77] Physical examination and imaging studies demonstrate masses that are usually indistinguishable from primary breast carcinoma. In most cases, core biopsy is preferred to FNA for pathological diagnosis since molecular studies and immunohistochemistry may play an important role in differentiating primary and metastatic tumours.[84] Treatment is directed at the primary malignancy. Prognosis is poor, with 80% of patients dying within 1 year.[77]

MALE BREAST CANCER

Epidemiology

The British physician John of Arderne reported the first case of male breast cancer (MBC) in the 14th century.[85] MBC accounts for 1% of all breast cancers in Western countries and only 0.1% of male cancer deaths.[86] The prevalence of MBC increases with age. The average age of diagnosis is about

10 years later than in women, but MBC can occur at any age. The incidence has remained stable over the past 40 years.[87] The average delay from onset of symptoms to diagnosis is 22 months.[88]

Risk factors

Alterations in estrogen and testosterone balance appear to play a role in the aetiology of MBCs. An elevated risk of developing MBC has been documented in men with a history of undescended testes, congenital inguinal hernia, orchiectomy, orchitis, testicular injury or infertility.[89,90] Males with Klinefelter's syndrome, which is characterised by gynaecomastia, small firm testes and a 47XXY karyotype, have a 50-fold increased risk of developing breast cancer.[91,92] Obesity and cirrhosis, which cause a hyperestrogenic state, are also linked to an elevated risk of developing MBC.[90,93] Gynaecomastia, once thought to be a risk factor, is now no longer believed to increase the risk of developing MBC.[88,90] Other risk factors include a history of radiation exposure, as in female breast cancer.[90]

Family history is an important risk factor. Between 15 and 20% of male patients with breast cancer have a family history of the disease.[94] The odds ratio for MBC increases with a positive family history and the risk increases as the number of affected first-degree relatives increases and as the age of diagnosis in affected relatives decreases.[94] These factors probably reflect an increasing risk of both *BRCA1* and *BRCA2* mutations. Inherited mutations such as *BRCA1* and *BRCA2* predispose men to developing breast cancer. Male carriers of *BRCA2* have a 6.3% cumulative risk of developing breast cancer.[95,96] In families with hereditary breast cancer, the presence of MBC increases the likelihood of having a *BRCA2* mutation. The number of MBCs attributable to *BRCA2* varies among populations and is 4% in the USA. However in Iceland, the 'founder effect' *BRCA2* mutation is present in 40% of MBCs.[96,97] More recent studies suggest that the risk of MBC is roughly equivalent in those with either *BRCA1* or *BRCA2* mutations.[99,99]

Clinical presentation

Of men with MBC, 85% present with a painless mass.[100] Nipple retraction, nipple ulceration, nipple discharge, and pain are other presenting signs and symptoms and 40–50% of men have nipple involvement due to the central location of most tumours.[101] The time from the onset of symptoms to diagnosis is longer in men and, as a result, men often present at later stages.

Differential diagnosis

Gynaecomastia, abscess, metastatic disease and sarcomas are the main conditions that should be excluded when diagnosing a breast mass in males. Physical examination and FNA or core biopsy are the most useful methods for differentiating MBC from other causes of breast masses in men.

Diagnosis

The work-up of a breast mass is similar in men and women, although imaging studies are less important in men. Physical examination characterises the size, shape and location of the mass, as well as the presence of nipple discharge, nipple retraction and skin changes. Examination of the axillary, supraclavicular and infraclavicular nodes should also be performed. A diagnostic mammogram and/or focused ultrasound can be used to characterise the lesion, but rarely obviates the need for a histological diagnosis. Since treatment is usually by mastectomy, imaging studies can often be omitted. As in women, diagnosis by needle biopsy, either core biopsy or FNA, is preferred to excisional biopsy.[102,103] Symptoms and abnormal laboratory values should guide the need for a metastatic work-up.

Pathology

Almost all pathological types of breast cancer found in women have been described in men. Most MBCs (90%) are invasive and of these, 80% are infiltrating ductal carcinoma and 5% are papillary.[104] Invasive lobular carcinoma represents only 1% of MBCs, probably due to the paucity of terminal lobules in the male breast. Paget's disease and inflammatory breast cancer are seen with similar frequency in men and women. Less common subtypes such as medullary, tubular, mucinous and squamous carcinomas have also been reported in men, but are found with lower frequencies than

seen in women. Of the 10% of MBCs that are non-invasive, almost all are DCIS.[104] Most are of the papillary subtype and are of low or intermediate grade.[105] Lobular carcinoma in situ is rare; when found, it is usually in conjunction with invasive lobular carcinoma.[101]

MBCs have a higher rate of estrogen receptor positivity than that in women when matched for age, stage and grade. Approximately 80% of MBCs are estrogen receptor positive and 75% are progesterone receptor positive.[88] There is limited information about erbB-2 or HER-2/neu over-expression in MBC, and its impact on prognosis is unclear. Data on other molecular markers found in female breast cancers, such as p53, bcl-2, cyclin D1 and epidermal growth factor receptor, is limited and their association with prognosis in MBC is inconclusive at this time.[106]

Prognosis

MBC is staged according to the AJCC or UICC staging system. As with female breast cancer, axillary lymph node status, tumour size, histological grade and hormone receptor status are significant prognostic factors in MBC.[107–110]

As in women, axillary lymph node status is the most important prognostic factor in MBC.[108] In one study of 335 cases, node-negative patients had a 90% 5-year survival rate while node-positive patients had a 65% 5-year survival rate.[107] The number of involved axillary nodes also predicts survival. The 10-year survival for patients with involvement of one to three nodes is 44% and this decreases to 14% in patients with four or more positive nodes.[108]

Histological grade of the tumour also predicts prognosis. Giordano et al.[88] reported 5-year survival for patients with grade 1 tumours of 76% compared with 66% for those with grade 2 tumours and 43% for those with grade 3 tumours. Hormone receptor status also appears to be associated with survival. Estrogen receptor-positive and progesterone receptor-positive tumours have significantly improved survival compared with estrogen receptor-negative and progesterone receptor-negative tumours.[111] Overall, stage for stage, MBC has the same prognosis as female breast cancer and the same factors predict outcome.

Treatment

Treatment of MBC is modelled on the treatment of female breast cancer. However, a retrospective review by Scott-Conner et al.[112] that compared treatment of matched MBC and female breast cancer patients found some significant differences. Males are less likely to have breast-conserving therapy than women, which would be expected given the anatomical considerations in the male breast. Men are also less likely to receive chemotherapy, and are less likely to receive radiation therapy if a lumpectomy is performed.

LOCAL THERAPY

Surgery is the primary therapy in MBC and mastectomy the most common procedure employed. Although breast-conserving surgery has been reported, the minimal amount of breast tissue in most male breasts and the central location of the majority of cancers do not make this a particularly attractive option. For stage I and II tumours, total mastectomy is the procedure of choice. If a small tumour is in proximity to the pectoralis major, it is reasonable to resect a small portion of the muscle with the specimen to ensure a negative margin. There is no longer any role for radical mastectomy. Locally advanced disease should be treated with neoadjuvant therapy followed by surgery. In most cases, this will allow a modified radical mastectomy to be performed. If the patient has clinically positive nodes, an axillary dissection should be done, as in women. If the axillary lymph nodes are clinically negative, SLNB can be performed. SLNB has been successfully performed in T1 and T2 tumours using a combination of preoperative lymphoscintigraphy, radioisotope tracer and isosulfan blue or patent blue V dye. The sensitivity and specificity are similar to that found in female breast cancer.[113,114]

ADJUVANT THERAPY

Endocrine therapy is indicated in hormone receptor-positive MBC. Single-institution trials have shown a survival benefit when tamoxifen is given to stage II and III breast cancers.[115] Small single-institution trials also indicate a survival benefit in men who receive cytotoxic chemotherapy.[116] The same guidelines used to make recommendations for women with breast cancer should be used for men.

No formal trials have been conducted to determine the indications for postmastectomy radiation in MBC, but a reduction in local recurrence with the use of radiation has been reported.[117] A recent retrospective review concluded that the indications for radiation therapy in MBC should be the same as for female breast cancer.[118]

Metastatic disease

Endocrine therapy is the mainstay of treatment for metastatic MBC. Orchiectomy and other ablative surgeries have been used to treat metastatic disease in the past. More recently, exogenous androgens, antiandrogens, steroids, estrogens, progestins, aminoglutethimide and tamoxifen have been reported to prolong survival.[115,119] Limited information is available on the effectiveness of the newer selective aromatase inhibitors. However, early reports indicate that aromatase inhibitors may not be as successful in men because they only block peripheral estrogen production, which accounts for 80% of estrogen production in men. The presence of an intact feedback loop to the hypothalamus can also lead to hyperstimulation of the testes during treatment with aromatase inhibitors, with increased circulating androgen levels. The remaining 20% of estrogen produced by the testes remains unopposed.[88] In hormone receptor-negative cancers, cytotoxic agents are the mainstay of therapy.[119]

REFERENCES

1. Paget J. On disease of the mammary areola preceding cancer of the mammary gland. St Barts Hospital Rep 1874; 10:87–9.

2. Vielh P, Validire P, Kheirallah S et al. Paget's disease of the nipple without clinically and radiologically detectable breast tumor. Histochemical and immunohistochemical study of 44 cases. Pathol Res Pract 1993; 189:150–5.

3. Lancer HA, Moschella SL. Paget's disease of the male breast. J Am Acad Dermatol 1982; 7:393–6.

4. Lagios MD, Westdahl PR, Rose MR, Concannon S. Paget's disease of the nipple. Alternative management in cases without or with minimal extent of underlying breast carcinoma. Cancer 1984; 54:545–51.

5. Kothari AS, Beechey-Newman N, Hamed H et al. Paget disease of the nipple: a multifocal manifestation of higher-risk disease. Cancer 2002; 95:1–7.

> With the increased interest in breast-conserving therapy for Paget's disease, this article highlights the importance of patient selection because of the high incidence of multifocality in Paget's disease.

6. Kister SJ, Haagensen CD. Paget's disease of the breast. Am J Surg 1970; 119:606–9.

7. Chaudary MA, Millis RR, Lane EB, Miller NA. Paget's disease of the nipple: a ten year review including clinical, pathological, and immuno-histochemical findings. Breast Cancer Res Treat 1986; 8:139–46.

8. Dixon AR, Galea MH, Ellis IO et al. Paget's disease of the nipple. Br J Surg 1991; 78:722–3.

9. Fu W, Lobocki CA, Silberberg BK et al. Molecular markers in Paget disease of the breast. J Surg Oncol 2001; 77:171–8.

10. Jacobeus HC. Paget's disease and its relationship to milk gland carcinoma. Virchows Arch Path Anat Physiol Klin Med 1904; 178:124–8.

11. Jahn H, Osther PJ, Nielsen EH et al. An electron microscopic study of clinical Paget's disease of the nipple. APMIS 1995; 103:628–34.

12. Ashikari R, Park K, Huvos AG et al. Paget's disease of the breast. Cancer 1970; 26:680–5.

13. Sakorafas GH, Blanchard K, Sarr MG, Farley DR. Paget's disease of the breast. Cancer Treat Rev 2001; 27:9–18.

14. Sakorafas GH, Blanchard DK, Sarr MG, Farley DR. Paget's disease of the breast: a clinical perspective. Langenbecks Arch Surg 2001; 386:444–50.

15. Jamali FR, Ricci A Jr, Deckers PJ. Paget's disease of the nipple–areola complex. Surg Clin North Am 1996; 76:365–81.

16. Kaelin CM. Paget's disease. In: Harris JR, Lippman ME, Morrow M, Osborne CK (eds) Diseases of the breast, 2nd edn. Baltimore: Lippincott Williams & Wilkins, 2000; pp. 277–83.

17. Rosen PP. Paget's disease of the nipple. In: Rosen PP (ed.) Rosen's breast pathology. Philadelphia: Lippincott–Raven, 1996; pp. 493–506.

18. Lucarotti ME, Dunn JM, Webb AJ. Scrape cytology in the diagnosis of Paget's disease of the breast. Cytopathology 1994; 5:301–5.

19. Smith KJ, Tuur S, Corvette D et al. Cytokeratin 7 staining in mammary and extramammary Paget's disease. Mod Pathol 1997; 10:1069–74.

20. Hitchcock A, Topham S, Bell J et al. Routine diagnosis of mammary Paget's disease. A modern approach. Am J Surg Pathol 1992; 16:58–61.

21. Ramachandra S, Gillett CE, Millis RR. A comparative immunohistochemical study of mammary and extramammary Paget's disease and superficial spreading melanoma, with particular emphasis on melanocytic markers. Virchows Arch 1996; 429:371–6.

22. Morris EA. Breast cancer imaging with MRI. Radiol Clin North Am 2002; 40:443–66.

23. Friedman EP, Hall-Craggs MA, Mumtaz H, Schneidau A. Breast MR and the appearance of the normal and abnormal nipple. Clin Radiol 1997; 52:854–61.

24. Marshall JK, Griffith KA, Haffty BG et al. Conservative management of Paget disease of the breast with radiotherapy: 10- and 15-year results. Cancer 2003; 97:2142–9.

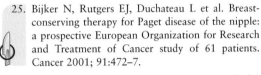

25. Bijker N, Rutgers EJ, Duchateau L et al. Breast-conserving therapy for Paget disease of the nipple: a prospective European Organization for Research and Treatment of Cancer study of 61 patients. Cancer 2001; 91:472–7.

> This is the largest prospective trial to date evaluating breast-conserving therapy in Paget's disease of the nipple with adequate follow-up.

26. Fu W, Mittel VK, Young SC. Paget disease of the breast: analysis of 41 patients. Am J Clin Oncol 2001; 24:397–400.

27. Kollmorgen DR, Varanasi JS, Edge SB, Carson WE III. Paget's disease of the breast: a 33-year experience. J Am Coll Surg 1998; 187:171–7.

28. Fourquet A, Campana F, Vielh P et al. Paget's disease of the nipple without detectable breast tumor: conservative management with radiation therapy. Int J Radiat Oncol Biol Phys 1987; 13:1463–5.

29. Polgar C, Orosz Z, Kovacs T, Fodor J. Breast-conserving therapy for Paget disease of the nipple: a prospective European Organization for Research and Treatment of Cancer study of 61 patients. Cancer 2002; 94:1904–5.

30. Stockdale AD, Brierley JD, White WF et al. Radiotherapy for Paget's disease of the nipple: a conservative alternative. Lancet 1989; ii:664–6.

31. Petrek JA. Pregnancy-associated breast cancer. Semin Surg Oncol 1991; 7:306–10.

> This is a key article in the PABC literature because it showed a similar survival in pregnant women compared with non-pregnant females with breast cancer. Prior to this, all women with PABC were thought to have a poor prognosis.

32. Antonelli NM, Dotters DJ, Katz VL, Kuller JA. Cancer in pregnancy: a review of the literature. Part II. Obstet Gynecol Surv 1996; 51:135–42.

33. National Cancer Institute. Breast cancer in pregnancy. Cancer-net. Available at http://www.cancer.gov/cancerinfo/pdq/treatment/breast-cancer-and-pregnancy#section_63

34. Gemignani ML, Petrek JA, Borgen PI. Breast cancer and pregnancy. Surg Clin North Am 1999; 79:1157–69.

35. Anderson JM. Mammary cancers and pregnancy. Br Med J 1979; 1:1124–7.

36. Zemlickis D, Lishner M, Degendorfer P et al. Maternal and fetal outcome after breast cancer in pregnancy. Am J Obstet Gynecol 1992; 166:781–7.

37. Woo JC, Yu T, Hurd TC. Breast cancer in pregnancy: a literature review. Arch Surg 2003; 138:91–8.

38. Ishida T, Yokoe T, Kasumi F et al. Clinico-pathologic characteristics and prognosis of breast cancer patients associated with pregnancy and lactation: analysis of case–control study in Japan. Jpn J Cancer Res 1992; 83:1143–9.

39. Jernstrom H, Lerman C, Ghadirian P et al. Pregnancy and risk of early breast cancer in carriers of BRCA1 and BRCA2. Lancet 1999; 354:1846–50.

40. King RM, Welch JS, Martin JK Jr, Coulam CB. Carcinoma of the breast associated with pregnancy. Surg Gynecol Obstet 1985; 160:228–32.

41. Ribeiro G, Jones DA, Jones M. Carcinoma of the breast associated with pregnancy. Br J Surg 1986; 73:607–9.

42. Scott-Conner CE, Schorr SJ. The diagnosis and management of breast problems during pregnancy and lactation. Am J Surg 1995; 170:401–5.

43. Guinee VF, Olsson H, Moller T et al. Effect of pregnancy on prognosis for young women with breast cancer. Lancet 1994; 343:1587–9.

44. Byrd BF Jr, Bayer DS, Robertson JC, Stephenson SE Jr. Treatment of breast tumors associated with pregnancy and lactation. Ann Surg 1962; 155:940–7.

45. Liberman L, Giess CS, Dershaw DD et al. Imaging of pregnancy-associated breast cancer. Radiology 1994; 191:245–8.

46. Ahn BY, Kim HH, Moon WK et al. Pregnancy- and lactation-associated breast cancer: mammographic and sonographic findings. J Ultrasound Med 2003; 22:491–7.

47. Gupta RK, McHutchison AG, Dowle CS, Simpson JS. Fine-needle aspiration cytodiagnosis of breast masses in pregnant and lactating women and its impact on management. Diagn Cytopathol 1993; 9:156–9.

48. Schackmuth EM, Harlow CM, Norton LW. Milk fistula: a complication after core biopsy. Am J Roentgenol 1993; 161:961–2.

49. Baker J, Ali A, Groch MW et al. Bone scanning in pregnant patients with breast carcinoma. Clin Nucl Med 1987; 12:519–24.

50. Hubbard AM, Crombleholme TM, Adzick NS et al. Prenatal MRI evaluation of congenital diaphragmatic hernia. Am J Perinatol 1999; 16:407–13.

51. Bonnier P, Romain S, Dilhuydy JM et al. Influence of pregnancy on the outcome of breast cancer: a case–control study. Societe Francaise de Senologie et de Pathologie Mammaire Study Group. Int J Cancer 1997; 72:720–7.

52. Keleher AJ, Theriault RL, Gwyn KM et al. Multi-disciplinary management of breast cancer concurrent with pregnancy. J Am Coll Surg 2002; 194:54–64.

53. Kilgore AR, Bloodgood JC. Tumors and tumor-like lesions of the breast in association with pregnancy. Arch Surg 1929; 18:2079–98.

54. Haagensen CD, Stout AP. Carcinoma of the breast: criteria for operability. Ann Surg 1943; 118:859–70.

55. Tretli S, Kvalheim G, Thoresen S, Host H. Survival of breast cancer patients diagnosed during pregnancy or lactation. Br J Cancer 1988; 58:382–4.

56. Duncan PG, Pope WD, Cohen MM, Greer N. Fetal risk of anesthesia and surgery during pregnancy. Anesthesiology 1986; 64:790–4.

57. Pedersen H, Finster M. Anesthetic risk in the pregnant surgical patient. Anesthesiology 1979; 51:439–51.

58. Morita ET, Chang J, Leong SP. Principles and controversies in lymphoscintigraphy with emphasis on breast cancer. Surg Clin North Am 2000; 80:1721–39.

59. Ebert U, Loffler H, Kirch W. Cytotoxic therapy and pregnancy. Pharmacol Ther 1997; 74:207–20.

60. Zemlickis D, Lishner M, Degendorfer P et al. Fetal outcome after in utero exposure to cancer chemotherapy. Arch Intern Med 1992; 152:573–6.

61. Berry DL, Theriault RL, Holmes FA et al. Management of breast cancer during pregnancy using a standardized protocol. J Clin Oncol 1999; 17:855–61.

   This article describes the largest series of patients treated with chemotherapy during pregnancy, with long-term follow-up of both the mother and infant.

62. Sood AK, Shahin MS, Sorosky JI. Paclitaxel and platinum chemotherapy for ovarian carcinoma during pregnancy. Gynecol Oncol 2001; 83:599–600.

63. De Santis M, Lucchese A, De Carolis S et al. Metastatic breast cancer in pregnancy: first case of chemotherapy with docetaxel. Eur J Cancer Care 2000; 9:235–7.

64. Isaacs RJ, Hunter W, Clark K. Tamoxifen as systemic treatment of advanced breast cancer during pregnancy: case report and literature review. Gynecol Oncol 2001; 80:405–8.

65. Nugent P, O'Connell TX. Breast cancer and pregnancy. Arch Surg 1985; 120:1221–4.

66. Kuper-Hommel MJ, Snijder S, Janssen-Heijnen ML et al. Treatment and survival of 38 female breast lymphomas: a population-based study with clinical

and pathological reviews. Ann Hematol 2003; 82:397–404.

67. Smith MR, Brustein S, Straus DJ. Localized non-Hodgkin's lymphoma of the breast. Cancer 1987; 59:351–4.

68. Ha CS, Dubey P, Goyal LK et al. Localized primary non-Hodgkin lymphoma of the breast. Am J Clin Oncol 1998; 21:376–80.

69. Brogi E, Harris NL. Lymphomas of the breast: pathology and clinical behavior. Semin Oncol 1999; 26:357–64.

70. Maddox JC, Evans HL. Angiosarcoma of skin and soft tissue: a study of forty-four cases. Cancer 1981; 48:1907–21.

This is the original article describing angiosarcoma of the skin and soft tissue and the largest series of patients with angiosarcoma.

71. Rao J, Dekoven JG, Beatty JD, Jones G. Cutaneous angiosarcoma as a delayed complication of radiation therapy for carcinoma of the breast. J Am Acad Dermatol 2003; 49:532–8.

This is an excellent review of all cases of angiosarcoma reported in the world's literature.

72. Cahan WG, Woodward KW, Higenbotham NL et al. Sarcoma arising from irradiated bone: report of 11 cases. Cancer 1948; 1:3–29.

73. Fineberg S, Rosen PP. Cutaneous angiosarcoma and atypical vascular lesions of the skin and breast after radiation therapy for breast carcinoma. Am J Clin Pathol 1994; 102:757–63.

74. Donnell RM, Rosen PP, Lieberman PH et al. Angiosarcoma and other vascular tumors of the breast. Am J Surg Pathol 1981; 5:629–42.

75. Stokkel MP, Peterse HL. Angiosarcoma of the breast after lumpectomy and radiation therapy for adenocarcinoma. Cancer 1992; 69:2965–8.

76. Ariel IM, Caron AS. Diagnosis and treatment of malignant melanoma arising from the skin of the female breast. Am J Surg 1972; 124:384–90.

77. Bartella L, Kaye J, Perry NM et al. Metastases to the breast revisited: radiological–histopathological correlation. Clin Radiol 2003; 58:524–31.

78. Balch CM, Buzaid AC, Soong SJ et al. Final version of the American Joint Committee on Cancer staging system for cutaneous melanoma. J Clin Oncol 2001; 19:3635–48.

79. Bedrosian I, Faries MB, Guerry D et al. Incidence of sentinel node metastasis in patients with thin primary melanoma (≤1 mm) with vertical growth phase. Ann Surg Oncol 2000; 7:262–7.

80. Essner R, Chung MH, Bleicher R et al. Prognostic implications of thick (≥4 mm) melanoma in the era of intraoperative lymphatic mapping and sentinel lymphadenectomy. Ann Surg Oncol 2002; 9:754–61.

81. Bohman LG, Bassett LW, Gold RH, Voet R. Breast metastases from extramammary malignancies. Radiology 1982; 144:309–12.

82. Amichetti M, Perani B, Boi S. Metastases to the breast from extramammary malignancies. Oncology 1990; 47:257–60.

83. Paulus DD, Libshitz HI. Metastasis to the breast. Radiol Clin North Am 1982; 20:561–8.

84. Hendrix MJ, Seftor EA, Kirschmann DA, Seftor RE. Molecular biology of breast cancer metastasis. Molecular expression of vascular markers by aggressive breast cancer cells. Breast Cancer Res 2000; 2:417–22.

85. Sheik O. Male breast cancer: factors influencing prognosis. Br J Cancer 1975; 30:13–35.

86. Weir HK, Thun MJ, Hankey BF et al. Annual report to the nation on the status of cancer, 1975–2000, featuring the uses of surveillance data for cancer prevention and control. J Natl Cancer Inst 2003; 95:1276–99.

87. La Vecchia C, Levi F, Lucchini F. Descriptive epidemiology of male breast cancer in europe. Int J Cancer 1992; 51:62–6.

88. Giordano SH, Buzdar AU, Hortobagyi GN. Breast cancer in men. Ann Intern Med 2002; 137:678–87.

This is an excellent overview of the risk factors, epidemiology and treatment of male breast cancer.

89. Mabuchi K, Bross DS, Kessler II. Risk factors for male breast cancer. J Natl Cancer Inst 1985; 7:371–5.

90. Thomas DB, Jimenez LM, McTiernan A et al. Breast cancer in men: risk factors with hormonal implications. Am J Epidemiol 1992; 135:734–48.

91. Jackson AW, Mulddal S, Ockey CH et al. Carcinoma of the male breast in association with Klinefelter syndrome. Br Med J 1965; 1:223–5.

92. Lynch HT, Kaplan AR, Lynch JF. Klinefelter syndrome and cancer. A family study. JAMA 1974; 229:809–11.

93. Braunstein GD. Diagnosis and treatment of gynecomastia. Hosp Pract (Off) 1993; 28(10A): 37–46.

94. Hill A, Yagmur Y, Tran KN et al. Localized male breast carcinoma and family history. An analysis of 142 patients. Cancer 1999; 86:821–5.

95. Friedman LS, Gayther SA, Kurosaki T et al. Mutation analysis of BRCA1 and BRCA2 in a male breast cancer population. Am J Hum Genet 1997; 60:313–19.

96. Thorlacius S, Olafsdottir G, Tryggvadottir L et al. A single BRCA2 mutation in male and female breast cancer families from Iceland with varied cancer phenotypes. Nat Genet 1996; 13:117–19.

97. Thorlacius S, Sigurdsson S, Bjarnadottir H et al. Study of a single BRCA2 mutation with high carrier

frequency in a small population. Am J Hum Genet 1997; 60:1079–84.

98. Thompson D, Easton DF. Cancer incidence in BRCA1 mutation carriers. J Natl Cancer Inst 2002; 94:1358–65.

99. Brose MS, Rebbeck TR, Calzone KA et al. Cancer risk estimates for BRCA1 mutation carriers identified in a risk evaluation program. J Natl Cancer Inst 2002; 94:1365–72.

100. Ribeiro G. Male breast carcinoma: a review of 301 cases from the Christie Hospital and Holt Radium Institute, Manchester. Br J Cancer 1985; 51:115–19.

101. Goss PE, Reid C, Pintilie M et al. Male breast carcinoma: a review of 229 patients who presented to the Princess Margaret Hospital during 40 years: 1955–1996. Cancer 1999; 85:629–39.

102. Westenend PJ, Jobse C. Evaluation of fine-needle aspiration cytology of breast masses in males. Cancer 2002; 96:101–4.

103. Pacelli A, Bock BJ, Jensen EA et al. Intracystic papillary carcinoma of the breast in a male patient diagnosed by ultrasound-guided core biopsy: a case report. Breast J 2002; 8:387–90.

104. Stalsberg H, Thomas DB, Rosenblatt KA et al. Histologic types and hormone receptors in breast cancer in men: a population-based study in 282 United States men. Cancer Causes Control 1993; 4:143–51.

105. Hittmair AP, Lininger RA, Tavassoli FA. Ductal carcinoma in situ (DCIS) in the male breast: a morphologic study of 84 cases of pure DCIS and 30 cases of DCIS associated with invasive carcinoma. A preliminary report. Cancer 1998; 83:2139–49.

106. Idelevich E, Mozes M, Ben Baruch N et al. Oncogenes in male breast cancer. Am J Clin Oncol 2003; 26:259–61.

107. Guinee VF, Olsson H, Moller T et al. The prognosis of breast cancer in males. A report of 335 cases. Cancer 1993; 71:154–61.

108. Cutuli B, Lacroze M, Dilhuydy JM et al. Male breast cancer: results of the treatments and prognostic factors in 397 cases. Eur J Cancer 1995; 31A:1960–4.

109. Ouriel K, Lotze MT, Hinshaw JR. Prognostic factors of carcinoma of the male breast. Surg Gynecol Obstet 1984; 159:373–6.

110. Salvadori B, Saccozzi R, Manzari A et al. Prognosis of breast cancer in males: an analysis of 170 cases. Eur J Cancer 1994; 30A:930–5.

111. Donegan WL, Redlich PN, Lang PJ, Gall MT. Carcinoma of the breast in males: a multi-institutional survey. Cancer 1998; 83:498–509.

112. Scott-Conner CE, Jochimsen PR, Menck HR et al. An analysis of male and female breast cancer treatment and survival among demographically identical pairs of patients. Surgery 1999; 126:775–80.

This is the largest retrospective case–control study of male and female breast cancer comparing treatment and survival.

113. Albo D, Ames FC, Hunt KK et al. Evaluation of lymph node status in male breast cancer patients: a role for sentinel lymph node biopsy. Breast Cancer Res Treat 2003; 77:9–14.

114. Port ER, Fey JV, Cody HS III, Borgen PI. Sentinel lymph node biopsy in patients with male breast carcinoma. Cancer 2001; 91:319–23.

115. Ribeiro G, Swindell R. Adjuvant tamoxifen for male breast cancer (MBC). Br J Cancer 1992; 65:252–4.

This article highlights the efficacy of endocrine therapy in male breast cancers, most of which are oestrogen receptor positive.

116. Patel HZ, Buzdar AU, Hortobagyi GN. Role of adjuvant chemotherapy in male breast cancer. Cancer 1989; 64:1583–5.

117. Schuchardt U, Seegenschmiedt MH, Kirschner MJ et al. Adjuvant radiotherapy for breast carcinoma in men: a 20-year clinical experience. Am J Clin Oncol 1996; 19:330–6.

118. Chakravarthy A, Kim CR. Post-mastectomy radiation in male breast cancer. Radiother Oncol 2002; 65:99–103.

119. Jaiyesimi IA, Buzdar AU, Sahin AA, Ross MA. Carcinoma of the male breast. Ann Intern Med 1992; 117:771–7.

Ten

Treatment of ductal carcinoma in situ

Nicola L.P. Barnes and
Nigel J. Bundred

BACKGROUND

The introduction of screening mammography has resulted in a marked increase in the detection of ductal carcinoma in situ (DCIS). Prior to the widespread use of breast screening, DCIS comprised less than 2% of newly diagnosed breast cancers. Since the introduction of national screening programmes, 25–30% of all screen-detected tumours are DCIS.[1] DCIS is a preinvasive breast cancer; the proliferations of malignant ductal epithelial cells remain confined by an intact basement membrane, with no invasion into the surrounding stroma.[2] Over 90% of DCIS currently diagnosed is impalpable, asymptomatic and detected by screening. These screening-detected cases are frequently small (<4 cm) and localised, and breast-conserving surgery is often possible. The remaining 10% present symptomatically, with a palpable breast lump, nipple discharge or Paget's disease of the nipple. If these symptoms are present, the underlying disease is usually extensive and frequently requires mastectomy. In the USA the number of new cases of DCIS increased by over fivefold (from 4901 cases to 28 958 cases) between 1983 and 1995 (maximally in women over 35 years of age),[3,4] but the actual population incidence of DCIS is unknown. Autopsy studies have shown varying prevalence rates, ranging from 0.2%[5] to 14%.[6] The sampling techniques and diagnostic criteria in these studies were not standardised and inadequate sampling of the breast tissue may have occurred. The actual population incidence of DCIS may well be higher than suggested by these methods.

RISK FACTORS, NATURAL HISTORY, PATHOLOGY AND RECEPTORS

Risk factors

Risk factors for the development of DCIS include a family history of breast cancer, older age at first childbirth and nulliparity.[7] Breast epithelial proliferation is increased by the use of the oral contraceptive pill[8] and hormone replacement therapy (HRT), particularly combined estrogen/progestogen HRT for over 5 years.[9] There is little evidence to date that either the oral contraceptive pill or HRT increases the risk of DCIS.[8] Two studies[10,11] have reported a relative risk of 1.4 for the development of DCIS following estrogen-only HRT preparations and a relative risk of 1.7–2.3 with estrogen and progestogen-containing preparations. Other studies have shown no increased risk following HRT use.[12,13]

Natural history

Although factors that pertain to an increased risk of developing DCIS have been identified, the natural history of this heterogeneous disease remains poorly understood. A review of DCIS recurrences and their primary lesions from the EORTC 10853 trial[14,15] found concordant histology (similar grade) in 62% of cases, and identical marker expression (estrogen receptor, progesterone receptor, p53 and c-erbB-2/HER-2/*neu*) in 63% of both invasive and non-invasive recurrences.[15] This high percentage of tumours with identical receptor profiles indicates that residual disease after initial treatment probably progresses to either further DCIS or invasive cancer. Retrospective studies of cases of low-grade DCIS misdiagnosed as benign found that, 20 years after local excision, approximately 33% of cases had developed an invasive cancer.[16] As not all cases of DCIS progress to invasive disease, detection by mammographic screening could lead to over-diagnosis and treatment of 'non-progressive DCIS', i.e. DCIS that would not have progressed to inva-sive disease if left untreated. A recent study used statistical modelling (Markov process model) to assess the probable extent of the overdiagnosis of non-progressive DCIS. This model estimates that a woman attending an incidence screen has a 166 times higher probability of having progressive DCIS or invasive cancer diagnosed than non-progressive DCIS;[17] in addition, although there is an element of overdiagnosis of non-progressive DCIS, this is small compared with the potential benefit of detecting more aggressive disease.

There is increasing evidence that the develop-mental pathways for low- and intermediate-grade DCIS are distinct from the development of high-grade DCIS. The initial development of low- and intermediate-grade DCIS compared with high-grade DCIS can be partly explained by reference to biological markers. In the sequence of progression from normal breast to DCIS, there is variable loss of chromosomal heterozygosity dependent on nuclear grade. Low- and intermediate-grade tumours show 16q loss, whereas there is 17p loss in high-grade lesions. It is likely that low-grade lesions arise from estrogen receptor-positive atypical ductal hyperplasia or lobular carcinoma in situ (LCIS) and progress to low-grade estrogen receptor-positive DCIS. High-grade lesions have no obvious precursor, unless they arise from usual ductal hyperplasia or atypical ductal hyperplasia that expresses 17p loss. The progression of well-differentiated/low-grade DCIS to poorly differentiated/high-grade DCIS or high-grade invasive cancer is an uncommon event.[15]

Pathology

CLASSIFICATION AND FEATURES

DCIS can be often classified into two major subtypes according to the presence or absence of comedo necrosis.[18] A tumour can be designated as comedo if atypical cells with abundant luminal necrosis fill at least one duct. The involved cells are large with pleomorphic nuclei and abnormal mitoses. The necrotic material often calcifies and is subsequently visible on mammography. Although reporting pathologists can state whether comedo necrosis is present, quantification of the number or percentage of involved ducts is subjective.

Non-comedo tumours encompass all other subtypes of DCIS.

- Solid: where tumour fills extended duct spaces.
- Micropapillary: where tufts of cells project into the duct lumen perpendicular to the basement membrane.
- Papillary: where the projecting tufts are larger than in the micropapillary type and contain a fibrovascular core.
- Cribriform: where the tumour takes on a fenestrated/sieve-like appearance.
- Clinging (flat): where there are variable columnar cell alterations along the duct margins. (There remains controversy as to whether clinging DCIS is truly an in situ cancer or whether it should be considered as hyperplastic rather than neoplastic.)

Rarer subtypes also exist, including neuroendocrine, encysted papillary, apocrine and signet cell.

The UK and EU-funded breast-screening pro-grammes use the system of low, intermediate and high nuclear grade to classify DCIS. This definition is based on the characteristics of the lesion as seen with a high-power microscope lens (×40) and uses a comparison of tumour cell size with normal epithelial and red blood cell size.[19]

- Low nuclear grade DCIS has evenly spaced cells with centrally placed small nuclei and few mitoses and the nucleoli are not easily seen.
- High nuclear grade DCIS has pleomorphic irregularly spaced cells with large irregular nuclei (often three times the size of erythrocytes), prominent nucleoli and frequent mitoses. It is often solid with comedo necrosis and calcification.
- Intermediate grade DCIS has features between those seen in low- and high-grade DCIS.

If a lesion contains areas of varying grade, it is awarded the highest grade present. A universally agreed classification system is yet to be established and will need to be observer independent and clinically relevant.

Traditionally, DCIS was thought of as a multicentric disease arising independently in multiple quadrants of the breast. Most cases of DCIS are now known to be unicentric.[20] Following extensive pathological sectioning of DCIS mastectomy specimens, only 1% show multicentric disease.[20] A **multicentric** tumour is defined as separate foci of tumour found in more than one breast quadrant, or more than 5 cm away from the initial primary. A tumour is considered **multifocal** if there are separate tumour foci in the same quadrant and close to the original tumour.[21] The local spread of DCIS is along the branching ducts (up to 20 or so) that form the glandular breast. The ducts, which are ill defined, often exceed the borders of a quadrant. Most DCIS is continuous along a given ductal segment, but poorly differentiated high-grade lesions can be multifocal.[22] These findings explain why most DCIS recurrences are at or near the site of the initial tumour,[23] but also why recurrences apparently remote from the initial lesion can exhibit similar genotypical and phenotypical characteristics to the primary lesion.[15]

As well as documenting pathological type and grade on the histology report, the pathologist often details the presence or absence of microinvasion. Microinvasion is an uncommon finding in DCIS and its classification is not standardised. However, as a general guide, microinvasion is a very small area of invasion (≤1 mm) that covers less than 0.5% of the histological slide area.[24] If microinvasion is detected histologically, a thorough examination of the entire specimen should be undertaken to exclude

other previously unnoticed areas of invasive cancer. Microinvasion confers a low risk of lymph node metastasis, approximately 2%.[25] Other lesions that can be mistaken for microinvasion include DCIS involving lobules, the branching of ducts, the distortion of ducts by acini or fibrosis, crush or cautery artefacts, and DCIS involving a benign sclerosing process (e.g. radial scar).[26–30]

LOBULAR CARCINOMA IN SITU

LCIS is a high-risk marker of invasive cancer but is not itself a premalignant lesion. It is often an incidental finding during breast biopsy and accounts for approximately 0.5% of symptomatic and 1% of screen-detected tumours. Ductal and lobular cells are anatomically contiguous in the ducto-lobular unit, but in situ ductal and lobular tumours show different pathological and clinical features. Patients developing LCIS tend to be younger and premenopausal, with bilateral and multicentric disease of lower grade and close to 100% estrogen receptor expression (**Table 10.1**).[30] Sometimes it is difficult to distinguish histologically between LCIS and DCIS and the pathology report should state this. The clinical interpretation of the report should take into account the increased risks from both tumour subtypes.

If LCIS is detected at core biopsy, the area of suspicion should be subjected to excision biopsy to confirm the diagnosis and exclude an adjacent invasive focus. If the LCIS is diagnosed coincidentally following excision of a coexisting lesion, no further treatment is necessary (even if the area of LCIS is not fully excised) and the patient should undergo regular outpatient review on a 'watch and wait' basis. The recent NSABP P-1 prevention trial showed a 56% reduction in risk of developing subsequent invasive cancer with tamoxifen.[31] Further studies are ongoing with raloxifene and aromatose inhibitors in patients with LCIS. Chemotherapy and radiotherapy have no place in the treatment of pure LCIS.

Receptors and markers

In order to advance our understanding of the development and behaviour of DCIS, there has been recent interest in cell receptor expression and signalling pathways controlling growth. These studies

Chapter Ten • Treatment of ductal carcinoma in situ

Table 10.1 • Comparative clinicopathological features of ductal carcinoma in situ (DCIS) and lobular carcinoma in situ (LCIS)

Clinicopathological feature	DCIS	LCIS
Age at diagnosis	54–58 years	44–47 years
Premenopausal	30%	70%
Absence of clinical signs	90%	99%
Mammographic findings	Micro-calcifications	None
Multicentric disease	30%	90%
Bilateral disease	12–20%	90%
Histological grade	65% high grade	90% low grade
Estrogen receptor status	65% positive	95% positive
Subsequent invasive disease	30–40%	25–30%
Ipsilateral–contralateral ratio	9:1	1:1

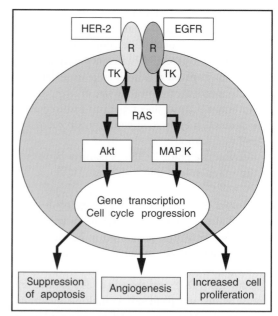

Figure 10.1 • The basic growth pathway in estrogen receptor-negative breast tumour cells. The estrogen receptor-positive signalling pathway is mediated via estrogen attaching to its receptor, which then moves down its concentration gradient to the cell nucleus. The presence of estrogen receptor in the cell nucleus subsequently increases gene transcription and expression of growth-promoting factors leading to increased cell proliferation and tumour growth. In cells that do not express estrogen receptors, the main signalling pathway for growth is via the epidermal growth factor (EGF)/c-erbB-2 receptor; this activates the RAS intracellular messenger, which increases cell proliferation and tumour growth via MAP kinase. RAS stimulation also leads to the suppression of the apoptosis cascade via Akt and BAD phosphorylation (an apoptotic protein). R, receptor; TK, tyrosine kinase; MAP K, MAP kinase.

have been mainly based on immunohistochemical assessment. They show that poorly differentiated high-grade comedo DCIS has low estrogen receptor expression, high rates of cell proliferation[32] (as expressed by Ki67, a nuclear antigen expressed in late G_1, S, G_2 and M phases of the cell cycle but not in the quiescent G_0)[33] and high rates of apoptosis,[34] and overexpresses c-erbB-2(HER-2/neu) and epidermal growth factor receptor (EGFR, a type 1 tyrosine kinase receptor).[32] Low-grade lesions have high estrogen receptor expression, with lower rates of cell proliferation[32] and apoptosis than high-grade lesions,[34] and they rarely express HER-2.[32] Progesterone receptor expression correlates with estrogen receptor expression in both low- and high-grade tumours.[32] In comparison, normal breast epithelium has low expression of estrogen receptor and progesterone receptor,[35] and a very low rate of apoptosis and HER-2 expression.

The increased rate of apoptosis seen in DCIS is lost on progression to invasive cancer, but the high proliferative rate is maintained.[36] Cyclin D1, an oncogene responsible for G_1 cell cycle proliferation/progression and induction of apoptosis, is over-

expressed in approximately 90% of in situ and invasive ductal cancers.[37] It also appears to be associated with a loss of differentiation (measured by p27[Kip1]).[38] In estrogen receptor-positive tumours, the driving force behind this increase in cell proliferation is the nuclear action of the activated estrogen receptor, which increases growth-promoting gene transcription. In estrogen receptor-negative tumours, the driving pathway is thought to be predominantly via EGFR/HER-2/RAS/MAP kinase activation (**Fig. 10.1**). This leads to a subsequent increase in transcription of both proliferative and, via Akt, anti-apoptotic genes. Activation of this pathway also induces the expression of cyclooxygenase

(COX)-2. COX-2 is an inducible enzyme that converts arachidonic acid to prostaglandins. It has been found to be overexpressed in up to 80% of DCIS.[39] COX-2-positive DCIS shows increased cell proliferation, and is related to increased tumour recurrence and decreased survival in invasive cancer.[40] Inhibition of COX-2 may be a potentially useful adjuvant therapy for estrogen receptor-negative DCIS.

In addition to alterations in cell proliferation and apoptosis, the development of neovascularisation is necessary for the growth of solid tumours. It is driven in part by angiogenic factors expressed in hypoxic areas of the tumour. Hypoxic areas of DCIS show a less well differentiated, more malignant phenotype of cells, with increased HIF-1α (a hypoxia-induced transcription factor), decreased estrogen receptor expression and increased expression of cytokeratin-19 (a breast stem cell marker).[28] It is felt that hypoxia-induced dedifferentiation could be a factor promoting tumour progression.[41]

PRESENTATION, INVESTIGATION AND DIAGNOSIS

Presentation

Over 90% of DCIS is detected at mammographic screening. Approximately 70% of these mammographically detected cases present as microcalcifications with no associated mass lesion. The calcifications may be heterogeneous, fine linear, branching, malignant or of indeterminate appearance. Microcalcifications with an associated mass lesion are identified in approximately 30% of DCIS mammograms.[42] Atypical mammographic features include circumscribed nodules, ill-defined masses, duct asymmetry and architectural distortion.[43] When diagnosed clinically, DCIS is often extensive or associated with a concurrent invasive tumour. It may present as a palpable mass, Paget's disease of the nipple or nipple discharge.[44]

Investigation and diagnosis

The importance of thorough clinical examination for detecting the above signs of DCIS or coexisting pathology should not be forgotten. In addition to clinical examination (often normal) and mammographic findings, diagnosis can only be confirmed by core biopsy, as cytology gives no information on stromal invasion. Image guidance to ensure the accuracy of sampling of these mainly impalpable mammographic lesions is vital. Mammographic magnification views are important in order to accurately delineate the extent of the microcalcifications.

STEREOTACTIC CORE BIOPSY AND VACUUM-ASSISTED BIOPSY

In the NHS breast-screening programme, the method of diagnosis is by stereotactic core biopsy with a 14G needle. Simple core biopsy is likely to be superseded by vacuum-assisted biopsy, which takes several contiguous biopsies during a single pass, and a metal clip can be inserted during the procedure to aid future localisation. Vacuum-assisted biopsy has higher sensitivity and specificity than core biopsy,[45,46] but it still underdiagnoses a coexisting invasive tumour in 10–20% of cases due to sampling error.[46] If the area of DCIS is extensive (>4 cm in size), multiple areas of the lesion need to be biopsied preoperatively to ensure that there is unlikely to be an invasive component to the disease and that all the microcalcifications are truly DCIS.

LOCALISATION-GUIDED BIOPSY

If the definitive histological diagnosis cannot be made with either core biopsy or vacuum-assisted biopsy, then an open biopsy will be necessary. Following mammographic magnification views, wires or radioactive tracers are used to localise the lesion and guide the surgeon during open biopsy. For extensive areas of microcalcification, bracketing wires, one at each extent of the area of concern, can be used to aid localisation and enable complete excision of the suspicious area. The excised specimen should be sent for immediate radiography, after careful orientation with Liga-clips, to confirm that all the microcalcification of concern has been excised. The guidelines of the British Association of Surgical Oncologists[47] recommend that 90% of diagnostic guided-biopsies for screen-detected abnormalities should weigh less than 20 g. Due to improved core biopsy diagnosis, wire-guided localisation procedures are usually therapeutic rather than diagnostic. However, the area of DCIS is often pathologically larger than mammographically suggested; this is especially true if magnification views are not used, and up to 30% of cases need re-excision to clear margins adequately.[48] Accurate orientation of the specimen is thus essential to minimise the volume of any re-excision.

TREATMENT: MASTECTOMY VERSUS BREAST-CONSERVING SURGERY

Mastectomy

Historically, DCIS was thought to be a multicentric disease, arising independently in multiple quadrants of the breast. Therefore, even after wide local excision became the accepted treatment for selected cases of invasive cancer, women with this preinvasive lesion were still undergoing mastectomy. The recurrence rate following mastectomy for DCIS is less than 1%.[49] As current evidence (see p. 151) points to DCIS being predominantly unicentric in origin, it is now recognised that mastectomy would be over-treatment for the majority of patients.[49] In 1983 mastectomy was performed for 71% of cases of DCIS in the USA but this had dropped to 44% by 1992.[50] A multidisciplinary consensus conference on the treatment of DCIS[1] recommends mastectomy for patients with large areas of DCIS (>4 cm), for multicentric disease and for patients where radiotherapy is contraindicated. Women should also be offered mastectomy if the excision margins are persistently involved following breast-conserving surgery and cavity re-excision. Women with DCIS requiring mastectomy are excellent candidates for skin-sparing mastectomy and immediate breast reconstruction.

Breast-conserving surgery

Breast-conserving surgery is now the treatment of choice for small localised areas of DCIS (<4 cm in diameter). These tumours often need to be radiologically localised preoperatively, as they are predominantly impalpable (see p. 153). The lesion should be excised in one piece if possible and orientated with Liga-clips. Before wound closure, the specimen should undergo radiography and the

results reported in order to ensure that all suspicious microcalcifications have been removed. Many surgeons use a four-quadrant cavity biopsy, with or without India ink staining to assess the surrounding breast. The pathologist must then assess the histological margin status, which should be clearly documented on the histology report. If the margins are close (<1 mm), the patient should undergo cavity re-excision, as clear margin status is a key prognostic factor. The DCIS consensus conference[1] agreed that the following criteria must be met before considering breast-conserving surgery without radiotherapy:

- tumour size must be less than 2 cm (pathological or mammographical);
- excision margins must be greater than 10 mm in each direction;
- the tumour must be of low or intermediate grade (grade I or II).

If these criteria cannot be met, adjuvant treatments, as discussed below, should be considered. The recommended treatment protocol for DCIS is shown in **Fig. 10.2**.

Axillary staging

The incidence of macroscopic lymph node metastasis in DCIS is less than 1%, and formal axillary staging in women with DCIS should be avoided.[51] Patients found to have positive lymph nodes (perhaps en bloc with the axillary tail at mastectomy) usually have occult invasive disease, and should be managed accordingly. Nodal micrometastases detected by immunohistochemistry have been reported in 5–14% of patients, although the prognostic relevance of this is unknown.[44] Sentinel node biopsy for DCIS is not currently indicated but is under investigation but may have a role in patients having mastectomy for DCIS.

RECURRENCE: RATES AND PREDICTORS

No trials have specifically evaluated breast-conserving surgery versus mastectomy in DCIS. The recurrence rate following mastectomy is known to be very low at less than 1%.[49] The overall

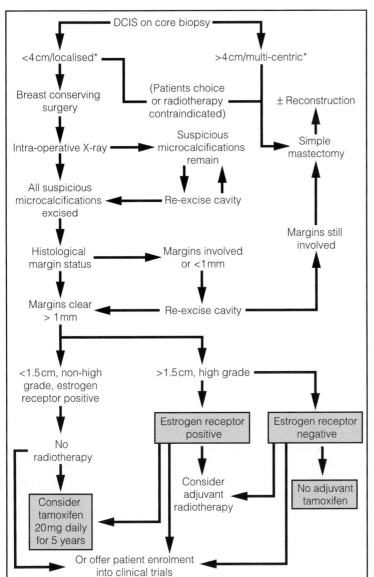

Figure 10.2 • Recommended treatment algorithm for ductal carcinoma in situ (DCIS).* Determined mammographically. Shaded boxes indicate those treatments suggested by the results of recent trials.[53,61]

recurrence for breast-conserving surgery alone is approximately 25% at 8 years follow-up, with up to 50% of recurrences (i.e. 12.5% of all cases) being invasive disease.[14,48,52,53] The women who develop invasive disease are at risk of metastatic spread. The remaining 50% of recurrences are in situ tumours, which by definition do not metastasise.[54] Reviews of clinical and pathological variables have demonstrated certain unfavourable tumour characteristics and these are outlined below.

Assessment of excision margins

A fundamental risk factor for recurrence is inadequate excision following breast-conserving surgery. This is judged as close (<1 mm) or involved margins[48] and/or failure to remove all suspicious microcalcifications.[55] Excision margin width has three times the power of tumour grade in predicting local recurrence.[56] The NSABP-B17, NSABP-B24 and

EORTC clinical trials all revealed that the presence of clear margins after local excision significantly decreased tumour recurrence.[14,57-59] On multivariate analysis of the EORTC trial, non-specified, close or involved margins conferred a hazard ratio of 2.07 (95% CI 1.35–3.16, P = 0.0008) compared with clear margins.[59] The NSABP-B24 trial found a covariate relative risk of 1.68 (95% CI 1.20–2.34) if the margins were involved. No prospective trials have looked at the optimum excision width required for in situ or invasive cancer. When considering the extent of surgical excision there has to be balance between minimising recurrence and an acceptable cosmetic outcome. A retrospective study by Chan et al.[48] reported that women with clear margins (judged as greater than 1 mm) had an 8.1% recurrence at a median follow-up of 47 months compared with 37.9% recurrence where excision margins were close (1 mm). There was no improvement in recurrence rates in more widely excised lesions.

High-grade/comedo tumours

High-grade tumours and tumours showing comedo necrosis are independent risk factors for recurrence. In a review of the EORTC 10853 trial,[59] high nuclear grade was found to have a hazard ratio of 2.23 (95% CI 1.41–3.51, P = 0.0011) for local recurrence, with 22% of high-grade tumours and 11% of intermediate-grade tumours developing either recurrent DCIS or invasive tumour. Comedo necrosis was also shown to be related to local recurrence, 18% of patients with comedo necrotic tumours developing recurrence (hazard ratio 1.80, 95% CI 1.08–3.00, P = 0.0183).

Histological type and tumour architecture

The degree of tumour differentiation is predictive of both local recurrence and metastatic disease. In the EORTC trial,[14,59] poorly differentiated tumours were at significantly higher risk of developing DCIS recurrence (hazard ratio 3.58, 95% CI 1.68–7.62, P = 0.0001) and metastasis (hazard ratio 6.65, 95% CI 1.46–30.22, P = 0.00083) than well-differentiated tumours. In this same trial, histological type was also strongly related to DCIS recurrence, though not to invasive recurrence. Both solid/comedo DCIS

(hazard ratio 4.40, 95% CI 2.28–8.48, P = 0.0001) and cribriform DCIS (hazard ratio 3.74, 95% CI 1.91–7.30, P = 0.0001) were found to be much more likely to recur than clinging or micropapillary tumours. Within the well-differentiated group, no tumours with clinging DCIS recurred.[59] It has been suggested that this well-differentiated clinging DCIS should be reclassified separately as 'columnar alteration with prominent apical snouts and secretion',[60] with debate as to whether this subtype would be more appropriately managed as atypical ductal hyperplasia or LCIS.

Age at diagnosis

A further risk factor for recurrence irrespective of tumour grade or type is a young age (<40 years) at diagnosis. The EORTC 10853 trial[14,59] found that women less than 40 years at diagnosis were more likely to recur (hazard ratio 2.54, 95% CI 1.53–4.23, P = 0.010) than older women. The NSABP B-24 trial[57] found that the rate of ipsilateral breast tumours (in the placebo population) in women aged 49 years or less at diagnosis was 33.3 per 1000, compared with 13.0 for those aged 50 and above. In the UK/ANZ DCIS trial,[61] only a small proportion (9.5%) of the women were less than 50 years old at diagnosis. The power of these results with regard to such a small subset may be limited, but of these younger women, 26% recurred after excision and tamoxifen compared with only 17% of women older than 50 years. Rodrigues et al.[62] studied women aged 42 years or less (mean age 38.5) or women aged 60 years or more (mean age 67.8) at diagnosis. They found that although there was no difference in tumour grade, comedo necrosis or overall histology (as also found in the EORTC trial) between the groups, c-erbB-2 was overexpressed in the younger patient population. Approximately 65% of the younger age group were c-erbB-2 positive compared with 38% of the older age group (P = 0.06). No significant difference was found between estrogen receptor, progesterone receptor, p53, Ki67, cyclin D1 or bcl-2 expression.

Tumour size and palpability

None of the major trials have found any statistical significance between recurrence and tumour size.

The NSABP-B17 trial[53] found that the size of mammographically detected tumours was not significant in predicting ipsilateral recurrence. However, when the researchers examined the clustering of microcalcifications in women whose mammograms did not show a tumour mass, they found that clustered microcalcifications greater than 10 mm (relative risk 2.06, 95% CI 1.36–3.10) or scattered calcifications (relative risk 2.41, 95% CI 1.40–4.16) had a significantly higher ipsilateral recurrence than clustered calcifications of 10 mm or less. The EORTC 10853 trial[59] found no difference in recurrence rates between tumours less than 10 mm in size and those 10–20 mm or greater than 20 mm in size ($P = 0.2127$). However, the tumours that were clinically apparent rather than mammographically detected were more likely to recur (covariate relative risk 2.17, 95% CI 1.53–3.08).[59]

Scoring systems

In order to bring together the most clinically relevant risk factors, Silverstein at al.[18] developed the Van Nuys Prognostic Index, with the aim of predicting which women would be at risk of recurrence following breast-conserving surgery. This numerical algorithm was derived from regression analysis of retrospective data pooled from patients with DCIS treated at two centres in the USA. The study was not randomised and used historical controls. The formula encompassed tumour size, margin width and pathological classification. The index has since been modified as the University of Southern California/Van Nuys Prognostic Index (USC/VNPI) and now includes patient age.[63] Each criterion is weighted with a score of 1, 2 or 3 and the individual scores combined to give an overall score from 4 to 12. Scores of 4–6, 7–9 and 10–12 are said to be at low, moderate and high risk of 5-year recurrence respectively. The data are skewed by the fact that 80% of large tumours (>4 cm) recurred, whereas in the UK these women would have undergone mastectomy. The value of the scoring system for a UK population, where the majority of cases of DCIS are small (<2 cm) and screen-detected (patients usually over 50 years old), may be limited. Boland et al.[56] were unable to demonstrate that size was a marker of recurrence in screen-detected DCIS in the UK.

Markers of recurrence

To improve the detection of specific patient groups at increased risk of recurrence, biological markers that could help determine recurrence potential in DCIS are being investigated. Provenzano et al.[64] found that estrogen receptor, progesterone receptor and bcl-2 negativity and HER-2 and p-21 positivity were associated with an increased risk of clinical recurrence. This was irrespective of tumour grade. Estrogen receptor, progesterone receptor, bcl-2 and HER-2 were found to be interdependent on each other, whereas p-21 was found to be independent of the above associations, which is thought to reflect the differing biological pathways of action between the markers. There has also been recent interest in another member of the type 1 tyrosine kinase receptor family, c-erbB-4/HER-4. Studies of invasive breast cancer have found that c-erbB-4 appears to have a protective effect against tumour recurrence. Tumours that showed coexpression of HER-2 and HER-4 had a better prognosis (reduced recurrence) than HER-2 positive HER-4 negative tumours.[65,66] The same has been demonstrated in DCIS.[67] A summary of the risk factors for DCIS recurrence is shown in **Box 10.1**.

ADJUVANT THERAPY

Radiotherapy

Three main trials have examined the value of radiotherapy following breast-conserving surgery for DCIS. The NSABP-B17,[53] EORTC 10853[14] and UK/ANZ DCIS[61] trials each studied a radiation dose of 50 Gy in 25 fractions. All found a significant reduction in ipsilateral recurrence following radiotherapy (**Table 10.2; Fig. 10.3**). The reduction was similar for both in situ and invasive recurrence. In the EORTC trial, DCIS recurrences reduced from 8% to 5% (hazard ratio 0.65, 95% CI 0.41–1.03) and invasive recurrences from 8% to 4% (hazard ratio 0.60, 95% CI 0.37–0.97) at 5 years follow-up.[14] An actual survival advantage following radiotherapy was not found in either the NSABP-B17 or EORTC 10853 trials (the UK/ANZ DCIS trial has had too few deaths to reach any conclusions). The DCIS consensus statement[1] and pathological review

Chapter Ten • Treatment of ductal carcinoma in situ

Box 10.1 • Risk factors for recurrence of ductal carcinoma in situ. Poor-prognosis tumours often possess multiple bad prognostic features, i.e. they tend to be poorly differentiated, high-grade, comedo tumours that are estrogen receptor negative and overexpress c-erbB-2

Excision margins	Margins ≤1 mm after breast-conserving surgery
Tumour grade	High grade (III)
Comedo necrosis	Present
Histological type	Poorly differentiated
Patient age	Younger age at diagnosis (≤40 years)
Biological markers	
Negativity	Estrogen receptor Progesterone receptor bcl-2 ?HER-4
Positivity	HER-2 p21 p53 Ki67 (high-percentage expression)
Patient presentation	Symptomatic
Tumour size	Not significant

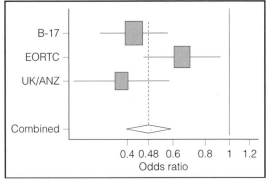

Figure 10.3 • Radiotherapy trials overview: ipsilateral ductal carcinoma in situ (DCIS) and invasive recurrences. This Forrest plot of the major randomised controlled trials of radiotherapy in DCIS (B17,[53] EORTC[14] and UK/ANZ[61]) shows a significant reduction in ipsilateral recurrence risk following radiotherapy for all trials, with a combined odds ratio for the reduction in recurrence of DCIS and invasive disease of 0.48 for all trials. From Trials of DCIS – results from clinical trials. Surg Oncol J 2003; 12:213–19, with permission.

of the EORTC trial suggested that completely excised low-grade DCIS has a recurrence rate of just 4% at 5 years, making adjuvant radiotherapy difficult to recommend due to the associated morbidity. In the USA, it is recommended that all patients who have undergone breast-conserving surgery for DCIS receive a course of radiotherapy.[53] In Europe, adjuvant radiotherapy is recommended for all high-grade DCIS. Intermediate- and low-grade DCIS is selected for adjuvant radiotherapy on an individual patient basis.

Endocrine therapy

Although radiotherapy reduces tumour recurrence following breast-conserving surgery, there is still an overall recurrence rate of 3–13%[14,53,61] at 5 years and research into the use of additional adjuvant therapies for DCIS remains important. The NSABP-B24 trial compared breast conserving-surgery and

radiotherapy with or without adjuvant tamoxifen. The study found that tamoxifen following breast-conserving surgery and radiotherapy was of benefit in reducing recurrence. There were 43% fewer invasive breast cancer events and 31% fewer non-invasive events in the tamoxifen-treated group.[53] The main advantage was in reducing invasive recurrence in the ipsilateral breast, although there was a significantly lower cumulative incidence of all breast cancer-related events in the tamoxifen group. In this trial, 30% of women were younger than 50 years at diagnosis and the reduction in recurrence was largely due to a 40% reduction in this younger age group, while there was only a 20% reduction in the age group greater than 50 years. A retrospective review of the NSABP-B24 results showed that tamoxifen was only beneficial in estrogen receptor-positive cases. The relative risk of recurrence of any breast cancer in the estrogen receptor-positive cohort was 0.41 (95% CI 0.25–0.65, $P = 0.0002$), whereas there was little benefit in the estrogen receptor-negative cases (relative risk 0.80, $P = 0.51$).[68] The UK/ANZ DCIS trial found that adjuvant tamoxifen reduced overall DCIS recurrence (hazard ratio 0.68, 95% CI 0.49–0.96, $P = 0.03$) but not invasive disease[61] (see **Table 10.2**).

Table 10.2 • Summary of major radiotherapy/tamoxifen clinical trials following breast-conserving therapy for ductal carcinoma in situ

	NSABP-17*		NSABP-24*		EORTC 10853[†]		UK/ANZ DCIS[‡]			
	BCS alone	BCS and XRT	BCS and XRT	BCS, XRT and tamoxifen	BCS alone	BCS and XRT	BCS alone	BCS and XRT	BCS and tamoxifen	BCS, XRT and tamoxifen
Number of patients	403	411	899	899	500	502	544	267	567	316
Number of local recurrences at median follow-up:										
43 months	64	28	–	–	–	–	–	–	–	–
48 months	–	–	–	–	83	53	–	–	–	–
53 months	–	–	–	–	–	–	119	22	101	21
74 months	–	–	130	84	–	–	–	–	–	–
90 months	140	47	–	–						
Local recurrence rates:										
4 year all recurrences	–	–	–	–	16%	9%	–	–	–	–
4 year invasive	–	–	–	–	8%	4%	–	–	–	–
5 year all recurrences	–	–	13%	8.2%	–	–	15%	3%	12%	3%
5 year invasive	–	–	7%	4.1%	–	–	5%	1%	5%	2%
8 year all recurrence	27%	12%	–	–	–	–	–	–	–	–
8 year invasive	13%	4%	–	–	–	–	–	–	–	–
Number of distant metastases	6	9	7	3	12	12	–	–	–	–
Total number of contralateral breast events	19	20	36	18	8	21	17	5	6	5
Number of contralateral invasive breast cancers	16	12	23	15	5	16	10	5	5	5
Bilateral event-free survival at:										
4 years	–	–	–	–	82%	86%	–	–	–	–
5 years	74%	84%	83%	87%	–	–	85%	97%	88%	97%
8 years	60%	75%	–	–	–	–	–	–	–	–

BCS, breast-conserving surgery; XRT, radiotherapy.

*Fisher ER, Dignam J, Tan-Chiu E et al. Pathologic findings from the National Surgical Adjuvant Breast Project (NSABP) eight-year update of Protocol B-17: intraductal carcinoma. Cancer 1999; 86:429–38.

[†]Julien J, Bijker N, Fentimen I et al. Radiotherapy in breast-conserving treatment for ductal carcinoma in situ: first results of the EORTC randomized phase III trial 10853. EORTC Breast Cancer Cooperative Group and EORTC Radiotherapy group. Lancet 2000; 355:528–33.

[‡]UK Coordinating Committee on Cancer Research (UKCCCR). Ductal carcinoma in situ (DCIS) Working Party on behalf of DCIS trialists in the UK, Australia and New Zealand. Radiotherapy and tamoxifen in women with completely excised ductal carcinoma in situ of the breast in the UK, Australia and New Zealand: randomised controlled trial. Lancet 2003; 362:95–103.

The UK/ANZ DCIS trial has not yet published a breakdown of tamoxifen response in relation to estrogen receptor status. A further study showing that response to tamoxifen is confined to estrogen receptor-positive DCIS also examined estrogen withdrawal (i.e. stopping HRT) in women with estrogen receptor-positive or -negative DCIS. There was a significant decrease in cell proliferation in the estrogen receptor-positive group but no change in proliferation was observed in estrogen receptor-negative tumours.[69] Results of the Canadian RTOG 98-04 trial comparing tamoxifen with or without radiotherapy following breast-conserving therapy are awaited.

In the randomised controlled trials, the rate of contralateral breast cancer after DCIS is 0.5% per year for 10 years. As tamoxifen can halve the risk of breast cancer in the contralateral breast, it could also be regarded as a chemopreventive agent. This could potentially justify its use in all estrogen receptor-positive women. However, approximately 60% of DCIS express HER-2. Estrogen receptor-positive tumours that also express HER-2 are often resistant to tamoxifen therapy but do respond to therapy with aromatase inhibitors. A comparison of tamoxifen with anastrozole (a third-generation aromatase inhibitor) after complete excision of DCIS is being tested in the IBIS II trial.

FOLLOW-UP AND PROGNOSIS

Following primary treatment for DCIS and radiological and pathological confirmation that there has been complete excision of all suspicious microcalcifications with clear margins, patients should be given the opportunity to participate in clinical trials. Follow-up in outpatient clinics, after the initial postoperative reviews, should be by annual bilateral two-view mammography to detect recurrence. Although most DCIS recurrence is impalpable, clinical examination is still important for detecting invasive recurrences, especially in the premenopausal breast. Breast cancer-specific mortality following breast-conserving surgery for DCIS is less than 2% at 10 years[3] and is not influenced by adjuvant radiotherapy.[7,70] This figure is comparable to that following mastectomy.

MANAGEMENT OF RECURRENCE

In situ recurrence

Patients with an in situ recurrence where the primary was treated with breast-conserving surgery alone can be offered re-excision (ensuring clear margins) followed by postoperative radiotherapy. Patients who have already received radiotherapy following their primary excision should be advised to have completion mastectomy. A skin-sparing mastectomy with a myocutaneous flap breast reconstruction gives excellent results.

Invasive recurrence

The management of invasive recurrence is again dependent on the initial therapy for DCIS. If the patient did not receive radiotherapy after initial DCIS excision, then wide local excision and radiotherapy may still be an option depending on the size and location of the invasive tumour. If wide local excision is not an option, then mastectomy and axillary staging is the treatment of choice, with adjuvant therapy dictated by standard protocol as for primary invasive cancers. Studies following salvage treatment for both in situ and invasive recurrences of DCIS have shown overall cause-specific survival rates in excess of 90% at 8 years after recurrence.[54]

DCIS OF THE MALE BREAST

DCIS accounts for 1.9–15% of breast cancers in men. It mainly presents clinically with symptoms of a retro-areola cystic-type mass or bloody nipple discharge. The clinical, rather than mammographic, detection possibly accounts for the different incidence of DCIS between men and women. The predominant histological subtypes in pure DCIS in men are papillary and cribrifrom, the standard treatment being total mastectomy with excision of the nipple–areola complex.[71] Pure DCIS is nearly all of low or intermediate grade; less than 3% of cases are high grade.[72] In a series of 114 patients, 84 with pure DCIS and 30 with DCIS and invasive cancer, there were no cases of high-grade comedo DCIS without an invasive tumour.[72] The percentage of men with DCIS that eventually develop an invasive cancer is not known.

THE FUTURE

Radiotherapy trials

The benefits of radiotherapy following breast-conserving surgery for DCIS are now clear, although clarification is needed as to which subsets of women definitely do or do not require radiotherapy. A UK trial has been proposed with the aim of studying the need for radiotherapy in women with estrogen receptor-positive low/intermediate-grade disease who are receiving adjuvant systemic hormonal therapy following local excision with clear margins.

Chemoprevention trials

The aim of adjuvant therapy for in situ breast cancer is the prevention of progression to invasive malignancy. The NSABP P-1 chemoprevention trial[73] compared tamoxifen to placebo in patients at high risk of breast cancer. The study reported a 49% reduction in incidence of invasive cancer and a 50% reduction of DCIS in the tamoxifen-treated group. The reduction in contralateral breast cancer was only seen in estrogen receptor-positive cases and no benefit was seen for estrogen receptor-negative patients. There is also interest into the potential use of aromatase inhibitors, which have a better side-effect profile than tamoxifen. The IBIS II trial, currently underway, randomises postmenopausal women with estrogen receptor-positive DCIS treated with breast-conserving surgery to receive tamoxifen (20 mg daily) or the aromatase inhibitor anastrozole (1 mg daily) for 5 years. It also stratifies women between anastrozole and placebo for high-risk postmenopausal chemoprevention. The NSABP B-35 trial will also compare tamoxifen versus anastrozole in postmenopausal women following breast-conserving surgery and radiotherapy for DCIS.[74]

The Canadian-based RTOG 98-04 trial is studying women with 'good-risk' DCIS (unicentric, low/intermediate grade, ≤2.5 cm) with clear margins following breast-conserving surgery, randomising them to receive tamoxifen alone or tamoxifen and radiotherapy.

National DCIS audit (Sloane Project)

The Sloane Project aims to audit all screen-detected DCIS in the UK over the course of 5 years. This will potentially collect data on 2000 cases per year. All 98 screening units in the country are expected to take part. For each case the clinical, pathological, radiological and treatment characteristics will be documented following the NHS Breast Screening Programme guidelines.

Novel therapies

A number of new classes of agent are being developed for use in chemoprevention or therapy for DCIS. The compounds targeted are selective blockers of either the estrogen receptor-dependent or the estrogen receptor-independent growth pathways (see **Fig. 10.1**) and include selective estrogen receptor down-regulators, new aromatase inhibitors (which prevent estrogen biosynthesis by inhibiting the conversion of adrenal androgens to estrogens), signal transduction inhibitors (e.g. EGFR tyrosine kinase inhibitors, RAS farnesylation transferase inhibitors, MAP kinase inhibitors), and COX-2 inhibitors. If disrupted, the RAS/MAP kinase pathway may have a strong chemopreventive/chemotherapeutic effect and is an important target pathway in estrogen-independent (estrogen receptor-negative) tumours. Treatment of human DCIS xenografts with the EGFR/tyrosine kinase inhibitor Iressa has been shown to inhibit cell proliferation and MAP kinase activation.[75] Farnesyltransferase inhibitors (e.g. R115777, which blocks the farnesylation step in the RAS activation pathway[76]) are also being investigated; HER-2 also signals via RAS activation and around 60% of DCIS express HER-2. Due to the possible protective effect of c-erbB-4 on recurrence (see p. 157), 'selective c-erb receptor' inhibition, rather than 'pan c-erb receptor' blockade, may be an ultimate goal when precise pathways of action are known.

COX-2 inhibitors (e.g. celecoxib) are also under investigation and have been shown to prevent tumour formation in *HER2* transgenic mice.[77] Further in vivo studies in animal models and randomised trials in patient populations with DCIS are underway.

Optimising treatment

Controversies regarding the optimum management of this heterogeneous preinvasive lesion still reign. The surgeon should ensure complete pathological and radiological excision of DCIS and discuss appropriate adjuvant therapy (radiotherapy or endocrine) with the patient in a multidisciplinary setting in order to minimise recurrence without overtreatment.

• Key points

- DCIS is a preinvasive breast tumour; the proliferation of malignant epithelial cells is confined within an intact basement membrane. The developmental pathway for low- and intermediate-grade DCIS is different from that for high-grade DCIS.
- DCIS accounts for approximately 25% of new screen-detected cancers.
- Small localized areas of DCIS (<4 cm) should be treated with breast-conserving surgery with or without radiotherapy. Larger lesions need to be treated by mastectomy. Axillary surgery should be avoided.
- Up to 13% of cases recur at 5 years following breast-conserving surgery and radiotherapy, 50% of which (i.e. up to 6.5% of all cases) may be invasive disease.
- The key factor for decreasing tumour recurrence is clear margins at the time of surgery.
- Bad prognostic factors include younger age at diagnosis (<40 years), poorly differentiated high-grade tumours, the presence of comedo necrosis, HER2 positivity and estrogen receptor negativity.
- Tamoxifen is not indicated after mastectomy for DCIS but is valuable in estrogen receptor-positive lesions subjected to wide local excision.

REFERENCES

1. Schwartz GF, Solin LJ, Olivotto IA et al. and the consensus conference committee. The consensus conference on the treatment of in situ ductal carcinoma of the breast, 22–25 April 1999. Cancer 2000; 88:946–54.

   This paper summarises the findings of a consensus conference panel consisting of approximately 30 experts in the field of DCIS and addresses issues of diagnosis and management of DCIS. The major findings are that the optimum treatment for small localised areas of disease is breast-conserving surgery and that axillary surgery is not indicated for DCIS.

2. Lagios MD. Heterogeneity of ductal carcinoma in situ of the breast. J Cell Biochem Suppl 1993; 17G:49–52.

3. Ernster VL, Barclay J, Kerlikowske K et al. Mortality among women with ductal carcinoma in situ of the breast in the population-based surveillance, epidemiology and end results program. Arch Intern Med 2000; 160:953–8.

4. Ernster VL, Barclay J. Increases in ductal carcinoma in situ (DCIS) of the breast in relation to mammography: a dilemma. J Natl Cancer Inst Monogr 1997; 22:151–6.

   This article reviews the diagnosis and treatment of DCIS in the USA, highlighting the dramatic increase in detection of DCIS with the advent of breast screening programmes.

5. Bartow SA, Pathak DR, Black WC et al. Prevalence of benign, atypical and malignant breast lesions in populations at different risk for breast cancer. A forensic autopsy study. Cancer 1987; 60:2751–60.

6. Neilsen M, Thomsen JL, Primsahl S et al. Breast cancer and atypia among young and middle-aged women: a study of 110 medicolegal biopsies. Br J Cancer 1987; 56:814–19.

7. Rakovitch E. Part 1. Epidemiology of ductal carcinoma in situ. Curr Probl Cancer 2000; 24:100–11.

8. Williams G, Anderson E, Howell A et al. Oral contraceptive (OCP) use increases proliferation and decreases oestrogen receptor content of epithelial cells in the normal human breast. Int J Cancer 1991; 48:206–210.

9. Hofseth LJ, Raafat AM, Osuch JR et al. Hormone replacement therapy with oestrogen or oestrogen plus medoxyprogesterone acetate is associated with increased epithelial proliferation in the normal post-menopausal breast. J Clin Endocrinol Metab 1999; 84:4559–65.

10. Schairer C, Byrne C, Keyl PM et al. Menopausal estrogen and estrogen–progestin replacement therapy and the risk of breast cancer (United States). Cancer Causes Control 1994; 5:491–500.

11. Longnecker MP, Bernstein L, Paganini-Hill A et al. Risk factors for in situ breast cancer. Cancer Epidemiol Biomarkers Prev 1996; 5:961–5.

12. Henrick JB, Kornguth PJ, Viscoli CM, Horwitz RI. Postmenopausal estrogen use and invasive versus in situ breast cancer risk. J Clin Epidemiol 1998; 51:1277–83.

13. Gapstur SM, Morrow M, Sellars TA. Hormone replacement therapy and risk of breast cancer with a favourable histology: results of the Iowa Women's Health Study. JAMA 1999; 281:2091–7.

14. Julien J, Bijker N, Fentimen I et al. Radiotherapy in breast-conserving treatment for ductal carcinoma in situ: first results of the EORTC randomized phase III trial 10853. EORTC Breast Cancer Cooperative Group and EORTC Radiotherapy group. Lancet 2000; 355:528–33.

> The results of a multicentre, randomised, controlled trial of 1010 patients with DCIS treated with breast-conserving surgery, randomised to receive no further treatment or radiotherapy. The study found that radiotherapy reduced overall invasive (40% reduction, P = 0.04) and non-invasive (35% reduction, P = 0.06) ipsilateral recurrences (median follow-up 4.25 years).

15. Bijker N, Peterse JL, Duchateau L et al. Histological type and marker expression of the primary tumour compared with its local recurrence after breast-conserving therapy for ductal carcinoma in situ. Br J Cancer 2001; 84:539–44.

> A review of 116 cases from the EORTC 10853 trial (local excision of DCIS plus or minus radiotherapy) that had recurred following initial treatment, comparing the histology of the primary DCIS and the recurrent disease. The authors found that there was concordant histology in 62% of cases and identical marker expression in 63%, concluding that primary DCIS and its recurrence were related by histology or marker expression and that local recurrence reflects growth of residual DCIS.

16. Page DL, Dupont WD, Rogers LW et al. Continued local recurrence of carcinoma 15–25 years after a diagnosis of low grade ductal carcinoma in situ of the breast treated only by biopsy. Cancer 1995; 76:1197–200.

17. Yen M-F, Tabár L, Vitak B et al. Quantifying the potential problem of over diagnosis of ductal carcinoma in situ in breast cancer screening. Eur J Cancer 2003; 39:1746–54.

18. Silverstein MJ, Lagios MD, Craig PH et al. A prognostic index for ductal carcinoma in situ of the breast. Cancer 1996; 77:2267–74.

19. Pathology Reporting in Breast Cancer, 2nd edn. Sheffield: National Health Service Breast Screening Programme Publications, Report No. 3, 1995; pp. 22–7.

20. Holland R, Hendriks JH, Vebeek AL et al. Extent, distribution, and mammographic/histological correlations of breast ductal carcinoma in situ. Lancet 1990; 335:519–22.

21. Steering Committee on Clinical Practice Guidelines for the Care and Treatment of Breast Cancer. The management of ductal carcinoma in situ (DCIS). Can Med Assoc J 1998; 158(suppl.):S27–S34.

22. Faverley DRG, Burgers L, Bult P et al. Three dimensional imaging of mammary ductal carcinoma in situ: clinical implications. Semin Diagn Pathol 1994; 11:193–8.

23. Holland PA, Ghandi A, Knox WF et al. The importance of complete excision in the prevention of local recurrence of ductal carcinoma in situ. Br J Cancer 1998; 77:110–14.

24. Silverstein MJ, Waisma JR, Gamagam P et al. Intraductal carcinoma of the breast. Clinical factors influencing treatment choice. Cancer 1990; 66:102–8.

25. Von Dongen JA, Harris JR, Peterse JL et al. In situ cancer. The EORTC consensus meeting. Lancet 1989; i:25–7.

26. Kerner H, Lichtig C. Lobular cancerisation: incidence and differential diagnosis with lobular carcinoma in situ of the breast. Histopathology 1986; 10:621.

27. Fisher ER. Pathobiological considerations relating to the treatment of carcinoma of the breast. CA 1996; 47:52.

28. Eusebi V, Collina G, Bussolati G. Carcinoma in situ in sclerosing adenosis of the breast. An immuno-cytochemical study. Semin Diagn Pathol 1989; 6:146.

29. Youngston BJ, Cranor M, Powell C, Rosen PP. Epithelial displacement in surgical breast specimens following needling procedures. Am J Surg Pathol 1994; 18:896.

30. Akashi-Tanaka S, Fukotomi T, Nanasawa T et al. Treatment of non-invasive carcinoma: fifteen-year results at the National Cancer Centre Hospital in Tokyo. Breast Cancer 2000; 7:341–4.

31. Dunn BK, Ford LG. Breast cancer prevention: results of the National Surgical Adjuvant Breast and Bowel Project (NSABP) breast cancer prevention trial (NSABP P-1: BCPT). Eur J Cancer 2000; 36(suppl. 4):49–50.

32. Millis RR, Bobrow LG, Barnes DM. Immuno-histochemical evaluation of biological markers in mammary carcinoma in situ: correlation with morphological features and recently proposed schemes for histological classification. Breast 1996; 5:113–22.

33. Sullivan RP, Mortimer G, Muircheartaigh IO. Cell proliferation in breast tumours: analysis of histological parameters Ki67 and PCNA expression. Ir J Med Sci 1993; 162:343–7.

34. Boland GP Knox WF, Bundred NJ. Molecular markers and therapeutic targets in ductal carcinoma in situ. Microsc Res Tech 2002; 59:3–11.

35. Shoker BS, Jarvis C, Clarke RB et al. Estrogen receptor-positive proliferating cells in the normal and pre-cancerous breast. Am J Pathol 1999; 155:1811–15.

36. Parton M, Dowsett M, Smith I. Studies of apoptosis in breast cancer. Br Med J 2001; 322:1528–32.

37. Weinstat-Saslow D, Merino MJ, Manrow RE et al. Overexpression of cyclin D mRNA distinguishes invasive and in situ breast carcinomas from non-malignant lesions. Nat Med 1995; 1:1257–60.

38. Zhou Q, Hopp T, Fuqua SA, Steeg PS. Cyclin D1 in breast pre-malignancy and early breast cancer: implications for prevention and treatment. Cancer Lett 2001; 162:3–17.

39. Soslow RA, Dannenberg AJ, Rush D et al. COX-2 is expressed in human pulmonary, colonic and mammary tumours. Cancer 2000; 89:2637–45.

40. Ristimaki A, Sivula A, Lundin J et al. Prognostic significance of elevated COX-2 expression in breast cancer. Cancer Res 2002; 62:632–5.

41. Helcynska K, Kronblad Å, Jögi A et al. Hypoxia induces a dedifferentiated phenotype in ductal carcinoma in situ. Cancer Res 2003; 63:1441–4.

42. Dershaw DD, Abramson MD, Kinne DW. Ductal carcinoma in situ: mammographic findings and clinical implications. Radiology 1989; 170:411–15.

43. Ikeda DM, Andersson I. Ductal carcinoma in situ: atypical mammographic appearances. Radiology 1989; 172:661–6.

44. Schuh ME, Nemoto T, Penetrante RB et al. Intraductal carcinoma. Analysis of presentation, pathologic findings, and outcome of disease. Arch Surg 1986; 121:1303–7.

45. Silverstein MJ, Parker R, Grotting JC et al. Ductal carcinoma in situ (DCIS) of the breast: diagnostic and therapeutic controversies. J Am Coll Surg 2001; 192:196–214.

46. Lee CH, Carter D, Philpotts LE et al. Ductal carcinoma in situ diagnosed with stereotactic core needle biopsy: can invasion be predicted? Radiology 2000; 217:466–70.

47. Blamey RW. The British Association of Surgical Oncology Guidelines for surgeons in the management of symptomatic breast disease in the UK (1998 revision). BASO Breast Speciality Group. Eur J Surg Oncol 1998; 24:464–76.

48. Chan KC, Knox WF, Sinha G et al. Extent of excision margin width required in breast conserving surgery for ductal carcinoma in situ. Cancer 2001; 91:9–16.

49. Silverstein MJ, Barth A, Poller DN et al. Ten year results comparing mastectomy to excision and radiation therapy for ductal carcinoma in situ of the breast. Eur J Cancer 1995; 31A:1425–7.

50. Fonseca R, Hartmenn L, Petersen I et al. Ductal carcinoma in situ of the breast. Ann Intern Med 1997; 127:1013–22.

51. Kitchen PR, Cawson JN, Krishnan CM et al. Axillary dissection and ductal carcinoma in situ of the breast: a change in practice. Aust NZ J Surg 2000; 70:419–22.

52. Ottesen GL, Graversen HP, Blichert-Toft M et al. Carcinoma in situ of the female breast. 10 year follow-up result of a prospective nationwide study. Breast Cancer Res Treat 2000; 62:197–210.

53. Fisher ER, Dignam J, Tan-Chiu E et al. Pathologic findings from the National Surgical Adjuvant Breast Project (NSABP) eight-year update of Protocol B-17: intraductal carcinoma. Cancer 1999; 86:429–38.

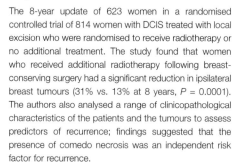

The 8-year update of 623 women in a randomised controlled trial of 814 women with DCIS treated with local excision who were randomised to receive radiotherapy or no additional treatment. The study found that women who received additional radiotherapy following breast-conserving surgery had a significant reduction in ipsilateral breast tumours (31% vs. 13% at 8 years, $P = 0.0001$). The authors also analysed a range of clinicopathological characteristics of the patients and the tumours to assess predictors of recurrence; findings suggested that the presence of comedo necrosis was an independent risk factor for recurrence.

54. Solin LJ, Fourquet A, Vincini FA et al. Salvage treatment for local recurrence after breast-conserving surgery and radiation as initial treatment for mammographically detected carcinoma in situ of the breast. Cancer 2001; 91:1090–7.

55. Waldman FM, DeVries S, Chew KL et al. Chromosomal alterations in ductal carcinomas in situ and their in situ recurrences. J Natl Cancer Inst 2000; 92:313–20.

56. Boland GP, Chan KC, Knox WF et al. Value of the Van Nuys Prognostic Index in prediction of recurrence of ductal carcinoma in situ after breast-conserving surgery. Br J Surg 2003; 90:426–32.

57. Fisher B, Dignam J, Wolmark N et al. Tamoxifen in the treatment of intraductal breast cancer: National Surgical Adjuvant Breast and Bowel Project B-24 randomised controlled trial. Lancet 1999; 353: 1993–2000.

Double-blind, randomised, controlled trial of 1804 women with completely or incompletely excised DCIS at breast-conserving surgery who were randomised to receive radiotherapy plus or minus tamoxifen. The women receiving tamoxifen had fewer breast cancer events at 5 years compared with placebo (8.2 vs. 13.4, $P = 0.0009$) mainly due to a decrease in invasive cancer in the ipsilateral breast. A retrospective review of the results (ref. 68) showed that this benefit was confined to oestrogen receptor-positive cases.

58. Fisher B, Constantino J, Redmond C et al. Lumpectomy compared with lumpectomy and radiation therapy for the treatment of intraductal breast cancer. N Engl J Med 1993; 328:1581–6.

59. Bijker N, Peterse JL, Duchateau L et al. Risk factors for recurrence and metastasis after breast conserving therapy for ductal carcinoma in situ: analysis of EORTC trial. J Clin Oncol 2001; 19:2263–71.

A review of 843 women of the 1010 randomised cases from the EORTC 10853 trial (local excision of DCIS plus or minus radiotherapy) that examined the clinico-pathological characteristics of the women. The authors found that clear margins were the most important factor in reducing local recurrence (hazard ratio 2.07, $P = 0.0008$). Patients with poorly differentiated DCIS were at higher risk of metastatic disease (hazard ratio 6.57, $P = 0.01$) and that other poor prognostic factors included young age (<40 years) at diagnosis (hazard ratio 2.14, $P = 0.02$) and symptomatic detection (hazard ratio 1.8, $P = 0.008$).

60. Fraser J, Raza S, Chorny K et al. Columnar alteration with prominent apical snouts and secretions: a spectrum of changes frequently present in breast biopsies with microcalcifications. Am J Surg Pathol 1998; 22:1521–7.

61. UK Coordinating Committee on Cancer Research (UKCCCR). Ductal carcinoma in situ (DCIS) Working Party on behalf of DCIS trialists in the UK, Australia and New Zealand. Radiotherapy and tamoxifen in women with completely excised ductal carcinoma in situ of the breast in the UK, Australia and New Zealand: randomised controlled trial. Lancet 2003; 362:95–103.

A 2 × 2 factorial design, randomised controlled trial of 1701 screen-detected patients with completely excised DCIS, randomised to receive tamoxifen, radiotherapy, both treatments or none. The authors found that radio-therapy reduced the incidence of both ipsilateral invasive recurrence (hazard ratio 0.45, $P = 0.01$) and DCIS recurrence (hazard ratio 0.36, $P = 0.0004$). Tamoxifen reduced overall DCIS recurrence (hazard ratio 0.68, $P = 0.03$) but not invasive disease. The trial has not yet published results with regard to oestrogen receptor status.

62. Rodrigues N, Dillon D, Parisot N, Haffty B. Differences in the pathologic and molecular features of intraductal breast carcinoma between younger and older women. Cancer 2003; 97:1393–403.

63. Silverstein MJ. The University of Southern California/Van Nuys Prognostic Index for ductal carcinoma in situ of the breast. Am J Surg 2003; 186:337–43.

Update of the original Van Nuys Prognostic Index, adding patient age to the existing criteria of tumour size, margin width, nuclear grade and comedo necrosis to aid prediction of recurrence in DCIS. The new formula was derived from recurrence data from a prospective database of 706 pure DCIS patients treated with breast-conserving surgery.

64. Provenzano E, Hopper JL, Giles GG et al. Biological markers that predict clinical recurrence in ductal carcinoma in situ of the breast. Eur J Cancer 2003; 39:622–30.

A nested case–control study within a population-based cohort of 95 cases of DCIS that attempted to identify subgroups of DCIS based on biological markers in relation to risk of recurrence. The authors found that HER2 positivity, bcl-2 negativity, and oestrogen and progesterone receptor negativity were all individually associated with an increased risk of recurrence, and the predictive value of these were independent of nuclear grade.

65. Witton CJ, Reeves JR, Going JJ et al. Expression of the HER1–4 family of receptor tyrosine kinases in breast cancer. J Pathol 2003; 200:290–7.

66. Suo Z, Risberg B, Kalsson M et al. EGFR family expression in breast carcinomas. C-erbB-2 and c-erbB-4 have different effects on survival. J Pathol 2002; 196:17–25.

67. Barnes NLP, Khavari S, Boland GP et al. Absence of HER4 expression predicts recurrence of ductal carcinoma in situ of the breast. Clin Cancer Res 2005; 11:2163–8.

68. Allred DC, Bryant J, Land S et al. Estrogen receptor expression as a predictive marker of the effectiveness of tamoxifen in the treatment of intraductal breast cancer: findings from NSABP Protocol B-24 (abstract). Breast Cancer Res Treat 2002; 76(suppl. 1):S36.

69. Boland GP, McKeowan A, Chan KC, Prasad R, Knox WF, Bundred NJ. Biological response to hormonal manipulation in oestrogen receptor positive ductal carcinoma in situ of the breast. Br J Cancer 2003; 89:277–83.

70. Allred DC, Mohsin SK, Fuqua SA. Histological and biological evolution of human premalignant breast disease. Endocr Relat Cancer 2001; 8:47–61.

71. Simmons RM. Male ductal carcinoma in situ presenting as bloody nipple discharge: a case report and literature review. Breast J 2002; 8:112–14.

72. Hittmair AP, Liniger RA, Tavassoli FA. Ductal carcinoma in situ (DCIS) in the male breast. A morphological study of 84 cases of pure DCIS and 30 cases of DCIS associated with invasive carcinoma: a preliminary report. Cancer 1998; 83:2139–49.

73. Fisher B, Constantino JP, Wickerman DL et al. Tamoxifen for prevention of breast cancer: report of the National Surgical Adjuvant Breast and Bowel

Project P-1 Study. J Natl Cancer Inst 1998; 90:1371–88.

74. Vogel VG, Constantino JP, Wickerham DL, Cronin WM. National Surgical Adjuvant Breast and Bowel Project Update: prevention trials and endocrine therapy of ductal carcinoma in situ. Clin Cancer Res 2003; 9(suppl.):495s–5 01s.

A summary of recent and proposed prevention trials and endocrine therapy trials for DCIS, including the BCPT P1 trial results showing that tamoxifen as chemoprevention decreases cases of invasive cancer (49%), DCIS (50%) and LCIS (56%) but only in oestrogen receptor-positive cases.

75. Chan KC, Knox WF, Ghandi A et al. Blockade of growth factor receptors in ductal carcinoma in situ inhibits epithelial proliferation. Br J Surg 2001; 88:412–18.

76. Johnston S. Farensyl transferase inhibitors: a novel targeted therapy for cancer. Lancet Oncology 2001; 2:18–26.

77. Masferrer JL, Leaky KM, Koki AT et al. Anti-angiogenic and anti-tumour activities of COX-2 inhibitors. Cancer Res 2000; 60:1306–11.

CHAPTER
Eleven

Systemic therapy in breast cancer

Susan Chua, Ander Urruticoechea and
Ian E. Smith

INTRODUCTION

Breast cancer was the first malignancy for which
effective systemic therapy was developed: Beatson[1]
reported the efficacy of ovarian ablation to control
advanced disease in 1896. Today there are more
forms of medical treatment available for breast
cancer than for all other common cancers combined,
and the list grows yearly (**Box 11.1**). These can be
broadly divided into the following categories: endocrine therapy, chemotherapy, bisphosphonates,
and signal transduction inhibitors (so far only
trastuzumab but with other agents on the horizon).

TREATMENTS

Endocrine therapy

Endocrine therapies are designed to counteract
the proliferative effects of estrogen in estrogen
receptor-positive breast cancer. Oophorectomy,
gonadotrophin-releasing hormone (GnRH) agonists
and aromatase inhibitors all reduce the level of
serum estrogen while tamoxifen and other antiestrogens competitively block the binding of estrogen
to its receptor.

TAMOXIFEN

Tamoxifen, a non-steroidal antiestrogen, is currently
the most widely used form of endocrine therapy for
breast cancer. It is a selective estrogen receptor
modulator because it has partial agonist activity in
some tissues, including bone, serum lipids and
endometrium, but has antagonist activity in breast
cancer tissue. The antitumour effect of tamoxifen
is mediated via competitive inhibition of estrogen
binding to estrogen receptors, thereby inhibiting the
expression of estrogen-regulated genes. This results
in a block in the G_1 phase of the cell cycle and a
decrease in tumour growth.[2] Tamoxifen may also
directly induce apoptosis.[3]

In general, tamoxifen is well tolerated. The most
common adverse effects are hot flushes (in up to
50% of women), vaginal discharge and irregular
menses.[4-6] These appear to be more prominent in
premenopausal/perimenopausal women and those
on prior hormone replacement therapy.

The most important toxicity is an approximate
doubling of the risk of endometrial cancer, which
equates to 80 excess cases per 10 000 tamoxifen-
treated women at 10 years. The Early Breast Cancer
Trialists' Collaborative Group (EBCTCG) analysed
data from 37 000 women involved in adjuvant
trials and demonstrated the incidence of endometrial cancer to be approximately twofold greater
in women receiving 1–2 years of tamoxifen and
approximately fourfold greater in women receiving
5 years of tamoxifen.[7] The National Surgical
Adjuvant Breast and Bowel Project (NSABP) B-14
study of 5–10 years of tamoxifen versus placebo
performed in 4063 women with estrogen receptor-
positive and node-negative breast cancer[8,9] also

Box 11.1 • Common systemic treatments of breast cancer

ENDOCRINE THERAPY	
Ovarian ablation	
Surgical oophorectomy	Gonadotrophin-releasing hormone agonists
Radiation ablation	
Selective estrogen receptor modulators	
Tamoxifen	Toremifene
Aromatase inhibitors	
Letrozole	Exemestane
Anastrozole	
Estrogen down-regulator	
Fulvestrant	
Estrogens	
Estradiol	Diethylstilbestrol
Progesterones	
Medroxyprogesterone acetate	Megestrol acetate
CHEMOTHERAPY	
Alkylating agents	
Cyclophosphamide	Carboplatin
Cisplatin	
Antimetabolites	
Capecitabine	Methotrexate
5-Fluorouracil	Gemcitabine
Tubulin active	
Docetaxel	Vincristine
Paclitaxel	Vinorelbine
Vinblastine	
Antibiotics	
Doxorubicin	Mitomycin C
Epirubicin	Mitoxantrone
Bisphosphonates	
Clodronate	Pamidronate
Ibandronate	Zoledronic acid
Signal transduction inhibitors	
Trastuzumab (Herceptin)	

found a 2.2 relative risk of developing endometrial cancer in the tamoxifen group. Similar results were seen in the NSABP P-1 prevention trial of high-risk women who were randomised to 5 years of tamoxifen or placebo. Tamoxifen did reduce the risk of breast cancer but increased the risk of endometrial cancer (relative risk 2.53).[10] The increase was seen mainly in women over 50 years of age.[10] There is no evidence that tamoxifen increases the risk of other solid tumours.[7,11,12]

Tamoxifen has also been associated with an increase in endometrial hyperplasia, endometrial polyps and ovarian cysts.[10] The value of gynaecological screening tests is still unproven.[13–15] Overall, the reduction in the development of recurrent breast cancer outweighs the risk of endometrial cancer. However, women on tamoxifen should be evaluated promptly if they experience any abnormal uterine bleeding.

Between 1 and 2% of women taking tamoxifen develop thromboembolism,[8,16] particularly if tamoxifen is given concurrently with chemotherapy.[17] The mechanism of action is not completely understood but tamoxifen decreases blood levels of antithrombin III and protein C.[18]

Retinopathy has been reported with high doses of tamoxifen in one trial,[19] although this has not been confirmed in other trials. No vision-threatening toxicity has been described but a slight increase in cataracts has been reported.[20,21]

There are benefits from tamoxifen. In postmenopausal women, tamoxifen increases bone mineral density of the axial skeleton and stabilises bone mineral density of the appendicular skeleton.[22,23] In premenopausal women, there may be a decrease in bone mineral density.[24] Tamoxifen reduces circulating total cholesterol and low-density lipoprotein levels,[25,26] which may partly explain the decrease in cardiovascular deaths seen in two large controlled trials.[27,28] This effect on cardiovascular deaths was not confirmed in the overview.[12] In the Swedish trial of postmenopausal women, less cardiovascular deaths were seen in those randomised to 5 years of tamoxifen compared with 2 years.[27]

OTHER SELECTIVE ESTROGEN RECEPTOR MODULATORS

Toremifene, the most widely tested drug for breast cancer after tamoxifen, is structurally very similar and has shown no clinical advantage over tamoxifen in terms of efficacy or adverse effects in randomised trials in advanced disease[29–31] and as adjuvant therapy.[32] Raloxifene, another selective estrogen receptor modulator, has less uterine agonist effects than tamoxifen and is currently being compared with tamoxifen in a major chemoprevention trial (STAR).[33] Clinical experience in breast cancer is limited.

FASLODEX

Faslodex (Fulvestrant or ICI 182780) is a pure steroidal antiestrogen devoid of agonist estrogen-like activity in breast and uterine tissues.[34] The in vitro binding affinity of faslodex for the estrogen receptor is approximately 100 times greater than that of tamoxifen; unlike tamoxifen, it suppresses estrogen-regulated gene expression.[35]

AROMATASE INHIBITORS

Aromatase inhibitors dramatically reduce estrogen production in postmenopausal women by inhibiting or inactivating aromatase, a cytochrome P-450 enzyme. Aromatase is located in subcutaneous fat, liver, muscle, brain, normal breast and breast cancer tissue.[36,37] Aromatase inhibitors are ineffective in premenopausal women because they produce an increase in gonadotrophin secretion, which results in reduced feedback of estrogen on the hypothalamus and pituitary. In some animal models aromatase inhibitors produce an increase in the weight of the ovaries.[38]

The first aromatase inhibitor developed for clinical use was aminoglutethimide (**Box 11.2**). A non-specific agent, it inhibited several enzyme systems including those involved with adrenal steroid metabolism. It had clinical efficacy[39] but adverse effects, particularly drowsiness and rash, limited its use. In the 1990s the so-called third-generation

aromatase inhibitors were developed with much greater potency and specificity than their predecessors. These include two subgroups: a steroidal analogue, exemestane, which binds irreversibly to aromatase and is an enzyme inactivator (type 1 inhibitor); and non-steroidal inhibitors that bind reversibly to the haem group of the enzyme (type 2 inhibitors), of which the main agents are anastrozole and letrozole.

These drugs are well tolerated with a remarkably low incidence of serious short-term adverse effects. The commonest of these include musculoskeletal pain, hot flushes, vaginal dryness and headache. A direct comparison of their adverse effects with tamoxifen is available from the Anastrazole or Tamoxifen Alone or in Combination (ATAC) trial (see **Table 11.5**).

PROGESTAGENS

Progestagens are derivatives of progesterone that have an antiestrogenic action and have been used extensively in the past for the treatment of metastatic disease. Megestrol acetate and medroxyprogesterone are the commonest agents used. The most common adverse effects are weight gain, increase in appetite, hypertension and fluid retention.[40] A more serious side effect is thromboembolism, which occurs in 4–5% of patients.[41] Uterine bleeding, hot flushes and oedema have also been associated with progestagens. Because of these adverse effects and the emergence of the third-generation aromatase inhibitors (see above), progestagens are used less than in the past but may still have a role as third-line hormonal agents.

OVARIAN ABLATION

Ovarian ablation was traditionally carried out surgically or by radiotherapy. It can now be easily performed by laparoscopy. GnRH agonists are increasingly used to achieve therapeutic ovarian suppression.

GONADOTROPHIN-RELEASING HORMONE AGONISTS

In premenopausal women, GnRH is released from the hypothalamus and binds to specific receptors in the pituitary gland, triggering the release of luteinising hormone (LH) and follicle-stimulating hormone (FSH) that stimulate the ovaries to produce estrogens, including estradiol. This mechanism

Box 11.2 • Classification of aromatase inhibitors

	Type 1 (steroidal)	Type 2 (non-steroidal)
First generation	None	Aminoglutethimide
Second generation	Formestane	Fadrozole
Third generation	Exemestane	Anastrozole, letrozole

is responsible for the production of up to 90% of circulating estradiol in premenopausal women. GnRH agonists over-stimulate and subsequently down-regulate GnRH receptors. Their effect is to produce an initial rise in LH and FSH in the first 7–10 days of treatment followed by a decrease after 14–21 days that leads to postmenopausal levels of progesterone and estradiol.[42,43] GnRH receptors have been demonstrated on the surface of human breast cancer cell lines and in human breast tumours, which may explain the direct antitumour action on breast cancer cells.[44] GnRH agonists have the advantage of reversibility over surgical and radiation-induced ovarian ablation.

Chemotherapy

Many cytotoxic agents are active in the treatment of breast cancer and more are being developed each year. Acute toxicities are summarised in **Box 11.3**. The details of the mechanism of action and toxicities of chemotherapy agents are complex and specialised; the interested reader is referred to more specialised reviews.[45–48]

LONG-TERM TOXICITIES OF CHEMOTHERAPY

The short-term adverse effects of chemotherapy are unpleasant and potentially dangerous but against this background long-term toxicities are surprisingly rare. In premenopausal women, the major impact of chemotherapy is early onset of ovarian failure and infertility.

The risk of ovarian failure is related to the patient's age and the total dose and type of chemotherapy.[49,50] A regimen comprising 6 months of cyclo-phosphamide, methotrexate and 5-fluorouracil (CMF) results in permanent ovarian failure in 70% of women over 40 years of age and 40% of younger women.[50] With a regimen of doxorubicin and cyclo-phosphamide (AC), the incidence of ovarian failure is approximately 13% of those less than 40 years old and 60% of those over 40 years.[51,52] Few data are available for taxanes. In older patients, the median onset of premature menopause is earlier and is more permanent.

Other problems related to early ovarian failure include menopausal symptoms such as hot flushes, night sweats, vaginal dryness, mood changes, sleep

Box 11.3 • Acute adverse effects of common chemotherapeutic agents

Myelosuppression

Infection

Nausea and vomiting

Mucositis

Diarrhoea

Neuropathy

Weight gain

Ovarian failure

Cardiac arrhythmias, cardiac failure

Thromboembolism

Alopecia

Lethargy

disturbances and psychological difficulties.[53] In this group of women there is also an increased risk of accelerated bone loss[54] and possibly an increased risk of cardiovascular disease. Consequently, these women should be advised to maintain an adequate diet of calcium and vitamin D, regular weight-bearing exercises and regular bone mineral density assessments. For these symptoms there are some effective non-hormonal interventions available.[55]

Another long-term adverse effect of chemotherapy is the increased risk of acute leukaemia and myelodysplasia. This is a rare but devastating complication of chemotherapy. The risk depends on the drug used, duration of therapy and the cumulative dose.[56] A review by the Canadian NCI group of 1545 women who had received adjuvant or neo-adjuvant chemotherapy showed a 1.7% conditional probability of leukaemia with cyclophosphamide, epirubicin and 5-fluorouracil (CEF) chemotherapy, a 0.4% probability with CMF chemotherapy and a 1.3% probability with AC chemotherapy.[57] Several other studies have shown that higher single doses (100–120 mg/m^2) or cumulative doses (720–800 mg/m^2) of doxorubicin are associated with roughly a 1% incidence of leukaemia.[56,58] Leukaemias associated with anthracyclines usually present 6 months to 5 years after treatment, whereas those associated with alkylating agents such as cyclophosphamide often present 5–7 years later and are often preceded by myelodysplasia.[59]

Cardiac toxicity is a complication of anthracycline-based chemotherapy and can occur as an acute, largely reversible, cardiotoxic effect or a dose-related cardiomyopathy. Risk factors for cardiomyopathy include a high cumulative dose, older age, pre-existing heart disease, a history of cardiac irradiation and coadministration of trastuzumab.[60–62] Continuous infusions or low-dose weekly administration decreases the risk of cardiomyopathy compared with bolus infusions. The incidence of cardiomyopathy in patients who have received a cumulative dose of 550 mg/m^2 of doxorubicin is 1–10%. Epirubicin is associated with less cardiac toxicity, with the risk of clinical cardiac impairment rising rapidly at doses of 900 mg/m^2 or above.[46] Symptoms usually respond well to conventional treatment of congestive heart failure.[63]

There is mounting evidence that adjuvant therapy may result in cognitive impairment. An analysis of five cross-sectional studies suggests an adverse effect.[64–68] The interpretation of these results has been confounded by several factors, such as different chemotherapy regimens, hormone therapy and timing of tests.[69]

Weight gain and an increase in percentage body fat has been observed in 50% or more women after chemotherapy, with weight gains ranging from 1.0 to 6.2 kg.[70,71] Premenopausal women appear to be more affected than postmenopausal women. The underlying cause is uncertain.

Bisphosphonates

Bisphosphonates are potent inhibitors of osteoclastic bone resorption and are effective in the treatment of hypercalcaemia of malignancy, postmenopausal osteoporosis and Paget's disease of the bone.[72] They are also now well established in the treatment of skeletal complications of breast cancer and multiple myeloma.[73,74] Bisphosphonates are characterised by a common phosphorus–carbon–phosphorus bond and are analogues of endogenous pyrophosphate in which the central oxygen atom is replaced by a carbon atom (**Fig. 11.1**). This substitution makes these drugs resistant to hydrolysis and allows the attachment of two side chains. One of these chains usually contains a hydroxyl moiety that gives these compounds high affinity for calcium crystals and bone mineral.

Bisphosphonates can be divided into two groups. Those resembling pyrophosphate (e.g. clodronate, etidronate) act as analogues of ATP and inhibit ATP-dependent intracellular enzymes. The second group are aminobisphosphonates (e.g. pamidronate, zoledronate), which inhibit enzymes of the mevalonate pathway and disrupt the signalling functions of key proteins.[75] Two bisphosphonates are available in an oral form (e.g. clodronate and ibandronate), while the rest are administered as an intravenous infusion (e.g. zoledronate and pamidronate).

Their main mechanism of action is inhibition of osteoclast activity. They bind avidly to exposed bone mineral around resorbing osteoclasts, resulting in high concentrations in resorption lacunae. On release from the bone surface, they are internalised by the osteoclast where they disrupt intracellular function and decrease bone resorption.[76]

ADVERSE EFFECTS

Bisphosphonates are generally well tolerated. In randomised controlled trials the incidence of adverse events was similar in the pamidronate and placebo groups.[77] All bisphosphonates can cause gastrointestinal side effects especially if given orally. Occasional patients have transient chills/pyrexia, myalgia, bone pain, malaise, arthralgia and hypocalcaemia but patients rarely have to discontinue treatment because of adverse effects. Pamidronate and zoledronate can cause renal impairment and this is partly related to the rate of administration.[78,79] No serious long-term adverse events have been reported even with prolonged use. However, mild anaemia and thrombocytopenia have been reported with chronic use.[80]

Trastuzumab (Herceptin)

The human epidermal growth factor receptor (HER)-2, also known as c-erbB-2 or HER-2/neu, plays an important role in normal cellular growth, differentiation and survival processes. Approximately 15–25% of breast cancers have HER-2 overexpression and this is associated with a worse disease-free survival (DFS) and overall survival (OS).[81–83]

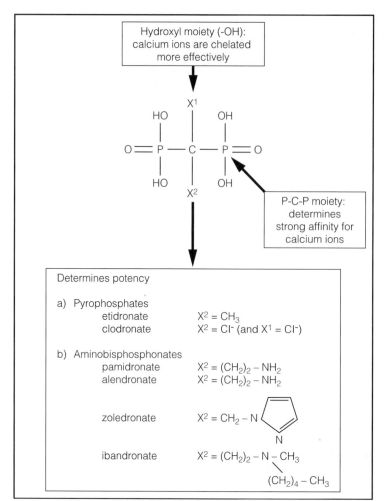

Figure 11.1 • Chemical structure of bisphosphonates.

The most commonly used test for determining HER-2 protein overexpression is an immuno-histochemical (IHC) assay, scored from 0 to 3+, with 3+ representing positive, 2+ weakly positive and 0 or 1+ negative. Interpretation of studies on HER-2 has been confounded by variability in anti-bodies and assay techniques and it is imperative that HER-2 assays are carried out in large-volume reference laboratories with appropriate quality controls. HER-2 can also be measured quantitatively by fluorescence in situ hybridisation (FISH), which provides a direct measure of gene amplification. This is considered the gold standard for evaluating HER-2 overexpression, and provides the best cor-relation with clinical response to trastuzumab: IHC3+ correlates well with FISH positivity, but only 20–24% of IHC2+ tumours are also FISH positive[84,85] (**Table 11.1**).

Trastuzumab (Herceptin) is a novel humanised monoclonal antibody that specifically targets HER-2 and achieves tumour regression in some patients with HER-2-positive metastatic breast cancer.[86] Benefit is only seen in IHC3+ or FISH-positive cancers.[84,85] In general, trastuzumab is well tolerated and does not have the typical adverse effects associated with chemotherapy, such as alopecia, myelosuppression, nausea and vomiting. The most common adverse effects are mild-to-moderate hypersensitivity infusion-related reactions; these are generally observed with the first infusion and are less frequent thereafter. A more serious adverse effect of trastuzumab is cardiotoxicity when given concurrently with or after

Table 11.1 • Concordance between immunohistochemistry (IHC) and fluorescence in situ hybridisation (FISH)

IHC	0	1+	2+	3+
FISH negative	207	28	67	21
FISH positive	7	2	21	176
Concordance	3%	7%	25%	89%

Modified from Mass R, Press M, Anderson S et al. Improved survival benefit from Herceptin (trastuzumab) in patients selected by fluorescence in situ hybridization (FISH) (abstract). Proc Am Soc Oncol 2001; abs. 85, with permission.

anthracyclines.[87] A retrospective evaluation from phase II studies showed that the incidence of cardiac dysfunction was 4% with trastuzumab alone, 27% when given with AC chemotherapy and 13% when given with paclitaxel after doxorubicin.[88,89] In most cases, cardiac function improved with standard treatment.

ADJUVANT THERAPIES

There is now convincing evidence that the majority of patients with early breast cancer benefit from adjuvant systemic therapy after surgery and its widespread use has played an important role in improving cancer survival outcomes in the UK during the last decade.[90]

Consensus conferences have provided useful clinical guidelines for the use of adjuvant therapy. The St Gallen Conference[91] in 2005 updated previous recommendations and these are summarised in **Tables 11.2** and **11.3**. These provide broad outlines for the use of adjuvant endocrine therapy and chemotherapy. Three new disease categories have been defined: 1) endocrine responsive, in which tumour cells express steroid hormone receptors; 2) endocrine response uncertain, in which the expression of steroid hormone receptors is quantitatively low or qualitatively uncertain; and 3) endocrine non-responsive, in which tumour cells have no detectable expression of steroid hormone receptors. Therefore, patients with endocrine responsive disease may be offered endocrine therapies alone, whereas chemotherapy alone will be offered to patients with

Table 11.2 • St Gallen's risk categories for patients with node-negative breast cancer

Risk category	Endocrine-responsive disease
Low risk	Node negative and *all* of the following: T ≤ 2 cm Histological grade 1 No peritumoral vascular invasion HER-2 negative Age ≥ 35 years
Intermediate risk	Node negative and *at least one* of the following: T > 2 cm Histological grade 2–3 Peritumoral vascular invasion HER-2 positive Age < 35 years *or* Node positive (1–3 nodes) *and* HER-2 negative
High risk	Node positive (1–3 nodes) *and* HER-2 positive *or* Node positive (≥ 4 nodes)

ER, estrogen receptor; PgR, progesterone receptor; T, pathological tumour size.
Modified from Goldhirsch et al.[91]

endocrine non-responsive disease. Those who have endocrine response uncertain disease will be offered a combination of chemotherapy and endocrine therapy.[92]

Selection of adjuvant treatment is influenced by a series of prognostic and predictive factors. Prognostic factors relate to the likelihood of disease relapse independent of treatment and include nodal status, tumour size, histological grade and age. Predictive factors relate to the likelihood of response to therapy; currently the main predictive factor is estrogen receptor status. HER-2 is emerging as both a prognostic and a predictive factor. Its amplification has adverse prognostic significance, particularly in node-positive disease. There is increasing evidence that it may also be a predictive factor for the selection of endocrine therapy: preliminary data from neoadjuvant trials and early breast cancers suggest that tumours which are positive for both estrogen receptor and HER-2 may respond better to aromatase inhibitors than to tamoxifen.[93,94]

Table 11.3 • St Gallen consensus recommendations for adjuvant treatment of patients with operable breast cancer

Risk group	Endocrine responsive	Endocrine response uncertain	Endocrine nonresponsive
Low risk	ET or none	ET or none	Not applicable
Intermediate risk	ET alone or chemotherapy → ET*	Chemotherapy → ET*	Chemotherapy
High risk	Chemotherapy → ET*	Chemotherapy → ET*	Chemotherapy

ET, endocrine therapy.
*Some forms of endocrine therapies apart from tamoxifen (which should be given sequentially) may be given concurrently with chemotherapy, e.g. ovarian suppression.
Modified from Goldhirsch et al.[91]

The risk–benefit ratio can often be subtle and the final choice should be influenced by the patient's own preference, following a careful and unbiased discussion of the options.

Adjuvant endocrine therapy

HORMONE RECEPTOR STATUS

Estrogen receptors are present in about 75–78% of breast cancers depending on the age group.[95] It is now widely accepted that patients whose tumours are estrogen receptor negative and progesterone receptor negative do not benefit from adjuvant endocrine therapy.[12] However, there are data to suggest that the small proportion of patients whose tumours are estrogen receptor negative but progesterone receptor positive can benefit from adjuvant endocrine therapy;[96] therefore progesterone receptor assessment should be undertaken in patients whose tumours are estrogen receptor negative.

TAMOXIFEN

The EBCTCG Oxford overview firmly established the clinical benefit of adjuvant tamoxifen in all women whose tumours are estrogen receptor positive or of unknown receptor status, with a 47% proportional reduction in recurrence and a 26% proportional reduction in mortality in women treated for 5 years[7] (**Table 11.4**). Proportional reductions in recurrence and mortality were similar for node-positive and node-negative tumours but the absolute improvements were greater in patients with node-positive tumours. These benefits were independent of age, menopausal status, dose of

tamoxifen and administration of chemotherapy. There was also a proportional reduction in contra-lateral breast cancers of 13, 26 and 47% after 1, 2 and 5 years of tamoxifen respectively. The degree of benefit was directly proportional to the level of estrogen receptor expression.[7]

Duration of tamoxifen

The current recommendation for the duration of tamoxifen therapy is 5 years. The EBCTCG overview compared 1, 2 and 5 years of tamoxifen and showed a significant trend towards a greater effect with longer treatment.[7] The proportional reductions in recurrence from 1, 2 and 5 years of tamoxifen after 10 years of follow-up were 21, 29 and 47% respectively. The corresponding proportional reductions in mortality were 12, 17 and 26% respectively.

The NSABP B-14 trial randomised patients with estrogen receptor-positive and node-negative breast cancer after 5 years of tamoxifen to placebo or more prolonged tamoxifen therapy.[9] At 7 years after re-randomisation there was no additional benefit from prolonged tamoxifen and there appeared to be a slight advantage in patients who discontinued tamoxifen after 5 years of treatment in DFS (82% vs. 78%, $P = 0.03$) and OS (94% vs. 91%, $P = 0.07$). Patients on prolonged treatment had more breast cancer recurrences and endometrial cancers but the differences were not statistically significant. Other trials have not supported the use of tamoxifen beyond 5 years.[97,98]

The issue of duration will not be completely resolved until the findings from two large British trials become available. In the Adjuvant Tamoxifen Treatment, Offer More? (aTTom) trial, patients

Table 11.4 • Benefits of adjuvant therapy

Age (years)	Treatment	RR (%)	Recurrence-free survival at 10 years (%)				RR (%)	Overall survival at 10 years (%)			
			Node negative		Node positive			Node negative		Node positive	
			Without treatment	With treatment	Without treatment	With treatment		Without treatment	With treatment	Without treatment	With treatment
<50	Combination chemotherapy	35	58	68	32	48	27	72	78	41	54
50–69	Combination chemotherapy	20	60	66	38	43	11	65	71	46	49
All ages (ER+)	Tamoxifen for 5 years	47	64	79	45	60	26	73	79	51	61

ER, estrogen receptor; RR, proportional reduction in recurrence.
Modified from Early Breast Cancer Trialists' Collaborative Group. Tamoxifen for early breast cancer: an overview of the randomised trials. Lancet 1998; 351:1451–67 and Early Breast Cancer Trialists' Collaborative Group. Polychemotherapy for early breast cancer: an overview of the randomised trials. Lancet 1998; 352:930–42.

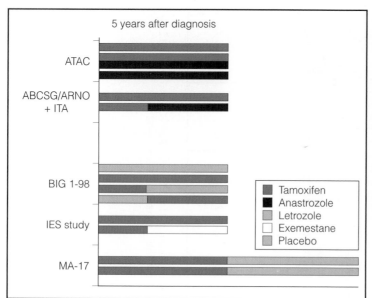

5 years after diagnosis

ATAC

ABCSG/ARNO + ITA

BIG 1-98

IES study

MA-17

Tamoxifen
Anastrozole
Letrozole
Exemestane
Placebo

Figure 11.2 • Outline of ongoing aromatase inhibitor adjuvant trials. ATAC (Arimidex or Tamoxifen Alone or in Combination), ABCSG/ARNO + ITA (Austrian Breast and Colorectal Cancer Study Group and the German Adjuvant Breast Cancer Group/Arimidex-Nolvadex Trial), BIG 1-98 (Breast International Group) Study, IES (Intergroup Exemestane Study) and MA-17 (study coordinated by the Canadian Breast Cancer Group). ATAC, ABCSG/ARNO + ITA, BIG 1-98 and IES are 5-year studies. The MA-17 randomised patients after 5 years of tamoxifen to 5 years of letrozole or placebo.

who have received tamoxifen for at least 2 years are randomly assigned to discontinuation of tamoxifen or at least another 3 years of tamoxifen.[99] In the Adjuvant Tamoxifen: Longer Against Shorter (ATLAS) trial, women who received tamoxifen for varying lengths of time are randomly assigned to discontinuation or continuation for another 5 years.[100]

AROMATASE INHIBITORS

Currently, there are at least 10 adjuvant trials comparing third-generation aromatase inhibitors with tamoxifen in postmenopausal women. These have been stimulated by encouraging results in metastatic disease that indicate superiority for letrozole and anastrozole. The long-term importance of these adjuvant trials is emphasised by the fact that almost 40 000 women are involved. These trials are directly comparing aromatase inhibitors with tamoxifen 1) upfront; 2) in combination; 3) as extended adjuvant therapy after 5 years of tamoxifen; or 4) in sequence. The format of these trial is summarised in **Fig. 11.2**. The largest and first to publish of these trials was the Anastrozole or Tamoxifen Alone or in Combination (ATAC) trial, which randomised 9366 postmenopausal women with invasive breast cancer (estrogen receptor positive or unknown) to 5 years of adjuvant anastrozole, tamoxifen or a combination of the two.[101] Approxi-

mately one-third had positive lymph nodes, two-thirds had tumours less than 2 cm and 21% had prior chemotherapy. Anastrozole achieved a small but significant benefit in DFS (3.3% improvement at 6 years, hazard ratio 0.83, 95% CI 0.73–0.94) in the hormone receptor-positive group compared with tamoxifen or the combination (**Fig. 11.3**). Patients treated with anastrozole also had a small but significant reduction in distant DFS (hazard ratio 0.86, 95% CI 0.74–0.99) but the latest analysis at 68 months has shown no difference in OS.

The second major upfront aromatase inhibitor trial (BIG 1-98) compared letrozole with tamoxifen in patients with receptor-positive breast cancer and the first results were presented at the St Gallen Conference 2005. This was a four-arm trial as follows: 1) tamoxifen for 5 years; 2) letrozole for 5 years; 3) tamoxifen for 2 years then letrozole for 3 years; 4) letrozole for 2 years then tamoxifen for 3 years. The primary core analysis simply compared upfront letrozole with tamoxifen, with patients in the crossover arms censored at the 2-year point. Median follow-up for this analysis was 26 months, with a predictive 5-year DFS for letrozole of 84% vs. 81.4% for tamoxifen (HR 0.81, $P = 0.003$). When deaths without breast cancer and second malignancies were taken out of the analysis, the HR for DFS was 0.79. These results (not yet published) are similar to those seen in the ATAC trial.

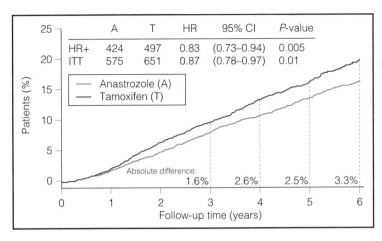

Figure 11.3 • Updated analysis from ATAC study showing the probability of recurrence in hormone receptor-positive (HR+) population. Disease-free survival includes all deaths as a first event. HR, hazard ratio; ITT, intention to treat.

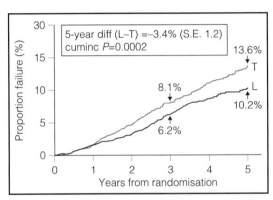

Figure 11.4 • Data from BIG 1-98 study showing cumulative incidence of breast cancer relapse in patients randomised to tamoxifen (T) or letrozole (L).

Letrozole is a more potent inhibitor of estrogen synthesis than anastrozole and results from these adjuvant trials are consistent with letrozole having a similar clinical efficacy to anastrozole. In both the ATAC and BIG 1-98 studies there were more fractures, less thromboembolic events and less endometrial cancer and other gynaecological problems in women receiving anastrozole or letrozole (**Table 11.5**).

Sequential adjuvant endocrine trials have shown that a switch to anastrozole after 2 years of tamoxifen therapy also improves event-free survival (**Fig. 11.5**). The Italian ITA trial and the ABCSG/ARNO study differ in that ITA only included node-positive patients while the other study included mainly patients with grade 1 or 3 tumours and no patient

received chemotherapy. The sequential use of exemestane therapy after 2–3 years of tamoxifen for the remainder of the 5 years has also recently shown a significant improvement over 5 years of tamoxifen alone, with an absolute benefit in DFS of 4.7% at 3 years.[210] (HR 0.73, $P < 0.01$; **Fig. 11.6**) There was a small but non-significant (at the pre-defined level of significance) excess of myocardial infarctions in the exemestane group, but a recent meta-analysis of all the aromatase inhibitor trials showed no excess of non-breast cancer deaths, indicating that this is unlikely to be a significant problem. A summary of the four major trials with aromatase inhibitors, their differences and end-points are summarised in **Table 11.6**.

The ATAC study suggested less benefit compared with tamoxifen in women who had prior adjuvant chemotherapy but other studies have not shown this. ATAC also suggested greater benefit for anastrozole in tumours that were estrogen receptor positive but progesterone receptor negative; results from other studies have not shown a greater advantage for aromatase inhibitors in this group over patients with estrogen and progesterone receptor-positive cancers (**Fig. 11.7**). Further work to identify who gains most from aromatase inhibitors continues.

As a result of this trial, the American Society of Clinical Oncologists (ASCO) conducted an evidence-based technology assessment on the role of aromatase inhibitors in the adjuvant setting.[102] The authors recommended that aromatase inhibitors should now be considered as part of adjuvant therapy

Table 11.5 • ATAC trial: adverse effects of anastrozole and tamoxifen

Adverse effect	Anastrozole (%)	Tamoxifen (%)	P value
Hot flashes	34.3	39.7	<0.001
Nausea and vomiting	10.5	10.2	0.7
Fatigue	15.6	15.2	0.5
Mood disturbance	15.5	15.2	0.7
Musculoskeletal disorder	27.8	21.3	<0.001
Vaginal bleeding	4.5	8.2	<0.001
Vaginal discharge	2.8	11.4	<0.001
Endometrial cancer	0.1	0.5	0.02
Fracture	5.9	3.7	<0.001
Hip	0.4	0.4	
Spine	0.7	0.3	
Wrist or radius	1.2	0.8	
Ischaemic cardiovascular	2.5	1.9	0.14
Ischaemic CNS	1.0	2.1	<0.001
Thromboembolic events	2.1	3.5	<0.001
Deep vein thrombosis and pulmonary embolus	1.0	1.7	0.02
Cataract	3.5	3.7	0.6

Modified from Baum M, Budzar AU, Cuzick J et al. Anastrozole alone or in combination with tamoxifen versus tamoxifen alone for adjuvant treatment of postmenopausal women with early breast cancer: first results of the ATAC randomised trial. Lancet 2002; 359:2131–9.

for all postmenopausal women with hormone receptor-positive disease. They also recommended that aromatase inhibitors should be considered in preference to tamoxifen in women with a past history of thromboembolism or who are intolerant of tamoxifen. A recent meta-analysis reported a significant survival advantage for regimens incorporating aromatase inhibitors compared with 5 years of tamoxifen, so the use of aromatase inhibitors is set to increase.

The MA-17 trial was a double-blind placebo-controlled trial[103] involving menopausal women with breast cancer who had completed 5 years of tamoxifen and randomised to a further 5 years of letrozole or placebo. This trial, involving over 5000 women, was stopped at its first interim analysis at 2.4 years follow-up at the recommendation of the independent data and safety monitoring committee after results indicated a significantly higher DFS in the letrozole group, with an estimated 4-year DFS of 93% vs. 87% with the placebo ($P \leq 0.001$). In the final updated analysis, the hazard ratios for DFS, distant DFS and OS in node-negative patients were 0.45 (95% CI 0.27–0.75), 0.63 (95% CI 0.31–1.27) and 1.52 (95% CI 0.76–3.06) respectively, while in node-positive patients the hazard ratios were 0.61 (95% CI 0.45–0.84), 0.53 (95% CI 0.36–0.78) and 0.61 (95% CI 0.38–0.98) respectively. The significant survival advantage in node-positive patients suggests that letrozole after 5 years of tamoxifen in estrogen receptor-positive postmenopausal patients will become standard of care for all but very low risk women after 5 years of tamoxifen (**Fig. 11.8**). A further randomisation in this trial after 10 years of adjuvant therapy will compare a further 5 years of letrozole and placebo. The fact that this trial was stopped early, albeit for valid ethical reasons, has created problems. The follow-up period was short, and since patients have been unblinded no long-term follow-up data will emerge.

The MA-17 trial has reminded clinicians that more breast cancer events develop 5–15 years after diagnosis and treatment than within the first 5 years and has shown that 5 years of adjuvant hormonal therapy is unlikely to be optimal. There was surprisingly little difference in adverse effects between the two groups, although low-grade hot flushes, arthritis, osteoporosis, arthralgia and myalgia were more frequent with letrozole; fracture rates were similar but there was less vaginal bleeding in the letrozole group. More importantly, there was a relative reduction in the frequency of contralateral breast cancer of 46%, comparable to that seen in previous studies with aromatase inhibitors and tamoxifen (**Fig. 11.9**).[12,101,104] Another similar maintenance trial, NSABP B-33, assessing the value of exemestane after tamoxifen, is now unlikely to be completed.[105]

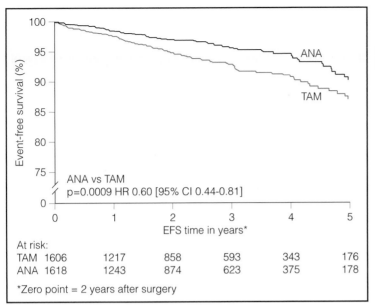

Figure 11.5 • Event-free survival from the ABCSG/ARNO study where patients were randomised to anastrozole or tamoxifen after 2 years of tamoxifen.

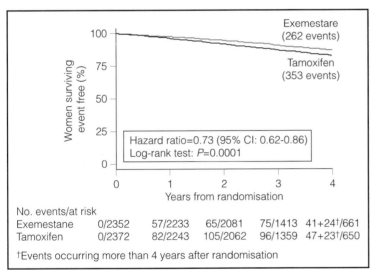

Figure 11.6 • Disease-free survival from the IES where patients were randomised to exemestane and tamoxifen after 2–3 years of tamoxifen.

ADJUVANT OVARIAN ABLATION IN PREMENOPAUSAL WOMEN

Five published trials have compared ovarian ablation with chemotherapy alone in the adjuvant setting. A brief summary of the results is given in **Table 11.7**. The Zoladex Early Breast Cancer Research Association (ZEBRA) trial[106] compared six cycles of CMF with 2 years of the GnRH agonist goserelin in 1640 premenopausal and perimenopausal patients with node-positive disease. In patients with estrogen receptor-positive cancers, both treatments were equivalent in terms of DFS (hazard ratio 1.01, 95% CI 0.84–1.20). Chemotherapy was superior in estrogen receptor-negative patients.

The Italian Breast Cancer Adjuvant Study Group (GROCTA) 02 trial[107] compared CMF versus ovarian suppression plus tamoxifen in 244 patients with estrogen receptor-positive breast cancers. After

Table 11.6 • A summary of four major adjuvant trials of aromatase inhibitors given as adjuvant treatment in the first 5 years after diagnosis.

	Follow up months	**% Node positive**	**% Chemo**	**HR primary endpoint**	**HR overall survival**
ATAC	68	34.0	21.3	0.83	0.97
BIG 1-98	35.5/25.8	41.3	25.3	0.81	0.86
IES	37.4 Post Tam	44.2	32.7	0.73	0.83
ABCSG/ARNO	28 Post Tam	25.9	0	0.60	0.76

ATAC (Arimidex or tamoxifen alone or in combination), BIG 1-98 (Breast International Group) Study, IES (Intergroup Exemestane Study) and ABCSG/ARNO Study (Austrian Breast and Colorectal Cancer Study Group and the German Adjuvant Breast Cancer Group/Arimidex-Nolvadex Trial).

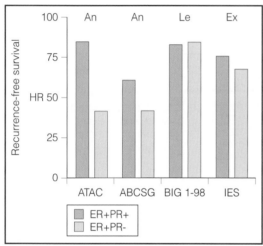

Figure 11.7 • Recurrence-free survival related to hormone receptor status in ATAC, ABCSG/ARNO, BIG 1-98 and IES studies. Patients were separated into those who had both [estrogen and progesterone receptors (ER+ PR+) or patients who were ER+ but PR–. HR, hazard rate; An, anastrazole; Le, letrozole; Ex, exemestane.

a median follow-up of 7 years no differences were found in DFS or OS (hazard ratio for relapse 0.95, 95% CI 0.62–1.46, $P = 0.48$; hazard ratio for death 0.71, 95% CI 0.38–1.31, $P = 0.3$).

The Austrian Breast and Colorectal Cancer Study Group (ABCSG) trial[108] compared CMF with goserelin plus tamoxifen in 1088 women with estrogen receptor-positive and/or progesterone receptor-positive tumours. The combination hormonal treatment was more effective than its chemotherapy counterpart in terms of DFS but

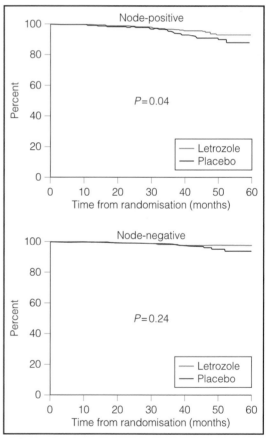

Figure 11.8 • Overall survival in the MA-17 study in which patients were randomised after 5 years of tamoxifen to letrozole or placebo. The median follow-up was 2.5 years. While overall survival was not improved in node-negative patients, there is the same reduction in local recurrences, new primaries and distant recurrences in node-negative patients as in node-positive patients.

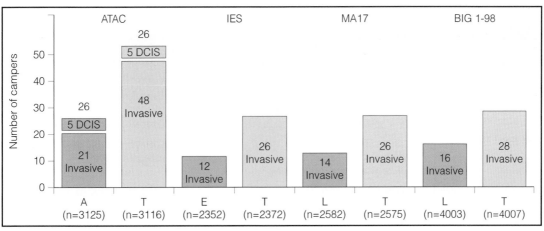

Figure 11.9 • The incidence of new (contralateral) breast primaries in the adjuvant aromatase inhibitor studies. DCIS, ductal carcinoma in situ.

Table 11.7 • Ovarian ablation versus chemotherapy in the adjuvant setting

Study (no. of patients)	Treatment arms	Results
ZEBRA[106] (1614)	A: CMF × 6 B: Goserelin (2 years)	DFS in ER+ patients: no difference
GROCTA 02[107] (244)	A: CMF × 6 B: OA + tamoxifen	DFS and OS: no difference
ABCSG 05[108] (1034)	A: CMF × 6 B: Goserelin (2 years) + tamoxifen (5 years)	OS: no difference DFS: longer with B ($P = 0.037$)
FASG 060[109] (333)	A: FEC 50 × 6 B: Triptorelin (3 years) + tamoxifen (3 years)	DFS and OS: no difference
TABLE[110] (600)	A: CMF × 6 B: Leuprorelin (2 years)	DFS: no difference

CMF, cyclophosphamide, methotrexate, 5-fluorouracil; DFS, disease-free survival; ER, estrogen receptor; FEC, 5-fluorouracil, epirubicin, cyclophosphamide; OA, ovarian ablation; OS, overall survival.

data are immature for OS and show no statistical difference between both groups.

A French study[109] compared triptorelin, another GnRH agonist, plus tamoxifen for 3 years with six cycles of 5-fluorouracil, epirubicin and cyclophosphamide (FEC) in 333 premenopausal women with hormone receptor-positive disease. No statistical differences were found in DFS or OS after 54 months median follow-up.

The Takeda Adjuvant Breast Cancer Study (TABLE)[110] compared six cycles of CMF with leuprorelin, another GnRH agonist, in 600 women (>90% estrogen receptor-positive cancers).

Progression-free survival was not significantly different between the arms.

Five trials have assessed the addition of medical ovarian ablation to chemotherapy and these are summarised in **Table 11.8**. The Zoladex in Premenopausal Patients (ZIPP) trial[111] evaluated the addition of goserelin to the standard treatment (surgery ± radiotherapy ± chemotherapy ± tamoxifen) in women under 50 years of age. At a median follow-up of 66 months, event-free survival was significantly longer for patients receiving goserelin (hazard ratio 0.8, 95% CI 0.70–0.92, P <0.001) as was OS (hazard ratio 0.82, 95% CI 0.61–0.99,

Table 11.8 • Medical ablation versus chemotherapy in the adjuvant setting

Trial (no. of patients)	Treatment arms	Results
ZIPP[111] (2710)	A: surgery ± RT ± chemotherapy ± tamoxifen B: A + goserelin	Goserelin addition: prolonged DFS ($P < 0.001$); prolonged OS ($P = 0.04$)
INT-0101[112] (1504)	A: CAF × 6 B: CAF + goserelin (5 years) C: CAF + goserelin (5 years)+ tamoxifen (5 years)	Tamoxifen addition: improved DFS ($P < 0.01$) Goserelin addition: no benefit
IBCSG VIII[113] (1063)	A: Goserelin (2 years) B: CMF × 6 C: CMF × 6 + goserelin (18 months)	Chemotherapy addition in ER+ patients: no benefit
De Matteis et al.[114] (92)	A: Epirubicin × 4 + CMF × 4 B: A + goserelin	Goserelin addition: no benefit
GOCSI Mam-1[115] (466)	A: CMF B: Doxorubicin → CMF C: CMF → goserelin + tamoxifen (2 years) D: Doxorubicin → CMF → goserelin + tamoxifen (2 years)	Goserelin + tamoxifen addition to chemotherapy: decreased relapse hazard ratio ($P = 0.04$); no change in survival ($P = 0.52$)

CAF, cyclophosphamide, doxorubicin, 5-fluorouracil; CMF, cyclophosphamide, methotrexate, 5-fluorouracil; DFS, disease-free survival; ER, estrogen receptor; OS, overall survival; RT, radiotherapy.

$P = 0.04$). Subgroup analysis suggested that goserelin had it greatest effect in estrogen receptor-positive patients not receiving chemotherapy.

The INT-0101 trial (organised by the Eastern Cooperative Oncology Group, South Western Oncology Group, and Cancer and Leukaemia Group B)[112] compared treatment with cyclophosphamide, Adriamycin and 5-fluorouracil (CAF) versus CAF plus goserelin (CAFZ) versus CAF plus goserelin plus tamoxifen (CAFZT). DFS after a follow-up of 6.2 years was 67, 70 and 77% respectively. The addition of tamoxifen was beneficial in patients with postmenopausal estrogen levels after chemotherapy, while the addition of goserelin was more beneficial in patients with premenopausal levels after CAF. There was a significant improvement in survival for the triple-therapy arm (CAFZT) over the other two arms (CAF and CAFT) ($P < 0.01$).

The International Breast Cancer Study Group (IBCSG) VIII trial[113] examined the benefit of adding chemotherapy to goserelin in patients with node-negative disease. The four treatment arms were as follows: CMF for six cycles; goserelin for 2 years; CMF for six cycles and goserelin for 18 months; and no treatment. The last arm was discontinued when the benefit for adjuvant treatment in node-negative patients was demonstrated. Recent data show that in patients with estrogen receptor-positive

tumours there is no difference in DFS between groups (81, 81 and 88% respectively).

A small, unpublished, peer-reviewed Italian study of 92 patients[114] showed that the addition of goserelin to chemotherapy with epirubicin provided no statistically significant benefit in terms of DFS or OS. The GOSCI trial[115] of 466 women examined the benefit of tamoxifen and goserelin in addition to chemotherapy. A decrease in relapse was seen in the arms that used endocrine treatment sequentially but there was no difference in terms of survival.

Prognostic significance of amenorrhoea after chemotherapy

In a recent update of the INT-0101 trial[112] with 9 years follow-up, a comparison was made between the outcome of patients achieving amenorrhoea after treatment in the chemotherapy-only arm and those who did not. The DFS was 59% in the former and 40% in the latter. This is consistent with other reports showing a lower incidence of disease-related events in patients rendered amenorrhoeic after chemotherapy.[106,108]

Tolerance of adjuvant GnRH agonists

A recent update of quality-of-life assessment from patients in the ZEBRA trial strongly suggested that, once chemotherapy is finished, there is no statistical difference in overall quality-of-life scores between patients receiving monthly goserelin for 2 years and those having no further treatment.[106] Nevertheless, hormone-related symptoms were significantly higher in the goserelin group.

One of the important adverse effects, particularly in the adjuvant setting, is the effect of goserelin on bone mineral density. In the ZEBRA trial, bone mineral density loss was greater with goserelin than with chemotherapy during the first 2 years of treatment; subsequently, partial recovery after cessation led this difference to disappear.[106]

Adjuvant chemotherapy

Axillary lymph node involvement remains the most powerful prognostic factor for recurrence, and women under the age of 70 with lymph node-positive disease should generally be offered adjuvant chemotherapy. In women with negative nodes, the decision to give chemotherapy depends on other prognostic factors. The St Gallen Conference guidelines divided women into three risk groups: low, intermediate and high, based on nodal status, hormone receptor status, tumour size, histological grade, age, HER-2 status, and peritumoral vascular invasion (see **Table 11.2**). These guidelines are not absolute, and serve to focus discussion with the patient on the risk–benefit balance.

The first effective adjuvant chemotherapy regimen, CMF, was developed in the 1970s.[116] For many years this was the mainstay of adjuvant treatment. The Oxford overview analysis of 47 trials, the majority of which used CMF-based regimens, established that adjuvant chemotherapy significantly reduces the risk of recurrence and death[12] (see **Table 11.4**). These results were significant irrespective of lymph node status, estrogen receptor status and tamoxifen use, but the degree of benefit was influenced by age and menopausal status. For all women under the age of 50, chemotherapy significantly improved the absolute 10-year survival by over 10% for those with node-positive disease (53% vs. 42%) and by around 6% for those with node-negative disease (78% vs. 71%). When results were analysed by age in decades, there was a strong trend towards younger women obtaining greater benefit. No significant benefit was demonstrated for patients over the age of 70 but the number of patients involved was small.

ANTHRACYLINES

The EBCTCG overview also showed a small but significant benefit in relapse-free survival and OS for anthracyclines compared with the more traditional CMF regimens.[12] Since this overview, other studies have confirmed the advantage of anthracycline-based therapy.[117–119,125,126] The National Cancer Institute of Canada MA.5 study[117] showed that six cycles of FEC was superior to six cycles of CMF, and the South Western Oncology Group trial 8897 showed a benefit of 5-fluorouracil, Adriamycin and cyclophosphamide (FAC) over CMF.[119] More recently, the UK NEAT study revealed superiority of epirubicin/CMF over CMF alone.[120] Anthracycline-based adjuvant chemotherapy is now standard care but the most effective combination of drugs, dose and duration of treatment remain uncertain and various regimens are currently used (**Box 11.4**).

Dose of anthracyclines

The two main anthracyclines in current use are Adriamycin (doxorubicin) and epirubicin. The Cancer and Leukaemia Group B (CALGB) 9344 trial randomised women with node-positive breast cancer to receive four courses of AC chemotherapy at one of three different Adriamycin dose levels (60, 75 or 90 mg/m^2), followed by four cycles of paclitaxel or nothing (see below).[121] This important dose-escalation trial showed no benefit for Adriamycin doses above 60 mg/m^2 and this dose should now be considered standard.

With epirubicin, a dose effect was shown in the French Adjuvant Study Group (FASG-05) trial that randomised lymph node-positive women with poor prognosis to six cycles of FEC 50 (epirubicin

Box 11.4 • Common adjuvant chemotherapy regimens

EC	Epirubicin, cyclophosphamide
AC	Adriamycin, cyclophosphamide
FEC	5-Fluorouracil, epirubicin, cyclophosphamide
FAC	5-Fluorouracil, Adriamycin, cyclophosphamide
AC and T	Adriamycin, cyclophosphamide followed by docetaxel/paclitaxel
CMF	Cyclophosphamide, methotrexate, 5-fluorouracil
Epi-CMF	Epirubicin, cyclophosphamide, methotrexate, 5-fluorouracil

50 mg/m^2) or six cycles of FEC 100 (epirubicin 100 mg/m^2).[122] A significant improvement in DFS (66.3 months vs. 54.8 months) and 5-year OS (77.4% vs. 65.3%) was seen in the FEC 100 group but there were significantly greater toxicities in the FEC 100 group, with more neutropenia, anaemia, nausea and vomiting, stomatitis, alopecia and grade 3 infections.

TAXANES

The potential importance of the taxanes as adjuvant therapy is emphasised by the large number of major trials currently running. Four important trials assessing the addition of a taxane to anthracycline chemotherapy in patients with lymph node-positive disease have been reported. In the CALGB 9344 trial, 3121 women who had received four cycles of AC chemotherapy at different dose levels (see above) were randomised to receive four further courses of paclitaxel (Taxol) or no further chemo-therapy.[121] The addition of paclitaxel resulted in a small but statistically significant improvement in DFS (absolute 5%, P = 0.0023) and OS (absolute 3%, P = 0.0064). So far in this trial the gain appears to be limited to patients with estrogen receptor-negative tumours who were not given tamoxifen.

After a median follow-up of approximately 64 months and 861 events, the NSABP B-28 trial reported preliminary results from a similarly designed trial. Around 3000 women were randomised to four courses of AC chemotherapy followed by four courses of paclitaxel versus four courses of AC chemotherapy alone;[123] 66% of patients were estrogen receptor positive and received tamoxifen but all women aged over 50 years were given tamoxifen regardless of estrogen receptor status. These results showed an absolute 4% significant improvement in DFS in the paclitaxel arm (72% vs. 76%, P = 0.008) but no difference in OS (both 85%, P = 0.46). These two trials are open to the criticism that efficacy differences could be explained by differences in treatment rather than by the addition of paclitaxel.

These two trials are open; the third trial, Breast Cancer International Research Group (BCIRG) 001, involved the other major taxane, docetaxel (Taxotere), used concurrently with an anthracycline rather than sequentially.[124] This trial randomised 1491 women to receive six cycles of standard FAC compared with six cycles of docetaxel, Adriamycin and cyclophosphamide (TAC). The second interim results, after a median follow-up of 55 months and 399 events, showed that there was a significant improvement in DFS (75% vs. 68%, P = 0.001) and OS (87% vs. 81%, P = 0.008) at 5 years for the TAC group. There was no difference in toxic deaths but the rate of febrile neutropenia was 24.7% in the TAC arm (despite prophylactic use of oral ciprofloxacin) compared with 2.5% in the FAC arm.

In the fourth trial, a French group (PACS01) compared six cycles of FEC using epirubicin 100 mg/m^2 (FEC 100) with three cycles of FEC followed by three cycles of docetaxel 100 mg/m^2 in women with node positive disease. The results showed a significant improvement in DFS in favour of the switch to docetaxel (5-year DFS 78.3% vs. 73.2%; HR 0.83; P = 0.012). Curiously, the benefit was significant in women over the age of 50 years but not for those under 50 years. There was also a small but significant OS advantage (90.7% vs. 86.7% 5-year OS; HR 0.77; P = 0.014).

There is an increasing body of evidence support-ing the use of taxanes in high-risk women in the adjuvant setting. The International Consensus Panel on the treatment of primary breast cancer[91] has for the first time included a taxane adjuvant regimen in the list of 'more effective regimens that may be preferred in patients at higher risk'. Further taxane trials, including the large UK TACT trial with over 4000 patients, should help to clarify this important issue. Meanwhile it should be noted that there is no evidence so far of the benefit of taxanes in patients with node-negative disease, and in this group of patients these drugs should only be used within the context of a trial.

DURATION OF TREATMENT

The EBCTG meta-analysis assessed five CMF-based trials and found no survival benefit for more than 6 months of treatment.[12] Two trials found equivalence between four cycles of AC and six cycles of CMF. The first study, the NSABP-B15 trial, involved lymph node-positive women with tamoxifen-resistant tumours. In the second study, the NSABP-B23 trial, women who were node nega-tive and had estrogen receptor-negative tumours were randomised to AC or CMF with or without tamoxifen. Other randomised trials have shown improved OS and DFS with more intensive anthracycline regimens such as FAC and FEC compared with CMF given for the same duration. Whether the apparent superiority of FAC/FEC over AC/EC results from the addition of a third drug (5-fluorouracil) or the longer duration of therapy (six to eight cycles of FEC/FAC vs. four cycles of AC) is unknown. However, the FASG-01 trial showed a significant benefit in DFS of six cycles of FEC 50 over three cycles of FEC 50 or 75, and improved OS with six cycles of FEC 50 over three cycles.[127]

The optimal timing of adjuvant chemotherapy after surgery remains uncertain. Treatment normally starts within a few weeks of surgery but it is unclear whether there is any gain from starting as early as possible and whether a delay has an adverse outcome. A retrospective study from a series of the IBCSG trials using CMF chemotherapy found a significant and clinically striking improvement in 10-year DFS in a small set of premenopausal patients with estrogen receptor-negative tumours who started within 21 days of surgery compared with those starting later (60% vs. 34%, $P = 0.0003$).[128] A recent review of more than 1100 patients from a prospectively maintained database treated with adjuvant chemotherapy at the Royal Marsden Hospital, including approximately 60% who had received anthracyclines,[129] showed no difference in either DFS or OS in patients starting chemotherapy within 21 days of surgery compared with those starting later.

DOSE DENSITY

Recent interest has surrounded accelerated (known as dose-dense) chemotherapy in which treatment is given at 2-week rather than 3-week intervals with granulocyte colony-stimulating factor (G-CSF) support to overcome the risk of neutropenic sepsis. A recent trial (the CALGB 974 trial) has shown that four courses of 2-weekly AC followed by four courses of 2-weekly paclitaxel (the accelerated arm) had improved efficacy over the same eight courses given conventionally at 3-week intervals in women with node-positive breast cancer, with 4-year DFS of 82% and 75% respectively.[130] In addition, the accelerated arm produced less neutropenic sepsis. Likewise an Italian trial, presented only as an abstract, has shown a similar increase in efficacy with reduced risk of neutropenic sepsis when six courses of FEC chemotherapy were given in accelerated fashion compared with the conventional approach.[131]

The shortened duration of adjuvant treatment with accelerated chemotherapy should be attractive to patients, and the reduced risk of neutropenic sepsis could save on resources. Further trials in this area are indicated.

Adjuvant bisphosphonates

Three adjuvant trials have investigated the use of bisphosphonates to prevent the appearance of bone metastases in women with early breast cancer; with conflicting results. The first trial[132] randomised 302 women with primary breast cancer and immunocytochemical evidence of cancer cells in a bone marrow aspirate to 2 years of clodronate 1600 mg daily or not. After nearly 5 years of follow-up, a reduction in the incidence of bone metastases, a trend to reduction in visceral metastases and an increase in OS were seen in the clodronate group.[132,133] The effect of clodronate decreased with longer follow-up.

The second trial[134] randomised 299 women with lymph node-positive breast cancer to 3 years of clodronate 1600 mg daily or control. This showed negative results; after a minimum of 5 years follow-up, significantly more bone metastases (26% vs. 18%) and non-skeletal metastases (45% vs. 27%) were seen in the clodronate group than the placebo group. OS was also significantly worse in the clodronate group (68% vs. 81%). However, there were imbalances in lymph node positivity, tumour size and progesterone receptor status between groups that could account, at least in part, for these unexpected results.

The third and largest trial randomised 1079 women to receive 2 years of clodronate 1600 mg daily or placebo starting within 6 months of surgery.[135] During the 2 years of treatment, there was a significant reduction in bone metastases in the clodronate group but at 5 years this effect was lost. No differences in recurrence of visceral metastases were seen. OS was significantly improved in the clodronate group.

The role of adjuvant clodronate remains uncertain, although the balance of evidence suggests clinical benefit. Further trials are now underway, including an NSABP study comparing 5 years of clodronate with placebo and a trial of the more potent bisphosphonate zoledronate (Zometa) also against placebo (AZURE). Recent results from the Austrian Breast Group comparing goserelin and tamoxifen with goserelin and anastazole has demonstrated that zoledronic acid can effectively counteracts the bone loss associated with treatment.[211]

Adjuvant trastuzumab (Herceptin)

Given the adverse prognosis associated with HER-2 overexpression and the established efficacy of trastuzumab in metastatic breast cancer, there has been much interest in the use of trastuzumab in the adjuvant setting. Four large, multicentre, randomised adjuvant trials involving more than 12 000 women continue to assess whether trastuzumab given after anthracycline chemotherapy or sequentially with a non-anthracycline regimen (Taxotere and carboplatin) can improve DFS and OS. Three of the four trials have recently reported preliminary results showing an approximate 50% reduction in relapse. The combined NSABP-B31 and NCCTG-N9831 trials, comparing AC followed by either paclitaxel alone or paclitaxel in combination with weekly trastuzumab, reported an absolute DFS advantage of 18% (HR 0.48, $2P = 3 \times 10^{-12}$) and an absolute OS of 4% (HR 0.67, $2P = 0.015$) at a median follow-up of 2 years.[212] In the NSABP-B-31 trial, more patients discontinued due to cardiac toxicity in the combined arm compared to the paclitaxel alone arm (4.1% vs. 0.7%) but there were no cardiac deaths in the combined arm.

In the HERA (Herceptin adjunct) trial, 5100 HER-2-positive patients were randomised to standard adjuvant systemic treatment with or without trastuzumab every 3 weeks for 12–24 months. Follow-up at 1 year showed a significant 46% reduction in the risk of recurrence and a 33% reduction in the risk of death. These are similar figures to the event-free survival in the NSABPB31 and Intergroup N9831 trial for the adjuvant trastuzumab (HR 0.67, $P = 0.015$), and a better overall survival (HR 0.45, $P = 3 \times 10^{-12}$). Trastuzumab should now be considered as part of the adjunct therapy regimen for all patients with HER-2-positive breast cancer. Any unanswered questions regarding the duration of treatment, long-

term safety, cardiac toxicity and ideal combinations will hopefully be revealed in the future with the maturity of these trials.

NEOADJUVANT MEDICAL THERAPY

Neoadjuvant (also called preoperative or primary) medical therapy has been increasingly used over the last decade. One of the main clinical aims is to downstage large cancers in order to avoid mastectomy and achieve conservative surgery. Clinical trials are also investigating whether short-term markers of tumour response predict long-term outcome of treatment.

Neoadjuvant endocrine therapy

Several trials using tamoxifen as an alternative to surgery in older women have shown high rates of short-term tumour regression but poor long-term local control.[136] In a small non-randomised study of older women with large primary cancers, neoadjuvant anastrozole, letrozole and exemestane have shown a higher response rate than those previously reported with tamoxifen.[137,138] Recently, two randomised trials comparing an aromatase inhibitor with tamoxifen as neoadjuvant therapy prior to surgery have been published. In the first, letrozole was compared with tamoxifen for 4 months before surgery in older patients with hormone receptor-positive large breast cancers requiring mastectomy or presenting as locally advanced disease.[139] Letrozole achieved a significantly higher rate of regression than tamoxifen (55% vs. 36%), with more patients achieving tumour regressions sufficient to allow breast-conserving surgery. An intriguing additional observation in this trial was the finding in a subgroup of patients whose tumour overexpressed HER-2 or HER-1 that the response to letrozole was very much higher than to tamoxifen (88% of 17 patients vs. 21% of 19 patients).

Recently, results have been presented from a second trial involving 330 patients in which neoadjuvant anastrozole was compared with tamoxifen or a combination of both for a period of 3 months prior to surgery.[140] This trial was a neoadjuvant version of ATAC and one of the main aims was to test whether short-term clinical or biological endpoints could act as surrogate markers for long-term outcome as identified in the ATAC trial itself. In contrast to the letrozole trial, patients with tumours of 2 cm or greater, not necessarily requiring mastectomy, were included in this trial There was no significant difference in the overall clinical response rates between the three arms, but in the 124 patients deemed by the surgeon to require mastectomy prior to neoadjuvant therapy, anastrozole achieved a significantly higher conversion rate to breast-conserving surgery than tamoxifen (47% vs. 22%, P = 0.03). This was also numerically higher than the conversion rate with the combination arm (26%). As in the neoadjuvant letrozole trial, anastrozole showed a numerically higher response rate than tamoxifen in patients whose tumours overexpressed HER-2. Only two patients also overexpressed HER-1 in this trial and these were not analysed separately. A small neoadjuvant trial from Russia has shown significantly better response rates with exemestane than with tamoxifen.

These results suggest that aromatase inhibitors are more effective than tamoxifen as neoadjuvant therapy in reducing the need for mastectomy and they also appear to be more effective specifically in patients whose tumours overexpress HER-2.[93] Letrozole is the agent of choice as it is the only drug with a product licence for neoadjuvant use.

Neoadjuvant chemotherapy

Neoadjuvant chemotherapy has high activity in early breast cancer, with overall objective response rates higher than for patients with metastatic disease, ranging from 70 to more than 90%, and pathological complete remission rates of approximately 20%.[141]

The two most influential neoadjuvant chemotherapy trials have been carried out by the NSABP. In the first, almost 1500 patients were randomised to receive neoadjuvant or adjuvant AC. At 5 years follow-up, OS rates were 80% for both arms, with DFS rates at 67% for both arms.[142] Other smaller trials have shown similar findings and a few have shown a small DFS benefit for the neoadjuvant approach; importantly, none have shown that neoadjuvant chemotherapy adversely effects survival.[141] The NSABP B-18 trial showed that the chances of conservative surgery rather than mastec-

tomy were increased with neoadjuvant chemotherapy (67% vs. 60% of patients treated conservatively, P = 0.002) and these findings have been confirmed in a smaller Royal Marsden trial (22% requiring mastectomy vs. 10% in the neoadjuvant group, P <0.003).[143]

In the second NSABP trial, B-27, three treatments were compared: (i) four courses of neoadjuvant AC followed by surgery; (ii) four courses of neoadjuvant AC followed by four courses of docetaxel and then surgery; (iii) four courses of neoadjuvant AC followed by surgery and then four courses of docetaxel.[144] Preliminary results show significantly higher clinical response and pathological complete remission with the addition of docetaxel to AC, but long-term outcome data are not yet available. A German trial of comparable design has shown similar benefit from the addition of docetaxel.[145] This trial and a smaller trial from Aberdeen have demonstrated that patients responding to four courses of cyclophosphamide, vincristine, Adriamycin and prednisolone and subsequently randomised to four further courses of docetaxel achieved a higher overall response rate and pathological remission rate than those receiving four cycles of the same chemotherapy.[146]

A novel schedule of continuous 5-fluorouracil with epirubicin and cisplatin achieved a high overall response rate of 98% and complete remission rate of over 60% in a pilot study.[147] However, a subsequent randomised trial of this schedule versus conventional AC has shown no significant difference in overall response rate, pathological complete remission or 5-year survival.[148]

At present, neoadjuvant chemotherapy remains a useful tool for trying to avoid mastectomy in patients presenting with large breast primaries and is also standard therapy for inflammatory breast carcinoma and for younger patients presenting with other forms of locally advanced disease. The rates of pathological complete response appear to be improved in patients with HER-2-positive cancers by combining chemotherapy and trastuzumab.

METASTATIC DISEASE

Although survival from breast cancer has been improving steadily over the last decade,[90] approximately 40% of patients with early breast cancer will eventually develop metastatic disease.[149] Median survival time after relapse is between 18 and 24 months[150] but many patients live for several years and a few survive a decade or more. The aims of treatment in metastatic breast cancer are to prolong life, to relieve symptoms and to maintain a good quality of life. Many drugs are now available for the treatment of breast cancer (see **Box 11.1**) and those not used as adjuvant therapy (the great majority) remain available for managing metastatic disease.

Endocrine therapy in metastatic disease

In general, endocrine therapy is used before chemotherapy in patients with hormone receptor-positive disease, unless the patient has life-threatening metastatic disease involving liver, lungs or the central nervous system. The reasons are, first, that such treatment tends to be simpler and is associated with fewer adverse effects than chemotherapy and, second, that response duration is usually considerably longer than with chemotherapy. The main evidence to support this practice comes from a meta-analysis of six trials.[151]

POSTMENOPAUSAL WOMEN

For many years, trials in postmenopausal women showed tamoxifen to be superior to, or at least as good as, all other endocrine agents including estrogens, progestagens, androgens and first- and second-generation aromatase inhibitors such as aminoglutethimide and formestane.[94] The advent of the third-generation aromatase inhibitors (anastrozole, letrozole and exemestane) has changed all this. In the 1990s, a series of trials showed anastrozole, letrozole and exemestane to be clinically superior to megestrol acetate as second-line therapy.[94]

Subsequently, three key trials have compared aromatase inhibitors with tamoxifen as first-line endocrine therapy. In the largest of these, letrozole was significantly superior to tamoxifen in terms of objective response rate, clinical benefit and time to disease progression.[152] The other two trials compared anastrozole with tamoxifen. The first showed clinical superiority of anastrozole in terms of time to disease progression.[153] The other, similar

in design, failed to show superiority for anastrozole but confirmed that it was at least as effective as tamoxifen.[154] Exemestane has also been compared with tamoxifen as first-line therapy in a randomised phase II study, which demonstrated a higher response rate (41% vs. 17%) and clinical benefit (defined as complete or partial response or stable disease for at least 6 months) with exemestane (57% vs. 42%).[155]

These trials indicate that aromatase inhibitors should now be considered standard first-line endocrine therapy for patients with advanced disease (assuming this has not already been used as adjuvant therapy). The data are more convincing for letrozole than for anastrozole, and indeed a randomised trial comparing the two in patients who failed tamoxifen suggested a small benefit in favour of letrozole; paradoxically, this was seen only in patients whose estrogen receptor status was unknown, with no difference emerging in patients with known estrogen receptor-positive tumours.[156]

The pure antiestrogen fulvestrant (Faslodex) has been compared with anastrozole in two large phase III trials, with no significant difference emerging between the two treatments.[157,158] Fulvestrant has only been compared with tamoxifen in two small trials, which randomised postmenopausal women to receive tamoxifen or fulvestrant prior to surgery. The first study[159] analysed the excised tumours for changes in proliferative index and estrogen receptor and progesterone receptor. Fulvestrant caused a decrease in both estrogen and progesterone receptors but tamoxifen only caused a decrease in estrogen receptor. Both drugs produced a similar decrease in the Ki-67 proliferative labelling index. The second study examined the cell turnover index, a composite measurement of both proliferation and apoptosis. Fulvestrant demonstrated a significant reduction in cell turnover index compared with tamoxifen.[160] However, in a direct comparison in the first-line setting, fulvestrant has shown no benefit over tamoxifen in terms of response rate or time to progression. The issue that needs to be addressed is what agent should be used after the failure of letrozole.

In a second-line endocrine therapy trial (SOFEA), fulvestrant alone after relapse on a non-steroidal aromatase inhibitor is being compared with fulvestrant in combination, with continuation of the aromatase inhibitor or exemestane alone as a third arm. This is based on experimental data suggesting that breast cancer cells may become exquisitely sensitive to very low doses of estrogen after prolonged estrogen withdrawal (as would occur on an aromatase inhibitor).

PREMENOPAUSAL WOMEN

In premenopausal patients, standard first-line therapies include tamoxifen and ovarian suppression and ovarian ablation. The medical option of ovarian suppression with a GnRH analogue is increasingly used instead of surgery and in particular instead of radiotherapy-induced ablation, following a trial showing a GnRH agonist to be similar in efficacy to surgical ablation.[161]

Recently, several small trials have examined the role of GnRH agonist plus tamoxifen versus either agent alone in the treatment of premenopausal women with metastatic disease.[162–165] Results from these trials have been combined in a meta-analysis that showed an increase in objective response rate, an improvement in progression-free survival and improved survival in women who received both agents.[165] However, there were some limitations to these findings. There was no formal cross-over of patients from the GnRH agonist to tamoxifen as second-line therapy in three of the four trials, toxicity data were not detailed and no quality-of-life information was gathered.

Finally, older endocrine agents including progestagens and high-dose estrogens are sometimes still used as third- and fourth-line endocrine therapy. In general, these are associated with more adverse effects (particularly high-dose estrogens) than the newer agents described above and also there are no good data at present on their efficacy in this setting.

Chemotherapy in metastatic disease

Systemic chemotherapy is generally used for metastatic disease in patients who have estrogen receptor-negative tumours, hormone-resistant disease or rapidly progressive disease. The impact of chemotherapy on survival in metastatic breast cancer has never been formally measured in a randomised trial, but circumstantial evidence suggests that for many patients the survival benefit is modest. It is therefore important to select treatments not just on the basis of efficacy but also with the aim of minimising toxicity. With conventional chemotherapy regimens, approximately 50% of patients achieve objective tumour regression but usually with duration of less than a year.[166] With new agents currently available, the opportunity has arisen for responses to second-line and even third-line chemotherapy but with each treatment the chance of response and its duration diminish.

ANTHRACYCLINES

Anthracycline-based chemotherapy is well established as a first-line option for patients with metastatic breast cancer when this has not been used as adjuvant treatment. In two meta-analyses, anthracycline-based regimens showed superiority over CMF-type therapy.[167,168] Thus for two decades, anthracyclines have been mainstay of palliative chemotherapy.

TAXANES

Both docetaxel and paclitaxel have been widely evaluated in the treatment of metastatic breast cancer after anthracycline use. Two large, prospective, randomised trials demonstrated that single-agent docetaxel significantly improved OS, time to disease progression and response rate compared with mitomycin C and vinblastine, and improved response rate and time to disease progression compared with methotrexate and 5-fluorouracil.[169,170] Single-agent paclitaxel also demonstrated similar response rate, progression-free survival and a trend in improved OS compared with CMF plus prednisone. Thus, the integration of this class of agents either alone[169] or in combination with other agents[171,172] in trials has shown improved OS of both untreated and refractory metastatic breast cancer compared with the groups without a taxane. Several different schedules and doses of taxanes have been investigated.

Not surprisingly, the combination of a taxane and an anthracycline has been widely investigated. Initially, difficulties were found using the combination of paclitaxel and doxorubicin. There was an increased incidence of severe neutropenia and gastrointestinal toxicity when given as prolonged infusions, and increased cardiotoxicity when they were given over a shorter period.[60,173] Changes in the schedule of administration of both drugs have resulted in the dose-limiting toxicity changing from cardiotoxicity to myelosuppression.

Six phase III trials comparing anthracycline/taxane combinations with anthracycline combinations without taxanes have been conducted[172,174–178] but only three have been published. The first was a phase II randomised study that compared doxorubicin and paclitaxel (AT) with FAC as first-line therapy. This showed a significant increase in response rate, time to disease progression and OS (22.7 vs. 18.3 months) in the AT arm.[172] The second randomised patients to AT (doxorubicin and docetaxel) or AC as first-line therapy.[174] Response rate (59% vs. 47%) and time to disease progression (37.3 vs. 31.9 weeks) were significantly better in the AT arm. Overall survival and quality-of-life measurements were similar. Febrile neutropenia, grade 3 diarrhoea and moderate asthenia were higher in the AT arm. In a similar study design by the European Organisation for Research and Treatment of Cancer (EORTC) that used paclitaxel instead of docetaxel in the AT arm, there were no significant differences in OS, response rate and time to disease progression.[175]

A recent meta-analysis of 20 randomised trials compared taxane-containing chemotherapy with non-taxane-containing chemotherapy. Taxane regimens appeared to significantly improve OS (hazard ratio 0.90, 95% CI 0.84–0.97, $P = 0.009$; HR 0.93, CI 0.86–1.00, $P = 0.05$), time to disease progression (hazard ratio 0.87, 95% CI 0.81–0.93, $P < 0.0001$; HR 0.92, CI 0.85–0.99, $P = 0.05$) and overall relapse (odds ratio 1.29, 95% CI 1.13–1.47, $P < 0.0001$, OR 1.34, CI 1.18–1.52, $P < 0.00001$). However, not all taxane-containing regimens were equally effective.[179]

CAPECITABINE

This is an effective agent in metastatic breast cancer, with the important advantages of oral availability and a low incidence of conventional toxicity including alopecia. It is a prodrug activated in the liver and perhaps also in the tumour itself by thymidine phosphorylase. Recently, in a phase III trial, the combination of capecitabine and docetaxel was shown to be superior to docetaxel alone in terms of response rate, time to disease progression and indeed OS.[171] However, it has been noted that

most patients receiving docetaxel alone did not subsequently go onto capecitabine and it is unclear whether the same survival results could have been achieved with sequential rather than concurrent treatment. This is an important issue, since this combination has not been widely used by oncologists because of a perceived high incidence of subjective and objective toxicities. As a palliative drug, capecitabine is in many ways more attractive as a single agent than in combination.

VINORELBINE

Vinorelbine is a semisynthetic vinca alkaloid that has significant clinical activity in metastatic breast cancer and the advantage of being generally well tolerated, with a low incidence of nausea, vomiting and alopecia. Its main toxicity is neutropenia. Recently, a combination of vinorelbine and epirubicin as neoadjuvant therapy has been shown to be as effective as the standard AC combination, with less severe nausea, vomiting and alopecia.[180] Vinorelbine is an undervalued drug in breast cancer.

GEMCITABINE

Gemcitabine has been widely used for some years in the treatment of lung cancer. It is a well-tolerated agent but does cause some bone marrow suppression. Important new data in metastatic breast cancer have shown that gemcitabine and paclitaxel as first-line therapy for metastatic disease is significantly superior to paclitaxel in terms of overall response rate (39.3% vs. 25.6 %, $P = 0.0007$), median time to disease progression (5.4 months vs. 3.5 months, $P = 0.0013$) and pain control. A series of further combinations are currently under study.[181]

PLATINUM SALTS

Cisplatin and carboplatin have not been widely used in the management of breast cancer but a series of small studies have suggested significant activity when used as first-line therapy.[182] Cisplatin has shown high activity in combination with epirubicin and continuous infusional 5-fluorouracil in advanced disease and as neoadjuvant therapy.[147,183] We have also used a combination of mitomycin C, vinblastine, cisplatin or carboplatin in patients with metastatic breast cancer, following conventional chemotherapy. Almost 30% of heavily pretreated patients achieved tumour regression, with good symptomatic relief (A. Urruticoechea, personal communication).

SEQUENTIAL OR COMBINATION CHEMOTHERAPY?

Traditionally, combination chemotherapy has been the rule in the treatment of metastatic breast cancer, but recently there has been evidence to suggest that sequential single agents may be as effective in terms of survival with the possibility of reduced toxicity.[184]

DURATION OF TREATMENT

The optimal duration of treatment for patients who have responsive disease remains unclear. Two randomised trials in patients who achieved a complete response to initial therapy showed a prolonged DFS from immediate treatment with a different chemotherapy regimen compared with observation and treatment on relapse.[185,186] Neither study demonstrated an improved OS and one of the studies actually showed a worse outcome.[186] No difference in survival was found between patients who had a partial response or stable disease and were randomised to receive a different chemotherapy regimen or observation[187] or high- or low-dose maintenance treatment.[188] Therefore there seems little survival benefit in giving prolonged maintenance chemotherapy for more than 6 months.

HIGH-DOSE CHEMOTHERAPY

A few years ago there was a vogue for high-dose chemotherapy with autologous stem-cell rescue, particularly in the USA. So far, a series of randomised trials have failed to show any benefit for this approach and there remains no indication for this outside a trial.[189,190]

Currently, there is no superiority of one particular regimen and therefore the patient's characteristics and tumour features should be used to guide an individual's treatment. It is important to note in reviewing these studies that improved response rate and time to disease progression does not necessarily correlate with improved OS or quality of life. Whether sequential or concurrent chemotherapy combinations are more effective or better tolerated remains to be determined. Similarly, whether two-drug or three-drug combinations are more effective than a single agent awaits the results of clinical trials. Those patients not previously exposed to an anthracycline or taxane in the adjuvant setting would be candidates for these two agents, especially if they were symptomatic or had visceral involvement.

Bisphosphonates in metastatic disease

Several randomised trials in patients with bone metastases have shown that bisphosphonates significantly reduce skeletal-related events including pathological fractures, spinal cord compression, hypercalcaemia and the need for intervention with radiotherapy or surgery by around 30–50%. They also reduce pain, but none of these trials have shown an improvement in survival.[191-196]

An early double-blind controlled trial of oral clodronate in 173 patients with bone metastases showed a significant reduction in hypercalcaemic episodes, incidence of vertebral fractures, rate of vertebral deformity and morbid skeletal events.[192] Two large, multicentre, phase III trials have shown that pamidronate in a dose of 90 mg by intravenous infusion every 3–4 weeks in addition to specific antineoplastic therapy significantly reduced the rate of skeletal complications and morbidity.[191,197,198] Mean pain and analgesic scores were also significantly lower with pamidronate.

Zoledronate is the most potent new-generation bisphosphonate and has demonstrated superiority over pamidronate in the treatment of hypercalcaemia of malignancy.[199] A large phase III trial involving 1648 patients compared zoledronate with pamidronate every 3–4 weeks in patients with myeloma or breast cancer with bone metastases.[78] This showed that zoledronate was as effective as pamidronate, and in patients with breast cancer zoledronate was significantly more effective in reducing the risk of skeletal-related events by 20% and by 30% in patients on hormonal therapy. The trial initially also set out to compare zoledronate in doses of 4 or 8 mg but renal toxicity was observed and found to be related to both dose and infusion duration. Consequently, the current recommended dose of zoledronate is 4 mg in a 15-minute infusion. This compares favourably with a 90-minute infusion for pamidronate.

Ibandronate is another highly potent bisphosphonate with both intravenous and oral formulations. A phase III placebo-controlled trial of 466 patients with metastatic breast cancer and bone metastases showed significant reduction in skeletal-related morbidity with intravenous ibandronate 6 mg.[200] A film-coated tablet has been developed and results from studies of this oral formulation are anticipated.

There is no agreed consensus on the optimal duration of bisphosphonate therapy. Most clinical trials treated patients for 2 years. Bisphosphonates are long-term supportive therapy and a recent review suggested that at least 6 months of treatment is needed to obtain benefit.[201] The ASCO guidelines advocate that intravenous bisphosphonates should be continued in conjunction with systemic therapy until there is significant clinical deterioration.[74]

At present, intravenous pamidronate and oral clodronate are the two most widely used bisphosphonates. Only a small percentage (<5%) of an oral dose of clodronate is absorbed and it is unclear whether oral clodronate is as efficacious as intravenous pamidronate or zoledronate. There are no prospective studies comparing oral and intravenous forms of bisphosphonates but, in general, less activity has been reported with oral administration than with intravenous use.[202]

Trastuzumab in metastatic disease

Trastuzumab is effective as single-agent therapy in patients with metastatic breast cancer overexpressing HER-2. It is now clear that only patients whose tumours are IHC3+ or FISH positive achieve benefit. Objective response rates are seen in less than 20% of patients who have received previous therapy,[203] but objective responses and clinical benefit are seen in almost 50% of patients with FISH-positive cancers when used as first-line treatment.[204]

The major clinical use of trastuzumab is in combination with chemotherapy. In a pivotal trial, the addition of trastuzumab to AC or taxol chemotherapy significantly improved not only response rate (50% vs. 32%, P <0.001) but also time to disease progression (7.4 vs. 4.6 months, P <0.001) and survival (25.1 vs. 20.3 months, P = 0.046).[89] This survival benefit was seen despite the subsequent sequential use of trastuzumab in around 70% of patients originally randomised to chemotherapy alone. The only major toxicity with trastuzumab was cardiac dysfunction in up to 28% of patients treated concurrently with AC and in patients who had previously received an anthracycline. In patients who developed overt cardiac failure, standard therapy was nearly always effective in achieving control. Recently, the combination of trastuzumab with docetaxel has also shown significant benefit in terms of response rate (61% vs. 36%, P = 0.001) and OS (24.1 vs. 13.2 months, P = 0.0001) compared with docetaxel alone.[205] In combination with vinorelbine, a response rate of 60–84% has been reported in several small non-randomised studies.[206–208] Other combinations are also under study, particularly platinum salts which appear to have a synergistic rather than an additive cytotoxic effect.[209]

The optimal duration of treatment with trastuzumab is unknown but there are anecdotal reports of a few patients remaining in remission for several years on treatment. Trials of trastuzumab as monotherapy or in combination have continued treatment as long as there is clinical benefit even after chemotherapy has stopped. Currently, a large randomised trial is addressing the question of whether trastuzumab should be continued or stopped at the time of starting second-line chemotherapy following disease progression with first-line treatment.

CONCLUSION

Many different forms of medical therapy are now available for the treatment of breast cancer and the options continue to increase. These changes have led to a significant improvement in the overall survival of women with early breast cancer, and have resulted in better symptom control as well as improved quality of life in advanced disease.

Acknowledgement

We should like to thank Alice Pedder for her skilled secretarial help in the preparation of this manuscript.

• **Key points**

Adjuvant therapies

- All patients having surgery for breast cancer should be considered for adjuvant therapy.
- Adjuvant treatments for women with ER positive disease include tamoxifen ± ovarian ablation (OA), for premenopausal women, and tamoxifen or aromatase inhibitors, for postmenopausal women.
- Adjuvant chemotherapy should be considered for patients at high risk of recurrence (positive nodes, large tumour, ER negative, age <35 years, HER-2 positive, peritumoral vascular invasion, histological grade 3).
- Anthrocycline-based chemotherapy is superior to CMF in the adjuvant setting.
- Taxanes should be considered in those with node-positive disease
- Adjuvant trastuzumab for at least 1 year should be considered in patients with HER-2 positive disease.

Metastatic therapies

- The aim in treating metastatic breast cancer is to palliate symptoms, improve quality of life and prolong survival.
- Endocrine treatments in premenopausal women include OA + tamoxifen → OA + letrozole/anastrazole → megestrol acetate.
- Endocrine treatments in postmenopausal women include letrozole/anastrazole → tamoxifen → exemestane → faslodex or megestrol acetate.
- Chemotherapy used includes anthrocyclines and taxanes, with no benefits for combination treatments.
- Bisphosphonates reduce skeletal morbidity.
- Trastuzumab is effective in patients with HER-2 positive (IHC 3 + or FISH +) tumours and is usually given with chemotherapy and continued until there is no further clinical benefit.

REFERENCES

1. Beatson JT. On the treatment of inoperable cases of carcinoma of the mamma: suggestions for a new method of treatment, with illustrative cases. Lancet 1896; ii:104–7, 162–5.

2. Osborne CK. Tamoxifen in the treatment of breast cancer. N Engl J Med 1998; 339:1609–18.

3. Ellis PA, Saccani-Jotti G, Clarke R et al. Induction of apoptosis by tamoxifen and ICI 182780 in primary breast cancer. Int J Cancer 1997; 72:608–13.

4. Fisher B, Redmond C, Wickerham DL et al. Systemic therapy in patients with node-negative breast cancer. A commentary based on two National Surgical Adjuvant Breast and Bowel Project (NSABP) clinical trials. Ann Intern Med 1989; 111:703–12.

5. Fisher B, Dignam J, Bryant J et al. Five versus more than five years of tamoxifen therapy for breast cancer patients with negative lymph nodes and estrogen receptor-positive tumors. J Natl Cancer Inst 1996; 88:1529–42.

6. Love RR, Cameron L, Connell BL et al. Symptoms associated with tamoxifen treatment in post-menopausal women. Arch Intern Med 1991; 151:1842–7.

7. Early Breast Cancer Trialists' Collaborative Group. Tamoxifen for early breast cancer: an overview of the randomised trials. Lancet 1998; 351:1451–67.

   Large meta-analysis establishing the use of 5 years of tamoxifen.

8. Fisher B, Costantino JP, Redmond CK et al. Endometrial cancer in tamoxifen-treated breast cancer patients: findings from the National Surgical Adjuvant Breast and Bowel Project (NSABP) B-14. J Natl Cancer Inst 1994; 86:527–37.

9. Fisher B, Jeong JH, Dignam J et al. Findings from recent National Surgical Adjuvant Breast and Bowel Project adjuvant studies in stage I breast cancer. J Natl Cancer Inst Monogr 2001; 30:62–6.

10. Kedar RP, Bourne TH, Powles TJ et al. Effects of tamoxifen on uterus and ovaries of postmenopausal women in a randomised breast cancer prevention trial. Lancet 1994; 343:1318–21.

11. Rutqvist LE. Re: second cancers after adjuvant tamoxifen therapy for breast cancer. J Natl Cancer Inst 1996; 88:1497–9.

12. Early Breast Cancer Trialists' Collaborative Group. Polychemotherapy for early breast cancer: an overview of the randomised trials. Lancet 1998; 352:930–42.

Pivotal meta-analysis establishing the benefit of adjuvant chemotherapy and the advantage of anthracyclines over CMF-based regimens.

13. Ascher SM, Imaoka I, Lage JM. Tamoxifen-induced uterine abnormalities: the role of imaging. Radiology 2000; 214:29–38.

14. Barakat RR, Gilewski TA, Almadrones L et al. Effect of adjuvant tamoxifen on the endometrium in women with breast cancer: a prospective study using office endometrial biopsy. J Clin Oncol 2000; 18:3459–63.

15. Bertelli G, Valenzano M, Costantini S et al. Limited value of sonohysterography for endometrial screening in asymptomatic, postmenopausal patients treated with tamoxifen. Gynecol Oncol 2000; 78:275–7.

16. Stewart HJ, Prescott RJ, Forrest AP. Scottish adjuvant tamoxifen trial: a randomized study updated to 15 years. J Natl Cancer Inst 2001; 93:456–62.

17. Pritchard KI, Paterson AH, Fine S et al. Randomized trial of cyclophosphamide, methotrexate, and fluorouracil chemotherapy added to tamoxifen as adjuvant therapy in postmenopausal women with node-positive estrogen and/or progesterone receptor-positive breast cancer: a report of the National Cancer Institute of Canada Clinical Trials Group. Breast Cancer Site Group. J Clin Oncol 1997; 15:2302–11.

18. Mannucci PM, Bettega D, Chantarangkul V et al. Effect of tamoxifen on measurements of hemostasis in healthy women. Arch Intern Med 1996; 156:1806–10.

19. Kaiser-Kupfer MI, Kupfer C, Rodrigues MM. Tamoxifen retinopathy. A clinicopathologic report. Ophthalmology 1981; 88:89–93.

20. Gorin MB, Day R, Costantino JP et al. Long-term tamoxifen citrate use and potential ocular toxicity. Am J Ophthalmol 1998; 125:493–501.

21. Paganini-Hill A, Clark LJ. Eye problems in breast cancer patients treated with tamoxifen. Breast Cancer Res Treat 2000; 60:167–72.

22. Kristensen B, Ejlertsen B, Dalgaard P et al. Tamoxifen and bone metabolism in postmenopausal low-risk breast cancer patients: a randomized study. J Clin Oncol 1994; 12:992–7.

23. Love RR, Mazess RB, Barden HS et al. Effects of tamoxifen on bone mineral density in postmenopausal women with breast cancer. N Engl J Med 1992; 326:852–6.

24. Powles TJ, Hickish T, Kanis JA et al. Effect of tamoxifen on bone mineral density measured by dual-energy x-ray absorptiometry in healthy premenopausal and postmenopausal women. J Clin Oncol 1996; 14:78–84.

25. Love RR, Newcomb PA, Wiebe DA et al. Effects of tamoxifen therapy on lipid and lipoprotein levels in postmenopausal patients with node-negative breast cancer. J Natl Cancer Inst 1990; 82:1327–32.

26. McDonald CC, Stewart HJ. Fatal myocardial infarction in the Scottish adjuvant tamoxifen trial. The Scottish Breast Cancer Committee. Br Med J 1991; 303:435–7.

27. Rutqvist LE, Mattsson A. Cardiac and thrombo-embolic morbidity among postmenopausal women with early-stage breast cancer in a randomized trial of adjuvant tamoxifen. The Stockholm Breast Cancer Study Group. J Natl Cancer Inst 1993; 85:1398–406.

28. Costantino JP, Kuller LH, Ives DG et al. Coronary heart disease mortality and adjuvant tamoxifen therapy. J Natl Cancer Inst 1997; 89:776–82.

29. Hayes DF, Van Zyl JA, Hacking A et al. Randomized comparison of tamoxifen and two separate doses of toremifene in postmenopausal patients with metastatic breast cancer. J Clin Oncol 1995; 13:2556–66.

30. Milla-Santos A, Milla L, Rallo L et al. Phase III randomized trial of toremifene vs tamoxifen in hormonodependent advanced breast cancer. Breast Cancer Res Treat 2001; 65:119–24.

31. Pyrhonen S, Valavaara R, Modig H et al. Comparison of toremifene and tamoxifen in post-menopausal patients with advanced breast cancer: a randomized double-blind, the 'nordic' phase III study. Br J Cancer 1997; 76:270–7.

32. Holli K. Tamoxifen versus toremifene in the adjuvant treatment of breast cancer. Eur J Cancer 2002; 38(suppl. 6):S37–S38.

33. Wickerham DL, Tan-Chiu E. Breast cancer chemo-prevention: current status and future directions. Semin Oncol 2001; 28:253–9.

34. Wakeling AE, Bowler J. ICI 182,780, a new antioestrogen with clinical potential. J Steroid Biochem Mol Biol 1992; 43:173–7.

35. Rajah TT, Dunn ST, Pento JT. The influence of antiestrogens on pS2 and cathepsin D mRNA induction in MCF-7 breast cancer cells. Anticancer Res 1996; 16:837–42.

36. Miller WR. Aromatase inhibitors: mechanism of action and role in the treatment of breast cancer. Semin Oncol 2003; 30(4 suppl. 14):3–11.

37. Nelson LR, Bulun SE. Estrogen production and action. J Am Acad Dermatol 2001; 45(3 suppl.): S116–S124.

195

References

38. Sinha S, Kaseta J, Santner SJ et al. Effect of CGS 20267 on ovarian aromatase and gonadotropin levels in the rat. Breast Cancer Res Treat 1998; 48:45–51.

39. Smith IE, Fitzharris BM, McKinna JA et al. Aminoglutethimide in treatment of metastatic breast carcinoma. Lancet 1978; ii:646–9.

40. Castiglione-Gertsch M, Pampallona S, Varini M et al. Primary endocrine therapy for advanced breast cancer: to start with tamoxifen or with medroxy-progesterone acetate? Ann Oncol 1993; 4:735–40.

41. Mattsson W. Current status of high dose progestin treatment in advanced breast cancer. Breast Cancer Res Treat 1983; 3:231–5.

42. Williams MR, Walker KJ, Turkes A et al. The use of an LH-RH agonist (ICI 118630, Zoladex) in advanced premenopausal breast cancer. Br J Cancer 1986; 53:629–36.

43. Cockshott ID. Clinical pharmacokinetics of goserelin. Clin Pharmacokinet 2000; 39:27–48.

44. Miller WR, Scott WN, Morris R et al. Growth of human breast cancer cells inhibited by a luteinizing hormone-releasing hormone agonist. Nature 1985; 313:231–3.

45. Partridge AH, Burstein HJ, Winer EP. Side effects of chemotherapy and combined chemohormonal therapy in women with early-stage breast cancer. J Natl Cancer Inst Monogr 2001; 30:135–42.

46. DeVita VT, Hellman S, Rosenberg SA. Cancer: principles and practice of oncology, 6th edn. Philadelphia: Lippincott, 2001.

47. Shapiro CL, Recht A. Side effects of adjuvant treatment of breast cancer. N Engl J Med 2001; 344:1997–2008.

48. Souhami R. Oxford textbook of oncology, 2nd edn. Oxford: Oxford University Press, 2003.

49. Bines J, Oleske DM, Cobleigh MA. Ovarian function in premenopausal women treated with adjuvant chemotherapy for breast cancer. J Clin Oncol 1996; 14:1718–29.

50. Goodwin PJ, Ennis M, Pritchard KI et al. Risk of menopause during the first year after breast cancer diagnosis. J Clin Oncol 1999; 17:2365–70.

51. Cobleigh MA, Bines J, Harris D et al. Amenorrhea following adjuvant chemotherapy for breast cancer (meeting abstract). Proc Am Soc Oncol 1995; 14:abs. 158.

52. Bryce CJ, Shenkier T, Gelmon K et al. Menstrual disruption in premenopausal breast cancer patients receiving CMF (IV) vs AC adjuvant chemotherapy (abstract). Breast Cancer Res Treat 1998; 50:284.

53. Ganz PA, Desmond KA, Leedham B et al. Quality of life in long-term, disease-free survivors of breast cancer: a follow-up study. J Natl Cancer Inst 2002; 94:39–49.

54. Howell SJ, Berger G, Adams JE et al. Bone mineral density in women with cytotoxic-induced ovarian failure. Clin Endocrinol 1998; 49:397–402.

55. Burstein HJ, Winer EP. Primary care for survivors of breast cancer. N Engl J Med 2000; 343:1086–94.

56. Arriagada R, Gutierrez J. Anthracyclines: is more better and/or more dangerous? Ann Oncol 2003; 14:663–5.

57. Crump M, Tu D, Shepherd L et al. Risk of acute leukemia following epirubicin-based adjuvant chemotherapy: a report from the National Cancer Institute of Canada Clinical Trials Group. J Clin Oncol 2003; 21:3066–71.

58. Bernard-Marty C, Mano M, Paesmans M et al. Second malignancies following adjuvant chemotherapy: 6-year results from a Belgian randomized study comparing cyclophosphamide, methotrexate and 5-fluorouracil (CMF) with an anthracycline-based regimen in adjuvant treatment of node-positive breast cancer patients. Ann Oncol 2003; 14:693–8.

59. Thirman MJ, Larson RA. Therapy-related myeloid leukemia. Hematol Oncol Clin North Am 1996; 10:293–320.

60. Gianni L, Munzone E, Capri G et al. Paclitaxel by 3-hour infusion in combination with bolus doxorubicin in women with untreated metastatic breast cancer: high antitumor efficacy and cardiac effects in a dose-finding and sequence-finding study. J Clin Oncol 1995; 13:2688–99.

61. Shan K, Lincoff AM, Young JB. Anthracycline-induced cardiotoxicity. Ann Intern Med 1996; 125:47–58.

62. Ewer MS, Gibbs HR, Swafford J et al. Cardiotoxicity in patients receiving transtuzumab (Herceptin): primary toxicity, synergistic or sequential stress, or surveillance artifact? Semin Oncol 1999; 26(4 suppl. 12):96–101.

63. Keefe DL. Anthracycline-induced cardiomyopathy. Semin Oncol 2001; 28(4 suppl. 12):2–7.

64. Schagen SB, Van Dam FS, Muller MJ et al. Cognitive deficits after postoperative adjuvant chemotherapy for breast carcinoma. Cancer 1999; 85:640–50.

65. Van Dam FS, Schagen SB, Muller MJ et al. Impairment of cognitive function in women receiving adjuvant treatment for high-risk breast cancer: high-dose versus standard-dose chemotherapy. J Natl Cancer Inst 1998; 90:210–18.

66. Brezden CB, Phillips KA, Abdolell M et al. Cognitive function in breast cancer patients receiving adjuvant chemotherapy. J Clin Oncol 2000; 18:2695–701.

67. Ahles TA, Saykin AJ, Furstenberg CT et al. Neuropsychologic impact of standard-dose systemic

chemotherapy in long-term survivors of breast cancer and lymphoma. J Clin Oncol 2002; 20:485–93.

68. Wieneke MH, Dienst ER. Neuropsychological assessment of cognitve functioning following chemotherapy for breast cancer. Psychooncology 1995; 4:61–6.

69. Phillips KA, Bernhard J. Adjuvant breast cancer treatment and cognitive function: current knowledge and research directions. J Natl Cancer Inst 2003; 95:190–7.

70. Demark-Wahnefried W, Winer EP, Rimer BK. Why women gain weight with adjuvant chemotherapy for breast cancer. J Clin Oncol 1993; 11:1418–29.

71. Irwin ML, McTiernan A, Baumgartner RN et al. Changes in body fat and weight after a breast cancer diagnosis: influence of demographic, prognostic, and lifestyle factors. J Clin Oncol 2005; 23: 774–782.

72. Theriault RL, Hortobagyi GN. The evolving role of bisphosphonates. Semin Oncol 2001; 28:284–90.

73. Berenson JR, Hillner BE, Kyle RA et al. American Society of Clinical Oncology clinical practice guidelines: the role of bisphosphonates in multiple myeloma. J Clin Oncol 2002; 20:3719–36.

74. Hillner BE, Ingle JN, Berenson JR et al. American Society of Clinical Oncology guideline on the role of bisphosphonates in breast cancer. American Society of Clinical Oncology Bisphosphonates Expert Panel. J Clin Oncol 2000; 18:1378–91.

75. Santini D, Vespasiani GU, Vincenzi B et al. The antineoplastic role of bisphosphonates: from basic research to clinical evidence. Ann Oncol 2003; 14:1468–76.

76. Rogers MJ, Frith JC, Luckman SP et al. Molecular mechanisms of action of bisphosphonates. Bone 1999; 24(5 suppl.):73S–79S.

77. Coukell AJ, Markham A. Pamidronate. A review of its use in the management of osteolytic bone metastases, tumour-induced hypercalcaemia and Paget's disease of bone. Drugs Aging 1998; 12:149–68.

78. Rosen LS, Gordon D, Kaminski M et al. Long-term efficacy and safety of zoledronic acid compared with pamidronate disodium in the treatment of skeletal complications in patients with advanced multiple myeloma or breast carcinoma: a randomized, double-blind, multicenter, comparative trial. Cancer 2003; 98:1735–44.

79. Zojer N, Keck AV, Pecherstorfer M. Comparative tolerability of drug therapies for hypercalcaemia of malignancy. Drug Saf 1999; 21:389–406.

80. Hortobagyi GN, Theriault RL, Porter L et al. Efficacy of pamidronate in reducing skeletal compli-

cations in patients with breast cancer and lytic bone metastases. Protocol 19 Aredia Breast Cancer Study Group. N Engl J Med 1996; 335:1785–91.

81. Slamon DJ, Clark GM, Wong SG et al. Human breast cancer: correlation of relapse and survival with amplification of the HER-2/neu oncogene. Science 1987; 235:177–82.

82. Liu Y, el Ashry D, Chen D et al. MCF-7 breast cancer cells overexpressing transfected c-erbB-2 have an in vitro growth advantage in estrogen-depleted conditions and reduced estrogen-dependence and tamoxifen-sensitivity in vivo. Breast Cancer Res Treat 1995; 34:97–117.

83. Press MF, Jones LA, Godolphin W et al. HER-2/neu oncogene amplification and expression in breast and ovarian cancers. Prog Clin Biol Res 1990; 354A:209–21.

84. Mass R, Press M, Anderson S et al. Improved survival benefit from Herceptin (trastuzumab) in patients selected by fluorescence in situ hybridization (FISH) (abstract). Proc Am Soc Clin Oncol 2001; 20:abs. 85.

85. Vogel CL, Cobleigh MA, Tripathy D et al. Superior outcomes with Herceptin (trastuzumab) (H) in fluorescence in situ hybridisation (FISH)-selected patients (abstract). Proc Am Soc Clin Oncol 2001; 20:abs. 86.

86. Harries M, Smith I. The development and clinical use of trastuzumab (Herceptin). Endocr Relat Cancer 2002; 9:75–85.

87. Sparano JA. Cardiac toxicity of trastuzumab (Herceptin): implications for the design of adjuvant trials. Semin Oncol 2001; 28(1 suppl. 3):20–7.

88. Baselga J. Clinical trials of Herceptin (trastuzumab). Eur J Cancer 2001; 37(suppl. 1):S18–S24.

89. Slamon DJ, Leyland-Jones B, Shak S et al. Use of chemotherapy plus a monoclonal antibody against HER2 for metastatic breast cancer that overexpresses HER2. N Engl J Med 2001; 344:783–92.

Pivotal study on the effectiveness of trastuzumab in HER-2-positive breast cancer. The first time an antibody has demonstrated clinical benefit in a non-haematological malignancy.

90. Peto R, Boreham J, Clarke M et al. UK and USA breast cancer deaths down 25% in year 2000 at ages 20–69 years. Lancet 2000; 355:1822.

91. Goldhirsch A, Glick JH, Gelber RD et al. Meeting highlights: international expert consensus on the primary therapy of early breast cancer. Ann Oncol 2005; 16:1569–83.

92. Albain KS, Green S, Ravdin PM et al. Adjuvant chemohormonal therapy for primary breast cancer should be sequential instead of concurrent: initial results from intergroup trial 0100 (SWOG-8814) (abstract). Proc Am Soc Oncol 200;

93. Ellis MJ, Coop A, Singh B et al. Letrozole is more effective neoadjuvant endocrine therapy than tamoxifen for ErbB-1- and/or ErbB-2-positive, estrogen receptor-positive primary breast cancer: evidence from a phase III randomized trial. J Clin Oncol 2001; 19:3808–16.

Clinical evidence of the cross-talk between HER-receptor family and the estrogen receptor pathways favouring the mechanism of action of aromatase inhibitors.

94. Smith IE, Dowsett M. Aromatase inhibitors in breast cancer. N Engl J Med 2003; 348:2431–42.

95. Li CI, Daling JR, Malone KE. Incidence of invasive breast cancer by hormone receptor status from 1992 to 1998. J Clin Oncol 2003; 21:28–34.

96. Bardou VJ, Arpino G, Elledge RM et al. Progesterone receptor status significantly improves outcome prediction over estrogen receptor status alone for adjuvant endocrine therapy in two large breast cancer databases. J Clin Oncol 2003; 21:1973–9.

97. Stewart HJ, Prescott RJ, Forrest AP. Scottish adjuvant tamoxifen trial: a randomized study updated to 15 years. J Natl Cancer Inst 2001; 93:456–62.

98. Tormey DC, Gray R, Falkson HC. Postchemotherapy adjuvant tamoxifen therapy beyond five years in patients with lymph node-positive breast cancer. Eastern Cooperative Oncology Group. J Natl Cancer Inst 1996; 88:1828–33.

99. Earl HM, Gray R, Kerr D et al. The optimal duration of adjuvant tamoxifen treatment for breast cancer remains uncertain: randomize into aTTom. Clin Oncol (R Coll Radiol) 1997; 9:141–3.

100. ATLAS trial: NIH clinical trial. ATLAS trial office. N Engl J Med 2003; 11-12-0003. www.cancer.gov/clinical trials/ATLAS

101. Baum M, Budzar AU, Cuzick J et al. Anastrozole alone or in combination with tamoxifen versus tamoxifen alone for adjuvant treatment of postmenopausal women with early breast cancer: first results of the ATAC randomised trial. Lancet 2002; 359:2131–9.

The first trial to support an advantage in the use of aromatase inhibitors over tamoxifen in the adjuvant setting.

102. Winer EP, Hudis C, Burstein HJ et al. American Society of Clinical Oncology technology assessment on the use of aromatase inhibitors as adjuvant therapy for postmenopausal women with hormone receptor-positive breast cancer: Status report 2004. J Clin Oncol 2005; 23:619–29.

103. Goss PE, Ingle JN, Martino S et al. A randomized trial of letrozole in postmenopausal women after five years of tamoxifen therapy for early-stage breast cancer. N Engl J Med 2003; 349:1793–802.

104. King MC, Wieand S, Hale K et al. Tamoxifen and breast cancer incidence among women with inherited mutations in BRCA1 and BRCA2: National Surgical Adjuvant Breast and Bowel Project (NSABP-P1) Breast Cancer Prevention Trial. JAMA 2001; 286:2251–6.

105. Mamounas EP. Adjuvant exemestane therapy after 5 years of tamoxifen: rationale for the NSABP B-33 trial. Oncology (Huntingt) 2001; 15(5 suppl. 7): 35–9.

106. Jonat W, Kaufmann M, Sauerbrei W et al. Goserelin versus cyclophosphamide, methotrexate, and fluorouracil as adjuvant therapy in premenopausal patients with node-positive breast cancer: The Zoladex Early Breast Cancer Research Association Study. J Clin Oncol 2002; 20:4628–35.

107. Boccardo F, Rubagotti A, Amoroso D et al. Cyclophosphamide, methotrexate, and fluorouracil versus tamoxifen plus ovarian suppression as adjuvant treatment of estrogen receptor-positive pre-/perimenopausal breast cancer patients: results of the Italian Breast Cancer Adjuvant Study Group 02 randomized trial. J Clin Oncol 2000; 18:2718–27.

108. Jakesz R, Hausmaninger H, Kubista E et al. Randomized adjuvant trial of tamoxifen and goserelin versus cyclophosphamide, methotrexate, and fluorouracil: evidence for the superiority of treatment with endocrine blockade in premenopausal patients with hormone-responsive breast cancer. Austrian Breast and Colorectal Cancer Study Group Trial 5. J Clin Oncol 2002; 20:4621–7.

109. Roche H, Kerbrat P, Bonneterre J et al. Complete hormonal blockade versus chemotherapy in premenopausal early-stage breast cancer patients (Pts) with positive hormone-receptor (HR) and 1–3 node-positive (N+) tumor: results of the FASG 06 trial (abstract). Proc Am Soc Clin Oncol 2000; 19:abs. 279.

110. Wallwiener D, Possinger K, Bondar G et al. Leuprorelin acetate vs. CMF in the adjuvant treatment of premenopausal women with ER/PR-positive, node-positive breast cancer: interim results of the TABLE study (abstract). Proc Am Soc Clin Oncol 2001; 19:abs. 359.

111. Houghton J, Baum M, Rutqvist LE et al. The ZIPP trial of adjuvant zoladex in premenopausal patients with early breast cancer: an update at five years (abstract). Proc Am Soc Clin Oncol 2000.

112. Davidson NE, O'Neill A, Vukov A et al. Chemohormonal therapy in premenopausal node-positive, receptor positive breast cancer: An Eastern Cooperative Oncology Group phase III intergroup trial (E5188, INT-0101) (abstract). Proc Am Soc Clin Oncol 2003; 22:abs. 15.

113. Castiglione-Gertsch M, O'Neill A, Gelber R et al. Is the addition of chemotherapy always necessary in node negative (N–) pre/perimenopausal breast cancer patients (pts) who receive goserelin? First results of IBSCG trial VIII (abstract). Proc Am Soc Clin Oncol 2002; 21:abs. 149

114. De Matteis A, Moore HC, Nuzzo F et al. Hormono-therapy with goserelin depot after adjuvant chemo-therapy in premenopausal women with early breast cancer: is there any benefit? (Abstract) Ann Oncol 1998; 9(suppl. 4):11.

115. Bianco A, Costanzo R, Di Lorenzo G et al. The Mam-1 GOSCI trial: a randomised trial with factorial design of chemo-endocrine adjuvant treat-ment in node-positive (N+) early breast cancer (EBC) (abstract). Proc Am Soc Oncol 2001; 20:abs. 104.

116. Bonadonna G, Valagussa P, Rossi A et al. Ten-year experience with CMF-based adjuvant chemotherapy in resectable breast cancer. Breast Cancer Res Treat 1985; 5:95–115.

117. Levine MN, Bramwell VH, Pritchard KI et al. Randomized trial of intensive cyclophosphamide, epirubicin, and fluorouracil chemotherapy com-pared with cyclophosphamide, methotrexate, and fluorouracil in premenopausal women with node-positive breast cancer. National Cancer Institute of Canada Clinical Trials Group. J Clin Oncol 1998; 16:2651–8.

118. Bergh J, Wiklund T, Erikstein B et al. Tailored fluorouracil, epirubicin, and cyclophosphamide compared with marrow-supported high-dose chemo-therapy as adjuvant treatment for high-risk breast cancer: a randomised trial. Scandinavian Breast Group 9401 study. Lancet 2000; 356:1384–91.

119. Hutchins L, Green S, Ravdin PM et al. CMF versus CAF with and without tamoxifen in high-risk node-negative breast cancer patients and a natural history follow-up study in low-risk node-negative patients: first results of intergroup trial INT 0102 (meeting abstract). Proc Am Soc Clin Oncol 1998; 17:abs. 1.

120. Poole C, Earl HM, Dunn JA et al. NEAT (National Epirubicin Adjuvant Trial) and SCTBG BR9601 (Scottish Cancer Trials Breast Group) phase III adjuvant breast trials show a significant relapse-free and overall survival advantage for sequential ECMF (abstract). Proc Am Soc Clin Oncol 2003; 22:abs. 13.

First trial to report an advantage with additional taxane in adjuvant chemotherapy for node-positive women.

121. Henderson IC, Berry DA, Demetri GD et al. Improved outcomes from adding sequential paclitaxel but not from escalating doxorubicin dose in an adjuvant chemotherapy regimen for patients with node-positive primary breast cancer. J Clin Oncol 2003; 21:976–83.

122. French Adjuvant Study Group. Benefit of a high-dose epirubicin regimen in adjuvant chemotherapy for node-positive breast cancer patients with poor prognostic factors: 5-year follow-up results of French Adjuvant Study Group 05 randomized trial. J Clin Oncol 2001; 19:602–11.

123. Mamounas E, Bryant J, Lembersky BC et al. Paclitaxel (T) following doxorubicin/cyclophosphamide (AC) as adjuvant chemotherapy for node-positive breast cancer: results from NSABP B-28 (abstract). Proc Am Soc Clin Oncol 2003; 22:abs.12.

124. Martin M, Pienkowski T, Mackey J et al. TAC improves disease free survival and overall survival over FAC in node positive early breast cancer patients. BCIRG 001: 55 months follow-up (abstract). Breast Cancer Res Treat 2003; 82(suppl. 1):abs. 43.

125. Fisher B, Redmond C, Wickerham DL et al. Doxorubicin-containing regimens for the treatment of stage II breast cancer: the National Surgical Adjuvant Breast and Bowel Project experience. J Clin Oncol 1989; 7:572–82.

126. Mouridsen H, Jo A, Michae A et al. Adjuvant anthracycline in breast cancer. Improved outcome in premenopausal patients following substitution of methotrexate in the CMF combination with epirubicin (meeting abstract). Proc Am Soc Clin Oncol 1999; 18:abs. 254.

127. Fumoleau P, Kerbrat P, Romestaing P et al. Randomized trial comparing six versus three cycles of epirubicin-based adjuvant chemotherapy in premenopausal, node-positive breast cancer patients: 10-year follow-up results of the French Adjuvant Study Group 01 trial. J Clin Oncol 2003; 21:298–305.

128. Colleoni M, Bonetti M, Coates AS et al. Early start of adjuvant chemotherapy may improve treatment outcome for premenopausal breast cancer patients with tumors not expressing estrogen receptors. The International Breast Cancer Study Group. J Clin Oncol 2000; 18:584–90.

129. Shannon C, Ashley S, Smith IE. Does timing of adjuvant chemotherapy for early breast cancer influence survival? J Clin Oncol 2003; 21:3792–7.

130. Citron ML, Berry DA, Cirrincione C et al. Ran-domized trial of dose-dense versus conventionally scheduled and sequential versus concurrent combi-nation chemotherapy as postoperative adjuvant treatment of node-positive primary breast cancer: first report of Intergroup Trial C9741/Cancer and Leukemia Group B Trial 9741. J Clin Oncol 2003; 21:1431–9.

First report to demonstrate benefit from accelerated adjuvant chemotherapy with the use of G-CSF.

131. Venturini M, Aitini E, Del Mastro L et al. Phase III adjuvant trial comparing standard versus accelerated FEC regimen in early breast cancer patients. Results

from GONO-MIG1 study (abstract). Breast Cancer Res Treat 2003; 82(suppl. 1):abs. 12.

132. Diel IJ, Solomayer EF, Costa SD et al. Reduction in new metastases in breast cancer with adjuvant clodronate treatment. N Engl J Med 1998; 339:357–63.

133. Diel IJ, Solomayer EF, Gollan C et al (abstract). Proc Am Soc Clin Oncol 2000; 19:abs. 12.

134. Saarto T, Blomqvist C, Virkkunen P et al. Adjuvant clodronate treatment does not reduce the frequency of skeletal metastases in node-positive breast cancer patients: 5-year results of a randomized controlled trial. J Clin Oncol 2001; 19:10–17.

135. Powles T, Paterson S, Kanis JA et al. Randomized, placebo-controlled trial of clodronate in patients with primary operable breast cancer. J Clin Oncol 2002; 20:3219–24.

  The largest trial of adjuvant bisphosphonate use showing a temporary benefit. Other contradictory studies have followed this.

136. Cheung KL, Howell A, Robertson JF. Preoperative endocrine therapy for breast cancer. Endocr Relat Cancer 2000; 7:131–41.

137. Dixon JM. Neoadjuvant endocrine therapy. In: Miller WR, Santen RJ (eds) Aromatase inhibition and breast cancer. New York: Marcel Dekker, 2000; pp. 103–16.

138. Miller WR, Dixon JM. Endocrine and clinical endpoints of exemestane as neoadjuvant therapy. Cancer Control 2002; 9(2 suppl.):9–15.

139. Eiermann W, Paepke S, Appfelstaedt J et al. Preoperative treatment of postmenopausal breast cancer patients with letrozole: a randomized double-blind multicenter study. Ann Oncol 2001; 12:1527–32.

140. Smith IE, Dowsett M. Comparison of anastrozole vs tamoxifen alone and in combination as neoadjuvant treatment of estrogen receptor-positive (ER+) operable breast cancer in postmenopausal women: the IMPACT trial (abstract). Breast Cancer Res Treat 2003; 82(suppl. 1):abs. 1.

141. Smith IE, Lipton L. Preoperative/neoadjuvant medical therapy for early breast cancer. Lancet Oncol 2001; 2:561–70.

142. Fisher B, Bryant J, Wolmark N et al. Effect of preoperative chemotherapy on the outcome of women with operable breast cancer. J Clin Oncol 1998; 16:2672–85.

143. Makris A, Powles TJ, Ashley SE et al. A reduction in the requirements for mastectomy in a randomized trial of neoadjuvant chemoendocrine therapy in primary breast cancer. Ann Oncol 1998; 9:1179–84.

144. Bear HD, Anderson S, Brown A et al. The effect on tumor response of adding sequential preoperative docetaxel to preoperative doxorubicin and cyclophosphamide: preliminary results from National Surgical Adjuvant Breast and Bowel Project Protocol B-27. J Clin Oncol 2003; 21:4165–74.

145. von Minckwitz G, Raab G, Schuette M et al. Dose-dense versus sequential adriamycin/docetaxel combination as preoperative chemotherapy (pCHT) in operable breast cancer (T2–3, N0–2, M0): primary endpoint analysis of the GePARDUO study (abstract). Proc Am Soc Oncol 2002; 21:43a.

146. Smith IC, Heys SD, Hutcheon AW et al. Neoadjuvant chemotherapy in breast cancer: significantly enhanced response with docetaxel. J Clin Oncol 2002; 20:1456–66.

147. Smith IE, Walsh G, Jones A et al. High complete remission rates with primary neoadjuvant infusional chemotherapy for large early breast cancer. J Clin Oncol 1995; 13:424–9.

148. Smith IE, A'Hern R, Coombes G. et al. A novel continuous infusional 5-FU-based chemotherapy regimen compared with conventional chemotherapy in the neoadjuvant treatment of early breast cancer: 5 year results of the TOPIC trial. Ann Oncol 2004; 15:751–8.

149. O'Shaughnessy J, Twelves C, Aapro M. Treatment for anthracycline-pretreated metastatic breast cancer. Oncologist 2002; 7(suppl. 6):4–12.

150. Perez EA. Current management of metastatic breast cancer. Semin Oncol 1999; 26(4 suppl. 12):1–10.

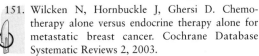

151. Wilcken N, Hornbuckle J, Ghersi D. Chemotherapy alone versus endocrine therapy alone for metastatic breast cancer. Cochrane Database Systematic Reviews 2, 2003.

  One of the major studies leading to the substitution of tamoxifen by aromatase inhibitors in the first-line treatment of metastatic breast cancer.

152. Mouridsen H, Gershanovich M, Sun Y et al. Superior efficacy of letrozole versus tamoxifen as first-line therapy for postmenopausal women with advanced breast cancer: results of a phase III study of the International Letrozole Breast Cancer Group. J Clin Oncol 2001; 19:2596–606.

153. Nabholtz JM, Buzdar A, Pollak M et al. Anastrozole is superior to tamoxifen as first-line therapy for advanced breast cancer in postmenopausal women: results of a North American multicenter randomized trial. Arimidex Study Group. J Clin Oncol 2000; 18:3758–67.

154. Bonneterre J, Thurlimann B, Robertson JF et al. Anastrozole versus tamoxifen as first-line therapy for advanced breast cancer in 668 postmenopausal women: results of the Tamoxifen or Arimidex Randomized Group Efficacy and Tolerability study. J Clin Oncol 2000; 18:3748–57.

155. Paridaens R, Dirix L, Lohrisch C et al. Mature results of a randomized phase II multicenter study

of exemestane versus tamoxifen as first-line hormone therapy for postmenopausal women with metastatic breast cancer. Ann Oncol 2003; 14:1391–8.

156. Rose C, Vtoraya O, Pluzanska A et al. Letrozole (Femara) vs. anastrozole (Arimidex): second-line treatment in postmenopausal women with advanced breast cancer (abstract). Proc Am Soc Clin Oncol 2002; 21:abs. 131.

157. Howell A, Robertson JF, Quaresma AJ et al. Fulvestrant, formerly ICI 182,780, is as effective as anastrozole in postmenopausal women with advanced breast cancer progressing after prior endocrine treatment. J Clin Oncol 2002; 20:3396–403.

158. Osborne CK, Pippen J, Jones SE et al. Double-blind, randomized trial comparing the efficacy and tolerability of fulvestrant versus anastrozole in postmenopausal women with advanced breast cancer progressing on prior endocrine therapy: results of a North American trial. J Clin Oncol 2002; 20:3386–95.

159. Robertson JF. ICI 182,780 (Fulvestrant): the first oestrogen receptor down-regulator. Current clinical data. Br J Cancer 2001; 85(suppl. 2):11–14.

160. Bundred NJ, Anderson E, Nicholson RI et al. Fulvestrant, an estrogen receptor downregulator, reduces cell turnover index more effectively than tamoxifen. Anticancer Res 2002; 22:2317–19.

161. Taylor CW, Green S, Dalton WS et al. Multicenter randomized clinical trial of goserelin versus surgical ovariectomy in premenopausal patients with receptor-positive metastatic breast cancer: an intergroup study. J Clin Oncol 1998; 16:994–9.

162. Klijn JG, de Jong FH, Blankenstein MA et al. Anti-tumor and endocrine effects of chronic LHRH agonist treatment (Buserelin) with or without tamoxifen in premenopausal metastatic breast cancer. Breast Cancer Res Treat 1984; 4:209–20.

163. Jonat W, Kaufmann M, Blamey RW et al. A randomised study to compare the effect of the luteinising hormone releasing hormone (LHRH) analogue goserelin with or without tamoxifen in pre- and perimenopausal patients with advanced breast cancer. Eur J Cancer 1995; 31A:137–42.

164. Boccardo F, Rubagotti A, Perrotta A et al. Ovarian ablation versus goserelin with or without tamoxifen in pre-perimenopausal patients with advanced breast cancer: results of a multicentric Italian study. Ann Oncol 1994; 5:337–42.

165. Klijn JG, Beex LV, Mauriac L et al. Combined treatment with buserelin and tamoxifen in pre-menopausal metastatic breast cancer: a randomized study. J Natl Cancer Inst 2000; 92:903–11.

166. Costanza ME, Weiss RB, Henderson IC et al. Safety and efficacy of using a single agent or a phase II agent before instituting standard combination chemotherapy in previously untreated metastatic breast cancer patients: report of a randomized study. Cancer and Leukemia Group B 8642. J Clin Oncol 1999; 17:1397–406.

167. A'Hern RP, Smith IE, Ebbs SR. Chemotherapy and survival in advanced breast cancer: the inclusion of doxorubicin in Cooper type regimens. Br J Cancer 1993; 67:801–5.

168. Fossati R, Confalonieri C, Torri V et al. Cytotoxic and hormonal treatment for metastatic breast cancer: a systematic review of published randomized trials involving 31,510 women. J Clin Oncol 1998; 16:3439–60.

169. Nabholtz JM, Senn HJ, Bezwoda WR et al. Prospective randomized trial of docetaxel versus mitomycin plus vinblastine in patients with metastatic breast cancer progressing despite previous anthracycline-containing chemotherapy. 304 Study Group. J Clin Oncol 1999; 17:1413–24.

170. Sjostrom J, Blomqvist C, Mouridsen H et al. Docetaxel compared with sequential methotrexate and 5-fluorouracil in patients with advanced breast cancer after anthracycline failure: a randomised phase III study with crossover on progression by the Scandinavian Breast Group. Eur J Cancer 1999; 35:1194–201.

171. O'Shaughnessy J, Miles D, Vukelja S et al. Superior survival with capecitabine plus docetaxel combination therapy in anthracycline-pretreated patients with advanced breast cancer: phase III trial results. J Clin Oncol 2002; 20:2812–23.

172. Jassem J, Pienkowski T, Pluzanska A et al. Doxorubicin and paclitaxel versus fluorouracil, doxorubicin, and cyclophosphamide as first-line therapy for women with metastatic breast cancer: final results of a randomized phase III multicenter trial. J Clin Oncol 2001; 19:1707–15.

173. Holmes FA, Madden T, Newman RA et al. Sequence-dependent alteration of doxorubicin pharmacokinetics by paclitaxel in a phase I study of paclitaxel and doxorubicin in patients with metastatic breast cancer. J Clin Oncol 1996; 14:2713–21.

174. Nabholtz JM, Falkson C, Campos D et al. Docetaxel and doxorubicin compared with doxorubicin and cyclophosphamide as first-line chemotherapy for metastatic breast cancer: results of a randomized, multicenter, phase III trial. J Clin Oncol 2003; 21:968–75.

175. Biganzoli L, Cufer T, Bruning P et al. Doxorubicin and paclitaxel versus doxorubicin and cyclo-phosphamide as first-line chemotherapy in metastatic breast cancer: the European Organization for Research and Treatment of Cancer 10961 Multicenter Phase III Trial. J Clin Oncol 2002; 20:3114–21.

176. Mackey JR, Paterson AH, Dirix L et al. Final results of the phase III randomized trial comparing docetaxel (T), doxorubicin (A) and cyclophosphamide (C) to FAC as first line chemotherapy (CT) for patients with metastatic breast cancer (abstract). Proc Am Soc Clin Oncol 2002; 21:abs. 137.

177. Luck H, Thomssen C, Untch M et al. Multicentric phase III study in first line treatment of advanced metastaic breast cancer (ABC). Epirubicin/paclitaxel (ET) vs epirubicin/cyclophosphamide (EC). A study of the Ago Breast Cancer Group (abstract). Proc Am Soc Clin Oncol 2000; 19:abs. 280.

178. Carmichael J. UKCCCR trial of epirubicin and cyclophosphamide (EC) vs. epirubicin and taxol (ET) in the first line treatment of women with metastatic breast cancer (MBC) (abstract). Proc Am Soc Clin Oncol 2001; 20:abs. 84.

179. Ghersi D, Wilcken N, Simes J et al. Taxane containing regimens for metastatic breast cancer. Cochrane Database Systematic Reviews 3, 2003.

180. Chua S, Smith IE, A'Hern R, Coombes G. et al. A randomised neoadjuvant chemotherapy trial of vinorelbine/epirubicin (VE) vs. standard doxorubicin/cyclophosphamide (DC) in patients with >3 cm diameter operable breast cancer (TOPIC2). Ann Oncol 2005; 16:1435–41

181. O'Shaughnessy J, Nag S, Calderiilo-Ruiz G et al. Gemcitabine plus paclitaxel (GT) versus paclitaxel (T) as first-line treatment for anthracycline pre-treated metastatic breast cancer (MBC): interim results of a global phase III study (abstract). Proc Am Soc Clin Oncol 2003; 22:abs. 25.

182. Smith IE, Talbot DC. Cisplatin and its analogues in the treatment of advanced breast cancer: a review. Br J Cancer 1992; 65:787–93.

183. Jones AL, Smith IE, O'Brien ME et al. Phase II study of continuous infusion fluorouracil with epirubicin and cisplatin in patients with metastatic and locally advanced breast cancer: an active new regimen. J Clin Oncol 1994; 12:1259–65.

184. Sledge GW, Neuberg D, Bernardo P et al. Phase III trial of doxorubicin, paclitaxel, and the combiation of doxorubicin and paclitaxel as front-line chemotherapy for metastatic breast cancer: an intergroup trial (E1193). J Clin Oncol 2003; 21:588–92.

185. Falkson G, Gelman RS, Pandya KJ et al. Eastern Cooperative Oncology Group randomized trials of observation versus maintenance therapy for patients with metastatic breast cancer in complete remission following induction treatment. J Clin Oncol 1998; 16:1669–76.

186. Peters WP, Jones RB, Vredenberg J et al. A large prospective, randomized trial of high-dose combination alkylating agents (CPB) with autologous cellular support (ABMS) as consolidation for patients with metastatic breast cancer acheiving complete remission after intensive doxorubicin-based induction therapy (AFM) (abstract). Proc Am Soc Clin Oncol 1996; 15:abs. 149.

187. Muss HB, Case LD, Richards F et al. Interrupted versus continuous chemotherapy in patients with metastatic breast cancer. The Piedmont Oncology Association. N Engl J Med 1991; 325:1342–8.

188. Falkson G, Gelman RS, Glick J et al. Metastatic breast cancer: higher versus low dose maintenance treatment when only a partial response or a no change status is obtained following doxorubicin induction treatment. An Eastern Cooperative Oncology Group study. Ann Oncol 1992; 3:768–70.

189. Stadtmauer EA, O'Neill A, Goldstein LJ et al. Conventional-dose chemotherapy compared with high-dose chemotherapy plus autologous hemato-poietic stem-cell transplantation for metastatic breast cancer. Philadelphia Bone Marrow Trans-plant Group. N Engl J Med 2000; 342:1069–76.

190. Berry DA, Broadwater G, Klein JP et al. High-dose versus standard chemotherapy in metastatic breast cancer: comparison of Cancer and Leukemia Group B trials with data from the Autologous Blood and Marrow Transplant Registry. J Clin Oncol 2002; 20:743–50.

191. Lipton A, Theriault RL, Hortobagyi GN et al. Pamidronate prevents skeletal complications and is effective palliative treatment in women with breast carcinoma and osteolytic bone metastases: long term follow-up of two randomized, placebo-controlled trials. Cancer 2000; 88:1082–90.

192. Paterson AH, Powles TJ, Kanis JA et al. Double-blind controlled trial of oral clodronate in patients with bone metastases from breast cancer. J Clin Oncol 1993; 11:59–65.

193. Holten-Verzantvoort AT, Kroon HM, Bijvoet OL et al. Palliative pamidronate treatment in patients with bone metastases from breast cancer. J Clin Oncol 1993; 11:491–8.

194. Rosen LS, Gordon D, Kaminski M et al. Zoledronic acid versus pamidronate in the treatment of skeletal metastases in patients with breast cancer or osteolytic lesions of multiple myeloma: a phase III, double-blind, comparative trial. Cancer J 2001; 7:377–87.

195. Body JJ, Lichinitser MR, Diel I et al. Double-blind placebo-controlled trial of intravenous ibandronate in breast cancer metatstatic to bone (abstract). Proc Am Soc Clin Oncol 1999; 18:abs. 2222.

196. Tripathy D, Lazarev A, Lichinitser MR et al. Oral ibandronate lowers the incidence of skeletal complications in breast cancer patients with bone metastases (abstract). Proc Am Soc Clin Oncol 2002.

197. Hortobagyi GN, Theriault RL, Lipton A et al. Long-term prevention of skeletal complications of metastatic breast cancer with pamidronate. Protocol 19 Aredia Breast Cancer Study Group. J Clin Oncol 1998; 16:2038–44.

Pivotal study showing the effectiveness of bisphosphonates in the treatment of bone metastases from breast cancer.

198. Theriault RL, Lipton A, Hortobagyi GN et al. Pamidronate reduces skeletal morbidity in women with advanced breast cancer and lytic bone lesions: a randomized, placebo-controlled trial. Protocol 18 Aredia Breast Cancer Study Group. J Clin Oncol 1999; 17:846–54.

199. Major PP, Coleman RE. Zoledronic acid in the treatment of hypercalcemia of malignancy: results of the international clinical development program. Semin Oncol 2001; 28(2 suppl. 6):17–24.

200. Body JJ, Diel IJ, Lichinitser MR et al. Intravenous ibandronate reduces the incidence of skeletal complications in patients with breast cancer and bone metastases. Ann Oncol 2003; 14:1399–405.

201. Ross JR, Saunders Y, Edmonds PM et al. Systematic review of role of bisphosphonates on skeletal morbidity in metastatic cancer. Br Med J 2003; 327:469.

202. Major PP, Lipton A, Berenson J et al. Oral bisphosphonates: a review of clinical use in patients with bone metastases. Cancer 2000; 88:6–14.

203. Cobleigh MA, Vogel CL, Tripathy D et al. Multinational study of the efficacy and safety of humanized anti-HER2 monoclonal antibody in women who have HER2-overexpressing metastatic breast cancer that has progressed after chemotherapy for metastatic disease. J Clin Oncol 1999; 17:2639–48.

204. Vogel CL, Cobleigh MA, Tripathy D et al. Efficacy and safety of trastuzumab as a single agent in first-line treatment of HER2-overexpressing metastatic breast cancer. J Clin Oncol 2002; 20:719–26.

205. Marty M, Cognetti F, Maraninchi D et al. Randomized phase II trial of the efficacy and safety of trastuzumab combined with docetaxel in patients with human epidermal growth factor receptor 2-positive metastatic breast cancer administered as first-line treatment: the M77001 study group. J Clin Oncol 2005; 23(19); 4265–74.

206. Burstein HJ, Harris LN, Marcom PK et al. Trastuzumab and vinorelbine as first-line therapy for HER2-overexpressing metastatic breast cancer: multicenter phase II trial with clinical outcomes, analysis of serum tumor markers as predictive factors, and cardiac surveillance algorithm. J Clin Oncol 2003; 21:2889–95.

207. Jahanzeb M, Mortimer J, Yunus F et al. Multicenter phase II trial of weekly navelbine plus herceptin in chemonaive patients with HER2 positive metastatic breast carcinoma (abstract). Proc Am Soc Clin Oncol 2001; 20:abs. 1986.

208. Burstein HJ, Kuter I, Campos SM et al. Clinical activity of trastuzumab and vinorelbine in women with HER2-overexpressing metastatic breast cancer. J Clin Oncol 2001; 19:2722–30.

209. Pegram MD, Lipton A, Hayes DF et al. Phase II study of receptor-enhanced chemosensitivity using recombinant humanized anti-p185HER2/neu monoclonal antibody plus cisplatin in patients with HER2/neu-overexpressing metastatic breast cancer refractory to chemotherapy treatment. J Clin Oncol 1998; 16:2659–71.

210. Coombes R, Hall E, Gibson L et al. A randomized trial of exemestane after two or three years of tamoxifen in postmenopausal women with primary breast cancer. N Eng J Med 2004; 350:1081–92.

211. Gnant M, Jakesz R, Mlineritsch B et al. Zoledronic acid effectively counteracts cancer treatment induced bone loss (CTIBL) in premenopausal breast cancer patients receiving adjuvant endocrine treatment with goserelin plus anastrazole versus goserelin plus tamoxifen: bone density subprotocol results of a randomised multicentre trial (ABSCG-12). Breast Cancer Res Treat 2004; 88(Suppl 1):S8.

212. Sledge G. Advances in monoclonal antibody therapy for breast cancer. Proc Am Soc Oncol 2005.

Twelve

Adjuvant radiotherapy in the management of breast cancer

Gillian Ross

INTRODUCTION

Radiotherapy has an key role in the reduction of risk of breast cancer recurrence. Importantly, results of recent clinical trials also suggest that successful locoregional tumour control may impact on overall survival. This chapter reviews the evidence base for current recommendations for adjuvant radiotherapy, and highlights areas of developments in practice.

What is radiotherapy?

Radiotherapy is the use of ionising radiation to kill cancer cells. When beams of X-rays pass through human tissue, the packets of energy (called photons) interact with tissue atoms and gradually lose momentum. The energy released within tissue damages critical molecules like DNA, producing strand breaks. Normal cells activate cell-cycle checkpoints, slowing progression to S phase, or mitosis, to enable DNA repair to occur. Most malignant cells are mutated in key cell-cycle genes (e.g. *p53*) and do not activate arrest of the cell cycle in the presence of radiotherapy-induced DNA damage. Tumour cells therefore pass on damaged DNA to daughter cells, usually activating apoptosis. Radiotherapy therefore exploits these key differences between normal and cancer cells.[1]

How is radiotherapy delivered?

Patients attend a treatment planning session before radiotherapy can begin. At this visit, the clinician marks the margins of the breast where radiation beams will be directed (**Fig. 12.1**). Treatment beams pass across the chest and through the breast tissue, efforts usually being made to minimise the amount of lung tissue included in the beam. This is important for avoiding radiation pneumonitis or long-term fibrosis. In the case of left-sided cancers, avoidance of cardiac irradiation is also important.

The unit of dose for radiotherapy is the Gray (Gy). Treatment courses vary between departments, but a commonly used schedule comprises 50 Gy given as daily treatments of 2 Gy over 5 weeks to the whole breast. In order to minimise patient attendance, especially in areas where geographical access to cancer centres is difficult, an alternative schedule of 40 Gy given in 15 treatments over 3 weeks is also commonly used. Minor variations on these dosing schedules are common, but treatment intensity is selected to give a high probablility of inactivating microscopic cancer cells while minimising adverse effects. To increase treatment intensity in the index quadrant of the tumour, it is common practice to deliver a 'boost' dose with electrons very focally. Electrons have the property of depositing their

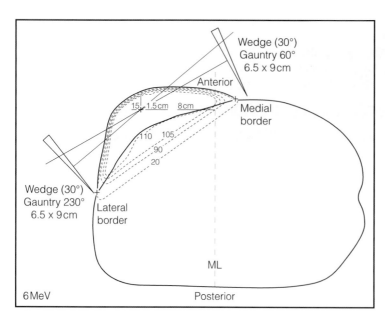

Figure 12.1 • Dose distribution for treatment of breast by tangential fields using an isocentric technique.

energy (i.e. DNA damage) within a few centimetres, and are used to increase the radiotherapy dose to the tumour bed. Typical boost doses range from 10 Gy in five fractions to 16 Gy in eight fractions.

Adverse effects

A principal effect of radiotherapy is to halt the process of division in dividing cells. In the breast area the overlying normal epidermis is affected by the radiotherapy, which suppresses cell proliferation throughout the course of treatment resulting in thinning, dryness and, in some cases, temporary moist desquamation of the skin. Blood vessels become more leaky and a varying degree of erythema develops. These effects usually resolve within 10–14 days of treatment. Increased pigmentation due to stimulation of melanocytes may last months. Simple skin care advice by an experienced radiographer or nurse is valuable during treatment. It is extremely uncommon for patients to feel unwell, and fatigue is not a problem unless the patient has had prior cytotoxic chemotherapy. Irradiation of lymph glands is recommended if there is nodal involvement on sampling, sentinel node biopsy and level I dissection and no further axillary surgery is planned. Irradiation of the supraclavicular fossa is indicated in patients with more than four

involved axillary lymph glands. If the axilla has been cleared, supraclavicular glands alone are treated. Irradiation of a fully dissected axilla should be avoided unless there is extensive extracapsular tumour extension into fat. In these circumstances, axillary and supraclavicular nodes are treated to maximise chances of achieving local tumour control, counselling the patient that postoperative irradiation in this circumstance increases the risk of treatment-related lymphoedema to approximately 40%.

RADIOTHERAPY AND BREAST CONSERVATION

The aims of breast conservation therapy using tumorectomy and adjuvant radiotherapy are to ensure survival equivalent to mastectomy, while optimising the cosmetic outcome and minimising risks of disease recurrence in the conserved breast. Since the 1970s, there have been six prospective randomised trials in which breast-conserving surgery (BCS) has been compared with mastectomy. The results are summarised in **Table 12.1**. These studies have confirmed the efficacy of BCS plus radiotherapy with respect to survival (**Fig. 12.2**). Differing surgical and radiotherapy techniques have resulted in rates of recurrence in the breast that vary from 4 to

Table 12.1 • Local recurrence rates in randomised trials comparing breast-conserving surgery (BCS) and radiotherapy (RT) with mastectomy

Reference	Trial	Follow-up (years)	Local recurrence (%)		Type of BCS
			Mastectomy	BCS + RT	
Sarrazin et al.[2]	Gustave-Roussy	10	9	7	2-cm margin
Veronesi et al.[3]	Milan	10	2	4	Quadrantectomy
Fisher et al.[4]	NSABP B-06	8	8	10	Lumpectomy
Lichter et al.[5]	NCI	8	6	20	Gross excision
Van Dongen et al.[6]	EORTC	8	9	13	1-cm margin
Blichert-Toft et al.[7]	Danish Breast Group	6	4	3	Wide excision

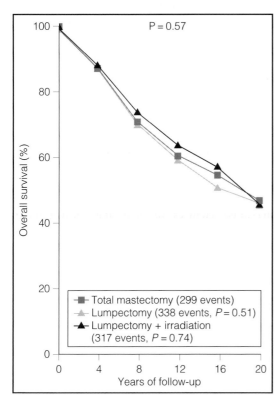

Figure 12.2 • Overall survival among 589 women treated with total mastectomy, 634 treated with lumpectomy alone and 628 treated with lumpectomy plus radiotherapy.

20% at 10 years. Despite undergoing a more radical surgical procedure, associated with significant rates of psychosexual morbidity, mastectomy still confers a risk of local recurrence of 2–9%.

Efforts have focused on refining and improving the outcomes. There is now a greater understanding of factors affecting risk of local recurrence, as well as quality of cosmesis, and greater awareness of techniques that help minimise treatment-related complications.

Risk factors for recurrence following BCS

The local recurrence rates observed in both randomised and retrospective studies range from 8 to 20% at 10 years. However, some of the longest follow-up has been obtained in retrospective studies. Kurtz et al.[8] have documented an incidence of recurrence that increased from 7% at 5 years to 14% at 10 years, rising to 20% at 20 years. The study group comprised 1593 women with stage I or II breast cancer that had been completely excised. Of the recurrences, 79% were in the vicinity of the tumor bed, but as time from treatment increased so the percentage of recurrences located elsewhere in the breast also increased. The majority of recurrences after 10 years were considered new tumours. Locoregional control was 88% at 5 years after salvage mastectomy and 64% after breast-conserving salvage procedures.

Factors that influence local recurrence include patient factors (e.g. young age), tumour factors (e.g. extensive intraductal component, lymphovascular invasion and grade) and treatment factors (e.g. resection margins, intensity of radiotherapy, and adjuvant systemic treatment). Tumour size and lymph node positivity are the most important predictive factors for overall survival, although neither has been shown to impact on local failure in the breast;[9,10] however, this may be difficult to ascertain due to competing risks of systemic failure in high-risk patients.

Pathological studies of the extent of microscopic invasive and in situ carcinoma that surrounds the macroscopic tumour in mastectomy specimens indicate that microscopic tumour extends some distance from the gross tumour. In T1 and T2 invasive cancers, microscopic extension may be present more than 2 cm from the tumour in more than 40% of patients.[11,12] This accords with the 42% probability of breast recurrence seen in the lumpectomy without radiotherapy treatment arm of NSABP-B06.[4,13] The principles behind modern BCS/radiotherapy are the surgical removal of enough breast tissue to ensure that the residual microscopic tumour burden is sufficiently low to be sterilised by moderate-dose adjuvant radiotherapy (Fig. 12.3). In all epithelial malignancies the total radiation dose required to control disease increases as tumour clonogen bulk increases. At the high radiation doses required to sterilise macroscopic disease or even large quantities of microscopic disease, there is very little therapeutic ratio in favour of tumour control over normal tissue damage. This leads to unacceptable late radiation effects in the breast and underlying chest wall. The 12% probability of ipsilateral breast recurrence in the adjuvant radiotherapy arm compared with 8% in the

mastectomy arm of NSABP B-06 suggests that moderate-dose radiotherapy can achieve acceptable local control when the margins of excision are microscopically free of tumour cells.[4,13]

Modern randomised controlled comparisons of BCS/radiotherapy and adjuvant radiotherapy with mastectomy indicate that breast preservation is not associated with any detriment to overall survival. However, local recurrence within the treated breast (3–20%) is generally more common than chest wall recurrence after mastectomy (4–9%) (see Table 12.1).[2–4,6,7,13,14]

Natural history of, and risk factors for, local recurrence

The natural history of local recurrence is protracted, with recurrence risks of 1–2% per year over at least 10 years following BCS/radiotherapy, most recurrences occurring within the index quadrant.[8,15] In contrast, postmastectomy recurrence tends to occur within 3 years of surgery.

The selection of patients for a BCS/radiotherapy strategy should take into account factors known to increase the risk of breast recurrence. Young patient age (<35–40 years) has been found to be a risk factor by several authors;[15–18] although youth correlates with the presence of adverse histopathological factors,[18] it independently signifies increased risk.[15]

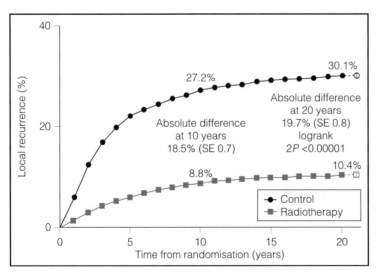

Figure 12.3 • Absolute effects of radiotherapy on isolated local recurrence as first event.

Retrospective analyses indicate that patients younger than 35 years also have an increased risk of recurrence following mastectomy.[19,20] The prospective trials of BCS/radiotherapy compared with mastectomy do not show any survival advantage for mastectomy in the subgroup of young patients. Youth is therefore not considered a contraindication to BCS/radiotherapy and adjuvant radiotherapy. Tumour multifocality, increasing tumour grade, vascular invasion, the presence of an extensive intraduct component (EIC) and the inadequacy of the surgical margins of excision have also been shown to be risk factors for breast recurrence on multivariate analyses. The increased risk of local recurrence associated with EIC is lost in multivariate analysis controlled for the presence of a tumour-free margin of excision.[15,21–24] The only one of these factors that is considered a definite contraindication to BCS/radiotherapy is macroscopic multifocality.

Importance of local recurrence

The effect of breast recurrence on overall survival is controversial. The apparent lack of detriment to survival of BCS/radiotherapy, despite an increased risk of ipsilateral breast recurrence, argues against any detrimental effect of local recurrence on survival.[2–4,6,7,13,14] More recently, the effect of prevention of local or regional recurrence on survival has been demonstrated in the 15-year follow-up results of two trials of postmastectomy radiotherapy[25,26] on long-term follow-up of BCS trials. This highlights the very long follow-up required to see differences in survival attributable to improvement in local disease control. This is especially the case in the context of BCS/radiotherapy, as local recurrence occurs later than that seen after mastectomy and this risk of recurrence continues for at least 10 years after treatment.[8,15] NSABP B-06 has shown that patients with local recurrence following BCS without radiotherapy have an increased risk of metastatic disease.[13] Touboul et al.[27] have found isolated local recurrence an independent risk factor for metastatic disease, with a relative risk of 9.9 (95% CI 5.5–18) after a mean follow-up of 7 years. It can be argued that these results may simply represent the effect of lead-time bias, as those with local recurrence may have early metastatic disease detected when they are restaged. However, others argue that it is intuitive that local recurrence can metastasise and compromise survival. The observed increases in distant metastasis associated with high rates of local recurrence may precede reductions in overall survival as observed in trials with 15-year follow-up.[28] Despite the controversy, it seems sensible to minimise the risk of local recurrence associated with breast conservation if this can be achieved with good cosmetic outcome. If not, one should consider mastectomy and breast reconstruction in those whose risk factors indicate a risk of local recurrence unacceptable to the individual patient.

Balance between optimal local control and cosmesis

Quadrantectomy was associated with a risk of local recurrence of 5.3% and lumpectomy of 13.3% in the Milan II trial, despite both being followed by radiotherapy. Microscopic involvement of the surgical margin by tumour occurred in 3% of the quadrantectomy group and 16% of the lumpectomy group, accounting for the excess local recurrence rate with lumpectomy. Cosmesis is significantly worse following quadrantectomy.[3] There is thus a balance between minimising the volume of breast tissue excised in order to maintain a good cosmetic result and removing sufficient tissue to allow maintenance of the radiation dose below that which leads to unacceptable late radiation damage, which itself compromises cosmesis.[29]

Margin status and local recurrence risk

The final surgical margin is a critical determinant of local recurrence risk, with actuarial recurrence rates of 2–5% for margin-negative groups and 16–21% for margin-positive groups.[18,21,22,24,30] More recent publications have suggested that although diffuse involvement of the margin is associated with an increased recurrence rate, focal involvement of the margin is not.[31–33]

Influence of systemic therapy on local recurrence following BCS

Chemotherapy alone does not reduce local recurrence risk after BCS.[4,13] Data on the effect of systemic therapy in addition to adjuvant radiotherapy on local recurrence is scarce. Retrospective series are confounded by competing risks, with those selected for systemic therapy more likely to develop distant disease before local recurrence. Treatment with adjuvant chemotherapy did seem to be associated with reduced risk of local failure following BCS/radiotherapy and radiotherapy in one study.[34] The analysis did not take into account the status of the surgical margin. Randomised data from NSABP B-13 indicates that in patients with clear margins adjuvant chemotherapy does appear to reduce risk of ipsilateral breast recurrence from 13.4% to 2.6% at 8 years.[35]

For patients with involved margins, a multivariate analysis of the Stanford series found the use of concurrent adjuvant chemotherapy to be independently associated with better local control in those with margins that were not more than 2 mm clear.[32] Other series including patients with involved margins have not found use of adjuvant chemotherapy to be associated with reduced risk of local recurrence.[18,24,27,30,36] Tamoxifen-like chemotherapy reduces local recurrence, and in postmenopausal women the new aromatose inhibitors appear to be better than tamoxifen in maintaining local control.

Optimising breast conservation with adjuvant radiotherapy

Current research is now focusing on optimising the physical delivery of radiotherapy to maintain benefits of treatment, with reduced late toxicity. Active studies are now addressing technical issues such as optimal dose fractionation and improved homogeneity of dose delivery by intensity modulation of beams. Given the increasing proportion of women receiving both adjuvant chemotherapy and radiotherapy we need to define the most efficacious sequencing based on evidence. Finally, as the UK Breast Screening Programme has identified a significant proportion of women with ductal carcinoma in situ or small (<2 cm) low-grade node-negative cancers, we need to carefully examine the role of adjuvant radiotherapy in such good-prognosis patients to be certain that treatment is efficacious.

POSTMASTECTOMY RADIOTHERAPY

Despite the widespread use of BCS in the management of early breast cancer, a significant number of patients are unsuitable for this approach and are offered mastectomy. Many women who are offered mastectomy rather than breast conservation tend to have larger tumours with adverse histopathological prognostic features. Despite the near complete removal of breast tissue that occurs at mastectomy, locoregional recurrence still occurs in 30–40% of women with these adverse prognostic features. The chest wall is the commonest site of locoregional recurrence and this is thought to arise from tumour that has involved dermal lymphatics. Unsurprisingly, the presence of tumour in axillary lymph nodes is the strongest indicator of risk of locoregional recurrence. High grade, tumour diameter over 4 cm and direct invasion of skin or pectoral fascia are also risk factors. Unlike breast recurrence following BCS, chest wall recurrence can only be controlled in about half of patients. Uncontrolled chest wall recurrence, which commonly progresses to encase the hemithorax, is one of the most distressing manifestations of advanced breast cancer and is difficult to satisfactorily palliate.

Adjuvant radiotherapy may be used following radiotherapy with two potential benefits: reduction in risk of locoregional recurrence and improved overall survival. A number of trials over the past 30 years have examined the effect of postoperative radiotherapy on these two endpoints. Many of the early trials were conducted before adjuvant systemic therapy had been shown to eradicate micrometastatic disease in some patients and before modern radiotherapy techniques that minimise normal tissue irradiation effects were widely used.

A meta-analysis published in 1987 of all randomised controlled trials started before 1975 showed that postmastectomy radiotherapy was associated with a 66% reduction in risk of locoregional recurrence.

However, radiotherapy was associated with an excess mortality in those living more than 10 years after randomisation. In this group the 25-year survival was 42% following radiotherapy and 51% following surgery alone. The excess mortality in the radiotherapy group was due to cardiac deaths (**Fig. 12.4**) and was balanced by a reduction in breast cancer mortality (**Fig. 12.5**). In 1995 the Early Breast Cancer Trialists' Collaborative Group[37] published a meta-analysis of randomised controlled trials started before 1985. This included 14 500 women randomised in 32 trials where primary surgery involved some form of mastectomy and 3000 women randomised in trials where surgery involved BCS. The use of radiotherapy was associated with a 66% reduction in risk of local recurrence. However, there was no difference in 10-year overall survival, being 40.3% for radiotherapy and 41.4% for surgery alone. There was a statistically significant difference in overall survival associated with use of adjuvant radiotherapy in

those treated by mastectomy and axillary sampling [odds reduction (OR) 14%, SD 7%, $P = 0.004$] compared with those treated by mastectomy alone (OR 3%, SD 4%, $P = $ NS) or mastectomy and axillary clearance (OR −3%, SD 4%, $P = $ NS).

Radiotherapy was associated with a reduced risk of death due to breast cancer (OR 0.94, 95% CI 0.88–1.00), i.e. zero to five fewer deaths due to breast cancer per 100 women treated. However, there was an increased risk of death from other causes (OR 1.24, 95% CI 1.09–1.42, $P = 0.002$). The relative increase in risk of death was the same at ages under 50 years, 50–59 years and over 60 years at the time of randomisation. However, the absolute excess risk of death associated with radiotherapy was greater in those aged over 60 at randomisation (4.2%) compared with those aged less than 50 (0.5%).[38]

Modern radiotherapy techniques recognise the importance of minimising the cardiac volume irradiated and use fractionated radiotherapy

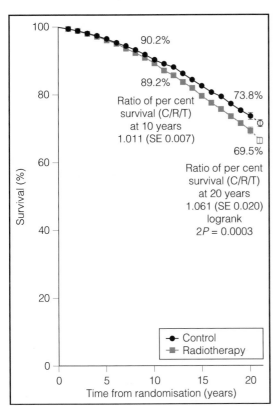

Figure 12.4 • Absolute effects of radiotherapy on non-breast cancer deaths.

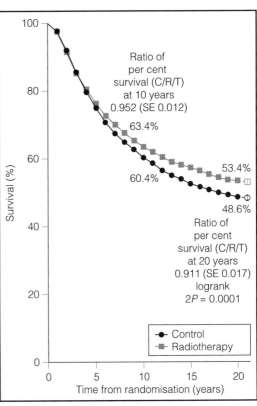

Figure 12.5 • Absolute effects of radiotherapy on breast cancer deaths.

regimens that reduce late normal tissue radiation effects.

Three large randomised trials have recently reported long-term results of postoperative radiotherapy after mastectomy in high-risk premenopausal women treated with cyclophosphamide, methotrexate and 5-fluorouracil (CMF) chemotherapy and high-risk postmenopausal women treated with tamoxifen. The Danish trial[25] included 1789 premenopausal women with pathologically positive axillary lymph nodes, tumour greater than 5 cm in diameter or invasion of the skin or the pectoral fascia. Following total mastectomy with stripping of the pectoral fascia and level I/II axillary dissection, patients received eight to nine cycles of CMF chemotherapy. Adjuvant radiotherapy was the randomised treatment and was delivered to the chest wall, axilla, supraclavicular and infraclavicular nodes and the internal mammary nodes using a cardiac-sparing technique. After a median follow-up of 114 months, the use of radiotherapy was associated with a 21% absolute reduction in risk of local recurrence (9% vs. 32%, P <0.001) and a 9% absolute increase in overall survival (P <0.001). The effect of radiotherapy on overall survival was irrespective of tumour size, node status, number of positive nodes or the histopathological grade.

The British Columbia trial[39] also examined the effect of postoperative radiotherapy in premenopausal women with pathologically involved axillary lymph nodes treated with modified radical mastectomy, including level I/II axillary dissection and six cycles of CMF chemotherapy. This group also irradiated the axilla, supraclavicular fossa and internal mammary chain (IMC). After 15-years follow-up the use of radiotherapy was associated with a 20% absolute reduction in risk of locoregional recurrence (13% vs. 33%, P = 0.003) and a 17% absolute increase in disease-free survival (50% vs. 33%, P = 0.007) and metastasis-free survival (51% vs. 34%, P = 0.006). Overall survival was improved by 8% at 15 years (54% vs. 46%, P = 0.007). Overall survival data were recently updated at the San Antonio Breast Cancer meeting and showed a statistically significant 30% reduction in risk of death (relative risk 0.7, P = 0.002) associated with use of radiotherapy. There was no difference in relative benefit of radiotherapy in those with one to three or more than three nodes involved. There was no excess cardiac morbidity or mortality in either of these trials.

These trials have received some criticism because the management of the axilla and the chemotherapy used was suboptimal, 3-weekly intravenous CMF being considered not as good as more modern anthracycline-containing regimens. In the absence of data showing a reduction of risk of death of equivalent magnitude for anthracycline-containing adjuvant regimens over CMF, it seems unlikely that the use of these regimens would negate the 30% reduction of risk of death gained by use of radiotherapy seen in these trials. Both of these trials demonstrate that prevention of locoregional recurrence reduces metastatic disease and death.

The effect of postmastectomy radiotherapy in postmenopausal women under 70 years of age treated with adjuvant tamoxifen has recently been reported by the Danish Breast Cancer Cooperative Group;[40] 1460 women were treated with total mastectomy and level I/II axillary dissection. All had pathologically positive axillary lymph nodes, tumours greater than 5 cm in diameter or involvement of skin or pectoral fascia. All received 30 mg tamoxifen daily for a year. Radiotherapy to the chest wall, axilla, supraclavicular/infraclavicular fossa and IMC was randomised. After a median follow-up of 119 months for survivors and 46 months for those that died, locoregional recurrence had occurred in 8% of the radiotherapy arm and 35% of the no radiotherapy arm. Radiotherapy was associated with a 9% absolute overall survival advantage at 10 years (45% vs. 36%, P = 0.03). There was no difference in proportionate benefit of radiotherapy in those with large or small tumours or with few or many positive nodes. The median number of nodes removed was seven. The proportionate benefit of radiotherapy was identical in those who had more or less than eight nodes removed. The benefit of radiotherapy on overall survival only became apparent more than 4 years after randomisation. There was no evidence of increased cardiac morbidity or mortality after 10 years of follow-up.

The duration of tamoxifen treatment and the absence of adjuvant chemotherapy would now be considered suboptimal. Whether the reduction in risk of local recurrence and subsequent improval in overall survival associated with radiotherapy would be nullified by use of tamoxifen for 5 years is unknown. One would have to demonstrate a sustained 27% absolute improvement in locoregional recurrence and 9% absolute improvement in survival compared with 1 year of tamoxifen alone to negate the observed advantage to radiotherapy.

These three randomised trials comprising 3500 women treated with more modern radiotherapy techniques and with adjuvant systemic therapy demonstrate very similar absolute improvements in locoregional recurrence and overall survival. Based on these data postmastectomy radiotherapy will prevent one death for every eleven women treated, and one locoregional recurrence for every three to five women treated.

RADIOTHERAPY AND POSTMASTECTOMY RECONSTRUCTION

Despite the success of conservative therapy for early breast cancer, many patients still require or choose mastectomy. For these patients the option of breast reconstruction offers improved cosmesis, body image and quality of life. The indications for postoperative radiotherapy are no different to those previously described for postmastectomy patients. It is clearly important to know how radiotherapy might impact on the success of the reconstruction. This will have implications for the advice and information given to such patients regarding the best timing and techniques for, and likely outcome of, the procedure. The target volume for radiotherapy after mastectomy should include the skin of the chest wall and the superficial fascia of the underlying muscles.

Implant reconstruction usually involves either prosthesis implantation only or a latissimus dorsi myocutaneous flap with an underlying implant. When surgery is followed by radiotherapy, there is often worsening of cosmesis and capsule formation around the implant. Implant removal is frequently recorded; overall surgical revision rates increase after radiotherapy and include capsulotomy, wound débridement and adjustment of implant position. Most implants that are removed because of capsule formation are successfully replaced, with a good outcome. In general, even with radiotherapy the proportion of patients with good or excellent cosmesis scores (albeit with various methods of assessment) is satisfyingly high.

Transverse rectus abdominis myocutaneous flap reconstruction is usually performed without pros-

thesis implantation. A number of studies have reported significantly increased complication rates (mostly flap failure and fat necrosis) in patients with a history of prior radiotherapy and a worse cosmetic outcome. There is little doubt that radiotherapy impacts on the outcome of implant reconstructions following mastectomy. It is likely that despite this the benefits of immediate reconstruction to the patient's overall quality of life are still significant and substantial. Furthermore, there is no evidence that delayed reconstruction improves the outcome. On this background it seems reasonable to advocate a policy of immediate reconstruction, preferably with a myocutaneous flap rather than an implant/expander alone even if the patient is likely to require radiotherapy. Clearly, the surgeon and the radiotherapist must do everything possible to lower the morbidity. The increased risk of capsule formation and implant removal must be made clear to the patient.

PARTIAL BREAST AND INTRAOPERATIVE RADIOTHERAPY

With screening identifying increasing numbers of patients with in situ or small cancers, there is an increasing interest in evaluating whether the positive effects of radiotherapy can be maintained by focusing treatment on the index breast quadrant alone, so-called partial breast radiotherapy. Techniques for partial breast radiotherapy include standard LINAC-based three-dimensional external beam therapy, radioactive implants (so-called 'brachytherapy') and intraoperative single-fraction treatment. The latter two approaches are being evaluated in two randomised studies against whole-breast radiotherapy in Europe.[41,42]

PALLIATIVE RADIOTHERAPY IN BREAST CANCER

Radiotherapy has a major role in symptom control in locally advanced breast cancer and metastatic disease. Women with locally advanced cancers unsuitable for surgery can have significant reduction in size of fungating or bleeding tumours by radiotherapy. Although low-dose treatments (e.g. 20 Gy in five fractions) can help achieve some tumour control, if the patient's life expectancy is longer than 6 months, then it is worth offering standard adjuvant therapy as 'high-dose' palliation, for example 50 Gy in 25 fractions (or its approximate biological equivalent) can gain long-term local control of bulk disease, especially if a boost dose to a smaller region of disease can be increased to 60–70 Gy.

Radiotherapy often produces rapid relief of bone pain in women with metastatic disease. Doses such as 8-Gy single treatments are appropriate for non-weight-bearing bones. Higher doses are required to achieve enough tumour regression to permit some bone remodelling and are more appropriate in disease involving vertebrae or major pelvic bones or femur. Treatment can significantly impact on

fracture rate or progression to overt spinal cord compression. It can be combined with early systemic therapy with bisphosphonates to reduce morbidity of bone metastases.

SUMMARY

Adjuvant radiotherapy has an established role in the reduction of risk of locoregional breast cancer recurrence, after both mastectomy and BCS. It may also impact on overall survival, adding to the benefits accrued by systemic adjuvant therapy. New developments include assessing the efficacy of partial breast irradiation in small cancers, and improving standard breast radiotherapy by intensity-modulated techniques.

Key points

- Radiotherapy after lumpectomy confers survival equivalent to mastectomy, with improved body image and is the standard of care for women wishing to preserve the breast.
- With proper attention to surgical margins, adjuvant radiotherapy should give local control rates of 95% or better at 5 years.
- Postmastectomy chest wall and nodal radiotherapy is offered routinely to women with high risk of locoregional relapse; risk factors include high grade, involvement of four or more nodes, dermal or pectoral infiltration.
- Future directions in breast radiotherapy research include adopting techniques aimed at minimising cardiac irradiation and defining the place of partial breast treatment.

REFERENCES

1. Perez CA, Brady LW. Principles and practice of radiation oncology, 4th edn. Philadelphia: Williams & Wilkins, Lippincott.

2. Sarrazin D, Lê MG, Arriagada R et al. Ten-year results of a randomized trial comparing a conservative treatment to mastectomy in early breast cancer. Radiother Oncol 1989; 14:177–84.

3. Veronesi U, Banfi A, Salvador B et al. Breast conservation is the treatment of choice in small breast cancer: long-term results of a randomized trial. Eur J Cancer 1990; 26:668–70.

4. Fisher B, Redmond C, Poisson R et al. Eight-year results of a randomized clinical trial comparing total mastectomy and lumpectomy with or without irradiation in the treatment of breast cancer. N Engl J Med 1989; 320:822–8.

5. Poggi MM, Danforth DN, Sciuto LC et al. Eighteen-year results in the treatment of early breast carcinoma with mastectomy versus breast conservation therapy: the National Cancer Institute Randomised Trial. Cancer 2003; 98:697–702.

6. van Dongen JA, Bartelink H, Fentiman IS et al. Randomized clinical trial to assess the value of breast-conserving therapy in stage I and II breast cancer, EORTC 10801 trial. J Natl Cancer Inst Monogr 1992; 11:15–18.

7. Blichert-Toft M, Brincker H, Andersen JA et al. A Danish randomized trial comparing breast-preserving therapy with mastectomy in mammary carcinoma. Preliminary results. Acta Oncol 1988; 27:671–7.

8. Kurtz JM Almaric R, Brandone H et al. Local recurrence after breast conserving surgery and

radiotherapy: frequency, time course and prognosis. Cancer 1989; 63:1912–17.

9. Clarke DH, Lê MG, Sarrazin D et al. Analysis of local–regional relapses in patients with early breast cancers treated by excision and radiotherapy: experience of the Institut Gustave-Roussy. Int J Radiat Oncol Biol Phys 1985; 11:137–45.

10. Halverson KJ, Perez CA, Taylor ME. Age as a prognostic factor for breast and regional nodal recurrence following breast conserving surgery and irradiation in stage I and II breast cancer. Int J Radiat Oncol Biol Phys 1993; 27:1045–50.

11. Ohtake T, Abe R, Kimijima I et al. Intraductal extension of primary invasive breast cancer treated by breast-conservative surgery: computer graphic three dimensional reconstruction of the mammary duct-lobular system. Cancer 1995; 76:32–45.

12. Holland R, Veling SH, Mravunac M et al. Histologic multifocality of Tis, T1–2 breast carcinomas: implications for clinical trials of breast-conserving surgery. Cancer 1985; 56:979–90.

13. Fisher B, Anderson S, Redmond CK et al. Reanalysis and results after 12 years of follow-up in a randomized clinical trial comparing total mastectomy with lumpectomy with or without irradiation in the treatment of breast cancer. N Engl J Med 1995; 333:1456–61.

14. Straus K, Lichter A, Lippman M et al. Results of the National Cancer Institute early breast cancer trial. J Natl Cancer Inst Monogr 1992; 11:27–32.

15. Fourquet A, Campana F, Zafrani B et al. Prognostic factors of breast recurrence in the conservative management of early breast cancer: a 25-year follow-up. Int J Radiat Oncol Biol Phys 1989; 17:719–25.

16. Kurtz JM, Spitalier JM, Amalric R et al. Mammary recurrences in women younger than forty. Int J Radiat Oncol Biol Phys 1988; 15:271–6.

17. Boyages J, Recht A, Connolly JL et al. Early breast cancer: predictors of breast recurrence for patients treated with conservative surgery and radiation therapy. Radiother Oncol 1990; 19:29–41.

18. Kurtz JM, Jacquemier J, Amalric R et al. Why are local recurrences after breast-conserving therapy more frequent in younger patients? J Clin Oncol 1990; 8:591–8.

19. Donegan W, Perez-Mesa C, Watson F. A biostatistical study of locally recurrent breast carcinoma. Surg Gynecol Obstet 1966; 122:529.

20. Matthews RH, McNeese MD, Montague RH et al. Prognostic implications of age in breast cancer patients treated with tumorectomy and irradiation or with mastectomy. Int J Radiat Oncol Biol Phys 1988; 14:659–63.

21. Anscher MS, Jones P, Prosnitz LR et al. Local failure and margin status in early-stage breast carcinoma treated with conservation surgery and radiation therapy. Ann Surg 1993; 218:22–8.

22. Gage I, Schnitt SJ, Nixon AJ et al. Pathologic margin involvement and the risk of recurrence in patients treated with breast-conserving therapy. Cancer 1996; 78:1921–8.

23. Solin LJ, Fowble BL, Schultz DJ et al. The significance of the pathology margins of the tumor excision on the outcome of patients treated with definitive irradiation for early stage breast cancer. Int J Radiat Oncol Biol Phys 1991; 21:279–87.

24. Borger J, Kemperman H, Hart A et al. Risk factors in breast-conservation therapy. J Clin Oncol 1994; 12:653–60.

25. Overgaard M, Hansen PS, Overgaard J et al. Post-operative radiotherapy in high-risk premenopausal women with breast cancer who receive adjuvant chemotherapy. Danish Breast Cancer Cooperative Group 82c Trial. N Engl J Med 1997; 337:949–55.

26. Ragaz J, Jackson SM, Le N et al. Adjuvant radiotherapy and chemotherapy in node-positive premenopausal women with breast cancer. N Engl J Med 1997; 337:956–62.

27. Touboul E, Buffat L, Belkacemi Y et al. Local recurrences and distant metastases after breast conserving surgery and radiation therapy for early breast cancer. Int J Radiat Oncol Biol Phys 1999; 43:25–38.

28. Hellman S. Stopping metastases at their source. N Engl J Med 1997; 337:996–7.

29. Wazer DE, DiPetrillo T, Schmidt-Ullrich R et al. Factors influencing cosmetic outcome and complication risk after conservative surgery and radiotherapy for early-stage breast carcinoma. J Clin Oncol 1992; 10:356–63.

30. Spivack B, Khanna MM, Tafra L et al. Margin status and local recurrence after breast-conserving surgery. Arch Surg 1994; 129:952–6; discussion 956–7.

31. Di Biase SJ, Komarnicky LT, Schwartz GF et al. The number of positive margins influences the outcome of women treated with breast preservation for early stage breast carcinoma. Cancer 1998; 82:2212–20.

32. Smitt MC, Nowels KW, Zdeblick MJ et al. The importance of the lumpectomy surgical margin status in long-term results of breast conservation. Cancer 1995; 76:259–67.

33. Peterson ME, Schultz DJ, Reynolds C et al. Outcomes in breast cancer patients relative to margin status after treatment with breast conserving surgery and radiation therapy. Int J Radiat Oncol Biol Phys 1999; 43:1029–35.

34. Rose MA, Henderson IC, Gelman R et al. Premenopausal breast cancer patients treated with

conservative surgery, radiotherapy and adjuvant chemotherapy have a low risk of local failure. Int J Radiat Oncol Biol Phys 1989; 17:711–17.

35. Fisher B, Dignam J, Mamounas HP et al. Sequential methotrexate and fluorouracil for the treatment of node-negative breast cancer patients with oestrogen-receptor negative tumours: eight-year results from NSAPB B-13 and first report of findings from NSABP B-10 comparing methotrexate and fluorouracil. J Clin Oncol 1996: 14:1982.

36. Ryoo MC, Kagan AR, Wollin M et al. Prognostic factors for recurrence and cosmesis in 393 patients after radiation therapy for early mammary carcinoma. Radiology 1989; 172:555–9.

37. Early Breast Cancer Trialists' Collaborative Group. Effects of radiotherapy and surgery in early breast cancer: an overview of the randomized trials. N Engl J Med 1995; 333:1444–55.

38. Cuzick J, Stewart H, Rutqvist L et al. Cause-specific mortality in long-term survivors of breast cancer who participated in trials of radiotherapy. J Clin Oncol 1994; 12:447–53.

39. Ragaz J, Jackson SM, Le N et al. Adjuvant radiotherapy and chemotherapy in node-positive premenopausal women with breast cancer. N Engl J Med 1997; 337:956–962.

40. Overgaard M, Jensen MB, Overgaard J et al. Post-operative radiotherapy in high-risk postmenopausal breast-cancer patients given adjuvant tamoxifen: Danish Breast Cancer Cooperative Group DBGG 82c randomised trial. Lancet 1999; 353:1641–8.

41. Keisch M. Partial breast radiotherapy. Breast Cancer Res 2005.

42. Ross GM. Partial breast radiotherapy: technically feasible but who will benefit? Breast Cancer Res 2005.

Thirteen

Palliative care in breast cancer

Janet Hardy

INTRODUCTION

As metastatic breast cancer is an incurable malignancy, the ability to palliate advanced disease is of major importance, particularly as around 14 000 women in the UK die of the disease each year. Palliative care is important not just in the terminal phase of disease but throughout the patient's illness. Chemotherapy, hormone therapy and radiotherapy are probably the most effective means of palliation in breast cancer, but it is not always possible or appropriate to deliver these treatment modalities. The common symptoms of breast cancer relate directly to the pattern of metastatic disease spread, and any treatment should always be delivered in conjunction with measures to control symptoms. Palliative care has the potential to improve the quality of life of women with metastatic breast disease.[1]

PAIN

Pain is the most common and certainly the most feared symptom in patients with cancer. However, chronic pain can be controlled in about 80% of patients if treated according to the analgesic guidelines of the World Health Organization (WHO). These are based on a three-step ladder approach whereby increasing severity of pain is matched by increasing strength of analgesia (**Fig.13.1**).[2] A systematic review has challenged the validity of those studies that have claimed to show the effectiveness of the WHO ladder, mainly on methodological grounds.[3] The weight of anecdotal evidence, however, does support the conclusion that this method provides a simple and effective means of controlling cancer pain in most patients.

Physicians need to become familiar with the use of a relatively small number of drugs in order to adhere to these guidelines. Analgesia at each step can be supplemented by the use of additive drugs or co-analgesics (see below). At each step of the ladder, drugs should be used up to the maximum dose and frequency prior to progression to the next step. The system is based on regular oral drug dosing rather than 'as-required' medication. It is illogical to use an alternate drug of the same strength if the previous drug on the same step has failed to control pain. Recommended drugs at each step are shown in **Fig. 13.2**. At step 1, paracetamol (acetaminophen) is used in preference to aspirin because of its relative lack of gastrointestinal toxicity.

Non-steroidal anti-inflammatory drugs (NSAIDs) are now also classed as step 1 analgesics rather than co-analgesics. They have proven efficacy in cancer pain[4] and are particularly useful in bone pain. There are many of these agents available. Apart from differences in cost and some differences in side-effect profile, there is little advantage of one NSAID over another. The analgesic effect is dose

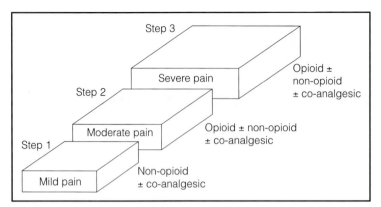

Figure 13.1 • WHO analgesic ladder.

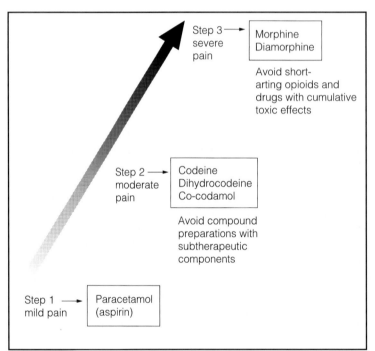

Figure 13.2 • Recommended analgesics at each step of the WHO analgesic ladder.

dependent up to a ceiling. The incidence of adverse effects (predominantly gastric and renal toxicity) increases with dose and chronic use.[4] Meta-analysis has shown NSAIDs to be as effective as, if not better than, paracetamol and to be more effective than several of the opioids traditionally used either alone or in combination at step 2 of the analgesic ladder.[4,5] Many are now available in slow-release preparations as well as suppository and elixir form (**Table 13.1**). It is important to remember that the prescription of an NSAID per rectum does not protect from gastrointestinal toxicity as this is a systemic effect. Other adverse effects include fluid retention and a reversible inhibition of platelet aggregation. All NSAIDs should be used with caution in elderly patients and in those with cardiac or renal impairment, and they should not be used in patients with low platelet counts. The selective cyclooxygenase (COX)-2 inhibitors (that inhibit only those prostaglandins contributing to the pain and swelling of inflammation and not those that are protective to the gut and kidneys) have been shown to be as effective as 'standard' NSAIDs with an improved gastrointestinal side-effect profile.[6]

Table 13.1 • Non-steroidal anti-inflammatory drugs (NSAIDs)

Drug	Usual oral dose	Comments
Naproxen*[†]	500 mg b.i.d.	Available as enteric-coated preparation
Diclofenac*[††]	50 mg t.i.d.	75- and 100-mg slow-release preparations available
Ibuprofen[†]	400 mg t.d.s. to 600 mg q.i.d.	Fewer side effects than other NSAIDs but weaker anti-inflammatory properties
Ketoprofen*	100–200 mg daily	Available as once-daily slow-release preparation
Sulindac	200 mg b.i.d.	Similar tolerance to naproxen
Indometacin*[†]	50 mg t.i.d.	Intermediate risk of gastrointestinal toxicity
Ketorolac[‡]	40 mg daily	Higher analgesic/anti-inflammatory ratio, can be given subcutaneously
Rofecoxib[†]	12.5–25 mg daily	Preferential cyclooxygenase (COX)-2 inhibitor
Celecoxib	100–200 mg b.i.d.	Preferential COX-2 inhibitor

*Available as suppository.
[†]Available as elixir/dispersable tablet.
[‡]Can be given subcutaneously (unlicensed route of delivery).

Unfortunately, long-term therapy with these agents increases the risk of cardiovascular and thrombotic adverse events. They should not be prescribed for patients at risk.

It has become clear that the previous ladder terminology of 'weak' and 'strong' opioids is misleading in that low-dose morphine produces effects indistinguishable from those of the opioids commonly used at step 2. All opioids are now classed together and separated only on the basis of those commonly used for mild to moderate pain at step 2 and those commonly used for moderate to severe pain at step 3.[7] Many of the opioids used at step 2 are available in combination preparations, e.g. co-proxamol (paracetamol and dextroproxyphene) and co-codamol (paracetamol and codeine). A common mistake at step 2 is to use combination analgesics that comprise low subtherapeutic doses of opioid, e.g. co-codaprin and co-codamol 8/500, which both contain only 8 mg codeine in combination with aspirin and paracetamol, respectively. Dihydrocodeine is a semisynthetic analogue of codeine and has the advantage of being available as an oral solution and as a delayed-release preparation that can be given twice daily rather than 4-hourly as with co-proxamol or co-codamol.

Although there are now a large number of alternative strong opioids available (see below), mor-

phine remains the opioid of choice at step 3.[8] There are a large number of preparations and strengths of morphine available (**Table 13.2**). When starting morphine, patients should ideally be prescribed one of the immediate-release preparations, e.g. Sevredol or Oramorph, that are given every 4 hours at a dose of 5–10 mg. The dose can then be increased every 24 hours or so until pain control is achieved. The total daily dose can then be given as a delayed-release preparation, either once or twice a day, e.g. 4-hourly 10 mg immediate-release morphine can be given as MST Continus 30 mg b.i.d. or as MXL capsules 60 mg once daily. A 'breakthrough dose,' which is equivalent to the 4-hourly dose (or one-sixth of the total 24-hour dose), can be given at any time in between planned doses for uncontrolled or 'breakthrough' pain. Patients should never be expected to wait the standard 4 hours for the next dose of morphine if they are in pain. The necessity for many breakthrough doses indicates that the baseline dose should be increased. It is unusual for patients to have to take delayed-release morphine more often than recommended. Very rarely, a patient may have to take MST Continus 8-hourly rather than 12-hourly, but this usually indicates that the baseline 12-hourly dose needs to be increased. There is no ceiling dose of morphine; the correct dose for any patient is the dose that controls the

Table 13.2 • Morphine formulations commercially available for routine use

IMMEDIATE-RELEASE ORAL PREPARATIONS	
Duration of action 4 hours	
Morphine sulphate oral solution, e.g. (Oramorph)	10 mg/5 mL (+ taste mask), suitable for dose titration
Concentrated oral morphine sulphate solution	100 mg/5 mL (no taste mask)
Morphine sulphate unit dose vials	10 mg/5 mL, 30 mg/5 mL, 100 mg/5 mL
Morphine tablets (Sevredol)	10, 20 and 50 mg tablets suitable for those patients who prefer tablets
Morphine suppositories	10, 15, 20, 30, 50 and 100 mg, similar bioavailability to oral morphine
DELAYED-RELEASE ORAL PREPARATIONS	
Duration of action 12 hours	
Morphine sulphate controlled-release tablets, e.g. MST Continus, Oramorph SR	Available in 5, 10, 30, 60, 100 and 200 mg strengths Suitable for patients with good pain control on a stable dose of morphine
Morphine sulphate slow-release suspension	Sachet of granules to mix with water: 20, 30, 60, 100 and 200 mg
Duration of action 24 hours	
Morphine sulphate controlled-release tablets, e.g. MXL capsules	Available in 30, 60, 90, 120, 150 and 200 mg capsules
Morphine sulphate injection	Diamorphine is usually preferred because of its greater solubility

pain. Most patients can be controlled on less than 30 mg 4-hourly, but the dose range is wide (5–500 mg 4-hourly). Guidelines for the prescription of morphine are shown in **Box 13.1** and in the document produced by the Expert Working Group of the European Association for Palliative Care (EAPC).[8] Patients are advised to take morphine regularly rather than 'as required', as morphine is a relatively poor analgesic when given orally in single doses. Morphine 6-glucuronide, an active morphine metabolite, is a potent analgesic but is produced in very small quantities after a single dose of morphine. It is thought that repeated dosing is necessary in order to allow accumulation of morphine 6-glucuronide to sufficient concentrations to provide analgesia and specifically to cross into the cerebrospinal fluid to reach central opioid receptors.[9]

Laxatives should always be prescribed with morphine as constipation is an inevitable adverse effect of the drug. Other adverse effects include nausea, vomiting and drowsiness, which usually resolve after a couple of days. Respiratory depression can be used to advantage to palliate breathlessness in a patient without pain, but in patients with pain this is not usually a problem. Pain does seem to provide physiological antagonism to the respiratory depressant effects of opioid analgesia. One explanation is that the respiratory centre receives nociceptive input that counterbalances the respiratory depressant potential of the opioid.[10] Dry mouth is unfortunately a common adverse effect that does not tend to resolve. Itch and hallucinations are rarer side effects, and are generally a contraindication to the continued use of the drug. An evidence-based review of the common adverse effects of morphine and how to manage them is presented in a report by the EAPC.[11]

Morphine toxicity is reflected by increasing drowsiness, miosis, myoclonic jerks and respiratory depression. This often reflects deteriorating renal function as morphine 6-glucuronide accumulates in renal failure. This situation can usually be managed by stopping the drug for a while and restarting at a lower dose given less frequently than 4-hourly. In severe toxicity the effect of morphine may be reversed

Box 13.1 • Guidelines for the prescription of morphine

1. Start with a low dose of immediate-release morphine

2. Prescribe a regular 4-hourly dose (with a double dose at night to avoid the middle-of-the night dose)

3. Prescribe the same dose to be given 'as required' for 'breakthrough' pain

4. Review after 24–36 hours and, if pain not controlled, increase 4-hourly dose by one-third, e.g. $10 \rightarrow 15 \rightarrow 20 \rightarrow 30 \rightarrow 40$ mg

5. Once the pain is controlled, convert to once or twice daily slow-release morphine preparations

6. Continue to supply appropriate 'breakthrough' doses equivalent to the 4-hourly dose in an immediate-release preparation

7. If pain control is lost, recalculate total daily dose required according to 'breakthrough' requirements

8. Always prescribe a laxative to be taken concurrently

9. Ensure that outpatients have a supply of antiemetics in case of opioid-induced nausea

10. Reassure the patient that most of the initial adverse effects, e.g. drowsiness, light-headedness and nausea, will pass

11. Ensure appropriate patient review

with naloxone, a synthetic opioid antagonist that competitively inhibits the effects of opioids.

Unfortunately, many patients equate morphine with the 'end of the road', and feel that if they agree to take morphine they are somehow 'giving up'. It is crucial therefore to explain that this is not the case and that morphine may in fact allow patients to live longer by allowing them greater activity and by relieving stress. Another common concern is a fear of addiction. Although patients can develop a physical dependence to morphine (as detected by a withdrawal syndrome when the drug is stopped suddenly), addiction encompasses psychological and behavioural factors that do not apply when morphine is taken for pain. There is no reason why a woman taking morphine cannot continue to undertake normal daily activities (including driving[12]), assuming her pain is under control.

When the oral route is not available, drugs must be delivered parenterally at step 3 (see below). Diamorphine is only available in the UK; morphine

and hydromorphone are used most commonly for subcutaneous and intravenous infusion in centres elsewhere. Fentanyl is a synthetic opioid that is available in a parenteral preparation and a transdermal delivery system. Skin patches are applied every 72 hours and a 'fentanyl depot' concentrates in the upper skin layers, from where the drug diffuses to the systemic circulation. The full clinical effects are not noted for 8–16 hours after application of the patch and persist for about 17 hours after patch removal. Fentanyl patches are therefore not suitable for patients with acute or changing pain as dose titration is difficult, but they do offer an alternate non-invasive parenteral approach for patients with chronic stable pain. Buprenorphine is also available in a transdermal delivery system and has the advantage of a smaller patch dose. Over recent years a number of new opioids and opioid preparations have become available for use in both malignant and non-malignant pain. Some of these are listed in **Table 13.3**, along with their respective advantages and disadvantages. Whereas the majority of patients are said to have good pain control using morphine and its derivatives according to the WHO guidelines, there has been much enthusiasm in recent times for opioid 'switching' or 'rotation'. The aim is to improve pain control with fewer adverse effects by changing a patient from one strong opioid to another. The exact mechanism underlying this phenomenon is not clear.[13] The most simplistic explanation is that changing to a new drug allows any toxic metabolites of the previous drug to dispel, with the result that the new drug is better tolerated. Others believe that because of the uncertainty surrounding opioid dose equivalents, opioid switching often results in a dose reduction, and hence a lessening of adverse effects. Switching between opioids complicates pain management and is only recommended with expert advice.[14]

Co-analgesics are drugs that have little intrinsic analgesic effect but, when taken with standard analgesia, can confer an additive benefit with respect to pain control at any step of the WHO ladder. Examples include the use of antidepressants and anticonvulsants for neuropathic pain (see below; **Table 13.4**). Corticosteroids are valuable co-analgesics in several pain situations. As well as their non-specific benefit in mood elevation and general well-being, they can often provide added analgesia

Table 13.3 • 'Alternative' strong opioids

Drug	Indication	Comments
Diamorphine	Nil by mouth Inability to take oral medications	Greater solubility than morphine allows injection of smaller volumes Drug option for subcutaneous strong opioid infusion
Fentanyl	When oral route not available or gut absorption poor	Available as a transdermal patch or parenteral preparation Less constipating than morphine
Methadone	Opioid rotation Neuropathic pain	Long half-life Unique dosing schedule Toxic metabolites can accumulate with prolonged use
Oxycodone	Intolerance to morphine Morphine 'phobia'	Synthetic analogue of morphine available in oral, rectal and parenteral formulations, no active metabolites
Hydromorphone	Opioid rotation	Analogue of morphine, with similar pharmacokinetic properties
Tramadol	WHO step 2 and 3 analgesic	Opioid and non-opioid analgesia by enhancement of serotoninergic and adrenergic pathways, therefore fewer opioid adverse effects
Pethidine	*Not* indicated in chronic pain because of short half-life	Less intense action at smooth muscle compared with morphine plus additional anticholinergic effects; toxic metabolites accumulate with prolonged use
Dextromoramide	Incident pain	Short half-life, duration of action 1–2 hours, unsuitable for regular analgesia in chronic pain

Table 13.4 • Co-analgesics

Indication	Appropriate agents	Comments
Bone pain	NSAIDs* Bisphosphonates	Anti-inflammatory action via inhibition of prostaglandin synthesis Potent inhibitors of osteoclast-mediated bone resorption
Neuropathic pain	Antidepressants, e.g. amitriptyline, dosulepin Anticonvulsants, e.g. sodium valproate, carbamazepine, gabapentin Antiarrhythmics, e.g. flecainide, mexiletine Corticosteroids	Analgesic effect via increased concentrations of serotonin in spinal cord; indicated for dysaesthetic, aching neuropathic pain Analgesic effect via stabilisation of neuronal membrane; indicated for shooting, lancinating pain Membrane stabilisers, usually used 'third line' Reduce perineuronal oedema
Soft-tissue inflammation	NSAIDs Corticosteroids Antibiotics	Useful for inflammatory breast tumours
Muscle spasm	Benzodiazepines Baclofen	Added anxiolytic effect Can be sedative

NSAID, non-steroidal anti-inflammatory drug.
*WHO step 1 analgesic.

for bone pain, neuropathic pain and inflammatory tumours. However, adverse effects after long-term use are significant and include proximal myopathy, Cushing's syndrome, oral *Candida*, glucose intolerance, sleep disturbance and even psychosis. Patients taking steroids should be monitored closely so that the drug can be discontinued if the desired symptomatic benefit is not achieved. If effective, maintenance doses should be kept as low as possible.[15]

Non-pharmacological means of pain control should also be considered. Acupuncture, transcutaneous electrical nerve stimulation (TENS), relaxation therapy, massage and distraction therapy can all benefit selected patients. Similarly, anaesthetic techniques for pain control, e.g. spinal opioid administration and neurolytic blocks, are indicated for the control of particularly difficult pain or where standard analgesia cannot be tolerated because of unacceptable adverse effects.

Factors that predict for difficult or poor pain control are neuropathic pain, incident pain (pain only on movement), high previous narcotic exposure, major psychological distress, high tolerance (necessitating rapid increase in dose) and a history of alcoholism or drug addiction.

SPECIAL CIRCUMSTANCES COMMON IN METASTATIC BREAST CANCER

Special pain situations

PAIN SECONDARY TO BONE METASTASES

Radiotherapy remains the treatment of choice for the palliation of metastatic bone disease (**Fig. 13.3**). Single fractions have been shown to be as effective as multiple fractions in the achievement of pain control,[16] and this is more acceptable to patients, especially those with a poor performance status. NSAIDs are specifically indicated in this situation and should be used as analgesics in their own right rather than as adjuncts to basic analgesia as described above.

Bisphosphonates are now considered part of the routine systemic treatment regimen of breast cancer. Their mechanism of action is complex and not fully understood, but they are known to be potent inhibitors of normal and pathological bone resorption. A recent systematic review has confirmed their role in the reduction of skeletal morbidity in breast cancer.[17] When given for more than 6 months, bisphosphonates significantly reduce the incidence of fractures (both vertebral and non-vertebral), hypercalcaemia and the need for radiotherapy. Studies that have lasted more than 12 months also show a reduction in the need for orthopaedic interventions. As well as a positive effect on the reduction of skeletal complications, bisphosphonates also have an analgesic effect. A Cochrane review[18] was limited by the methodological flaws and/or inconsistencies in many of the studies but was able to recommend that bisphosphonates be considered in addition to analgesia and radiotherapy when these

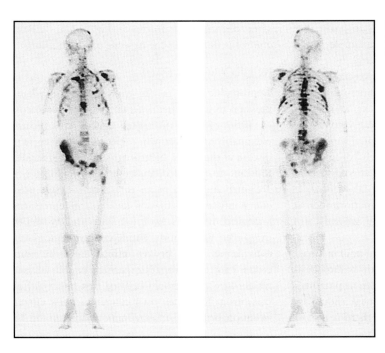

Figure 13.3 • Bone scan showing widespread metastases from breast carcinoma.

modalities alone are inadequate for the management of painful bone metastases. The maximum response is likely to be seen within 4 weeks. Unfortunately, there was insufficient evidence to recommend the most effective drug or route of delivery.

Infusional therapy is probably more effective for both analgesia and the prevention of complications, but is difficult for some patients because of the necessity of regular hospital visits. Oral therapy is more convenient for many patients despite the low oral bioavailability of the tablets and the dietary restrictions (patients are advised to take the tablets on an empty stomach at least 1 hour before eating). Optimal doses and schedules are still to be determined, but pamidronate 60–90 mg, zoledronic acid 4 mg every month or clodronate 1500 mg by intravenous infusion every 2 weeks is recommended for the palliation of bone pain. Zoledronate has the advantage of a short delivery time (infusion over 15 minutes), making it more convenient for outpatient treatment and it appears to be the most effective of the agents currently available. The drugs are generally well tolerated, apart from occasional gastrointestinal side effects. They are also cost-effective if the reduction in admission to hospital secondary to reduced skeletal complications is taken into account.

INCIDENT PAIN

Incident pain is a descriptive term for pain that occurs only on movement, for example when weight-bearing on a limb with a large lytic bone lesion.[19] It is difficult to control, especially when pain control at rest is satisfactory. Short-acting oral analgesics are recommended such as immediate-release morphine or Palfium, preferably given just prior to an anticipated activity. Fentanyl has a short half-life and is therefore another useful drug in this scenario. It can be delivered parenterally via a subcutaneous bolus or via the buccal mucosa. If tolerated, Entonox can be used in situations such as when dressings covering painful wounds are changed.

The most common cause of incident pain in breast cancer is a lytic bone metastasis or pathological fracture. Orthopaedic procedures such as pinning a femur or a total hip joint replacement should be undertaken prophylactically where there is loss of

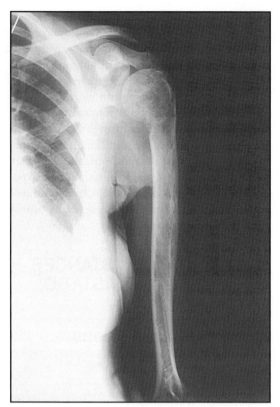

Figure 13.4 • Pathological fracture of a humerus that may have been prevented by prophylactic pinning.

integrity of bone cortex or as a palliative procedure after pathological fracture (**Fig. 13.4**).[20] Pain control is difficult in the absence of stabilisation.

NEUROPATHIC PAIN

Neuropathic pain results from damage or compression to a peripheral nerve. The most common example of this in breast cancer is brachial plexopathy after treatment of the axilla, or recurrent disease in the axilla. Neuropathic pain is classically resistant to standard analgesia and co-analgesics are often indicated at an early stage. Drugs used commonly in this situation include antidepressants and anticonvulsants. Although there are few studies in cancer pain, both antidepressants and anticonvulsants have proven effectiveness in non-cancer-related neuropathic pain. It is still unclear which drug class should be used first line.[21] All of these drugs have their own inherent adverse effects (sedation being the most common) and should be used with care. The doses required to achieve an analgesic effect are often well below the doses required to achieve their other effects, e.g. the analgesic effect of amitriptyline is seen well below its antidepressant effect. Second-line management of neuropathic pain with antiarrhythmics (e.g. flecainide) or N-methyl-D-aspartate antagonists (e.g. ketamine or methadone) is potentially hazardous and calls for the input of a specialist pain or palliative care team. Neurolytic blocks (e.g. intercostal or brachial plexus block) should be considered for neuropathic pain that does not respond to the measures described above.

LIVER CAPSULAR PAIN

Pain in the right upper quadrant is common in patients with liver metastases. This not only follows swelling of the liver capsule but may also be particularly severe after a bleed into a liver metastasis. NSAIDs can provide excellent analgesia and are often used in conjunction with opioids. Similarly, corticosteroids can reduce swelling, inflammation and pain in an enlarged liver. Dexamethasone should be started at an oral dose of about 8 mg daily and then reduced to the lowest effective dose to avoid adverse effects. A maintenance dose of 2–4 mg daily is often necessary to maintain control.

HEADACHE

In the scenario of metastatic breast cancer, especially if associated with vomiting, headache is often a sign of cerebral metastases. A trial of a NSAIDs in combination with paracetamol is indicated. It is often taught that codeine and strong opioids should be avoided in this situation because of the possibility of respiratory depression associated with hypercapnia leading to reflex cerebral vasodilation, a further increase in intracranial pressure and increased headache. However, this does not seem to be a problem in everyday practice and should not be cited as a contraindication to opioids. The prompt use of opioid analgesia can avoid dependence on corticosteroid therapy and reduce the inevitable adverse effects associated with long-term use.

SPIRITUAL PAIN

Pain is multifactorial and is exacerbated by added burdens such as fear, anxiety, anger, depression, sleep disturbance, uncertainty and other uncontrolled symptoms. These factors are often overlooked, with the main focus of pain control being on the physical aspects. It is important to address these aspects if 'complete' pain control is to be achieved. Simple measures such as explanation, reassurance, understanding and empathy can have profound pain-relieving effects.

Depression has been shown to have a significantly detrimental effect on survival in breast cancer.[22] Clinical depression must be actively sought and appropriately treated in all women with breast cancer. Similarly, anxiety may require specific treatment with anxiolytics (e.g. buspirone, diazepam, lorazepam). Buspirone hydrochloride has less addictive potential and should therefore be used in preference to diazepam for long-term use.

Dyspnoea

It is not always the malignancy that causes shortness of breath in a patient with metastatic breast cancer. Any other contributing causes, such as infection, pulmonary embolism or anaemia, should be excluded or treated appropriately. Tumour-specific causes include malignant pleural effusions, lymphangitis carcinomatosis, intrapulmonary metastases, pericardial effusions and constricting chest wall disease.

Breast cancer is the most common tumour that metastasises to the lung pleura in women. Treatment options are determined by the symptoms and performance status of the patient and the availability of systemic treatment. Guidelines for the aspiration of a malignant pleural effusion have been published by the British Thoracic Society.[23] Repeat pleural aspiration is recommended for the palliation of breathlessness in patients with a short life expectancy. Patients of better performance status are likely to benefit from intercostal tube drainage and intrapleural instillation of a sclerosant. Talc is the most effective sclerosant available and may be administered via thoracoscopy or an intercostal tube in the form of a 'talc slurry'.[24] Reported success rates are high (>80%). Tetracycline and bleomycin are alternative sclerosant agents. The most common adverse effects after administration are chest pain and fever. Small-bore catheters are no less effective than large-bore ones, with the potential advantage of reduced patient discomfort and ease of placement. Pleuroperitoneal shunts should be considered in a fit patient whose major problem is recurrent effusions.

Lymphangitis carcinomatosis is a common complication of metastatic disease. Patients present with gradually progressive shortness of breath and a dry cough. Auscultation of the chest is often non-contributory but a chest radiograph will show fine septal lines reflecting interstitial oedema. Lymphangitis is best palliated with corticosteroids, given at the lowest possible dose that controls symptoms. Corticosteroids can also relieve dyspnoea associated with intrapulmonary disease, almost certainly by reducing peritumour inflammation.

Dyspnoea is a subjective phenomena that can be described as an 'uncomfortable awareness of breathing'. It is not well correlated with objective measures of respiratory distress. The respiratory depressive effect of opioids can often be used to advantage in patients who are dyspnoeic, especially those without pain. There is now some evidence to support the use of oral opioids for the palliation of dyspnoea, whereas systematic review has failed to define a role for nebulised morphine.[25] Regular morphine used in conjunction with anxiolytics such as diazepam can calm both the patient and the respiratory drive. Opioids are also effective cough suppressants. Codeine is used most commonly, but the long half-life of methadone makes it the logical drug to use in the evening to control a nocturnal cough without leading to unacceptable daytime drowsiness. Lidocaine (lignocaine) or bupivacaine nebulisers are rarely required. A short course of palliative radiotherapy to an obstructed bronchus, especially if this is associated with haemoptysis, should be considered in those patients of adequate performance status.

Nausea and vomiting

The commonest cause of nausea and vomiting in metastatic breast disease is therapy, specifically chemotherapy and radiotherapy. Other common causes are hypercalcaemia, liver metastases and constipation.

Nausea and vomiting is often multifactorial in origin and a specific treatable cause may not be identified. There are a large number of antiemetics available that act at different receptor sites or via different mechanisms. The appropriateness of each in specific situations is shown in **Table 13.5**.

Table 13.5 • Antiemetics

Drug	Specific indication	Comments
Metoclopramide*	Treatment-related nausea and vomiting Gastric stasis	Dopamine antagonist ($5HT_3$ antagonist at high dose) Gastrokinetic, may induce acute dystonic reaction
Domperidone	Speeds gastric emptying and gut transit time	Available as suppository Gastrokinetic
Haloperidol*	Drug of choice for opioid-induced nausea and vomiting	Sedative at dose >3 mg daily Long half-life, can be given once or twice daily
Cyclizine*	Nausea and vomiting associated with bowel obstruction	Antihistamine; can cause dry mouth Will not exacerbate bowel colic
Levomepromazine (methotrimeprazine)*	If sedation is desirable	Powerful, broad-spectrum antiemetic, with activity at several different receptors
Prochlorperazine	Motion sickness	Phenothiazine derivative
Ondansetron* and granisetron	Chemotherapy- and radiotherapy-induced vomiting; also postoperative vomiting	Potent $5HT_3$-receptor antagonists
Corticosteroids*	Vomiting, secondary to raised intracranial pressure or liver metastases	Broad-spectrum antiemetic

*Can be given subcutaneously (unlicensed route).

Levomepromazine (methotrimeprazine) is a 'broad-spectrum' antiemetic acting at 5-hydroxytryptamine $(5HT)_2$, dopaminergic, cholinergic and histamine receptor sites.[26] It is a logical antiemetic to use when no specific cause can be identified. There is little evidence to support the use of the $5HT_3$-receptor blockers other than for chemotherapy- or radiotherapy-induced vomiting. Corticosteroids can often achieve control when all other antiemetics have failed, especially in the presence of metastatic liver disease. A cycle of protracted vomiting can be broken by giving antiemetics parenterally, e.g. via a continuous subcutaneous infusion. Drugs suitable for delivery by this route are shown in **Table 13.5**.

Anorexia and weight loss

Anorexia and weight loss are not as common in breast cancer as in many other advanced malignancies, e.g. carcinoma of the pancreas or lung. Corticosteroids improve appetite and general well-being, and there is some evidence that they result in non-fluid weight gain although this effect is likely to be short-lived.[27] Progestogens are used as hormonal therapy of breast cancer. Increased appetite and weight gain are well-documented adverse effects of these agents that can be used to advantage in metastatic disease.[28]

Sore mouth

One of the commonest causes of a sore mouth is a dry mouth, developing as a consequence of drugs, anticancer treatment or general debility. This in turn can lead to the development of oral infections with *Candida albicans*. Nystatin gives local control of oral thrush but is unlikely to eradicate the infection. A 5-day course of fluconazole is indicated, care being taken in patients with renal impairment. Most patients find amphotericin lozenges unpalatable as they are large and sticky. The underlying xerostomia must be corrected to avoid reinfection. Artificial saliva is the treatment of choice but must be used frequently. Chewing gum is effective if patients can tolerate it. Fluoride may stimulate saliva in some patients, and fluoride mouthwashes and toothpaste are recommended. Regular tooth brushing and mouth care should be encouraged to avoid infection. Many mouthwashes (e.g. chlor-hexidine gluconate) can exacerbate mouth dryness. Saliva stimulants (e.g. chewing gum), pilocarpine and parasympathomimetic agents (e.g. bethanechol) are under investigation.[29]

Abdominal distension

The commonest cause of abdominal distension in metastatic breast cancer is ascites, secondary to liver metastases or intraperitoneal disease. Abdominal paracentesis can lead to considerable relief and should be relatively painless when performed with a narrow-bore tube, e.g. a suprapubic catheter. Leaving a tube in situ provides a route of infection, and paracentesis is best repeated on an 'as-required' basis. The use of diuretics in this situation may serve only to dehydrate the patient and rarely results in satisfactory control of ascites.

Lymphoedema

Lymphoedema of the upper limb develops after recurrence in the axilla and as a complication of treatment (surgery and radiotherapy). It is associated with pain and often loss of mobility and function of the arm. This is a specialist treatment area requiring the input of specialised lymphoedema teams.

Diuretics may help, but meticulous skin care, massage, elevation of the limb, bandaging and use of support sleeves to prevent recurrence are other practical measures.[30] Oedematous limbs are prone to infection, and antibiotics should be prescribed at the earliest suggestion of cellulitis.

Swelling of the ankle often causes the patient great alarm even in the face of widespread metastatic disease. Hypoalbuminaemia, immobility and concurrent drugs as well as mechanical blockage by tumour exacerbate this condition. Diuretics, appropriate mobilisation and support hosiery remain the mainstay of treatment. Intravenous albumin supplementation provides only short-lasting benefit and is not generally recommended.

Wounds

Many women live with extensive locally recurrent malignancy for many months before they die of other complications of metastatic cancer. Chest wall disease can be most distressing, particularly because

Table 13.6 • Wound management

Type of wound	Management
Necrotic	
Brown/black hard dead tissue must be removed to allow granulation	Requires débridement by surgery, hydrocolloid gels, hydrogels and/or enzymes
Sloughy	
Yellow dead tissue must be removed to allow granulation	Hydrogels, hydrocolloid gel sheets and paste Alginate/hydrofibre dressings for high exudate
Infected	
Identified by clinical signs: pain, heat, swelling, redness	Hydrocolloid gel/hydrogels Alginates/hydrofibre or foam cavity dressing for high exudate Change dressings daily Consider systemic (*not* topical) antibiotics Irrigate with 0.9% saline, avoid topical antiseptic agents
Malodorous	
	Consider systemic antibiotics if malodour is related to infection Metronidazole gel and primary and secondary dressings of choice Charcoal dressing can absorb odour
Granulating	
Pink/red appearance, bleeds easily, requires protection	Avoid frequent changes of dressings Hydrocolloid gel/hydrogels plus hydrofibre/alginates or foam cavity dressing for high exudate Hydrocolloid sheets Hydrogel sheets
Bleeding wounds	
	Initial management with pressure dressings Then consider adrenaline (epinephrine) soaks, tranexamic acid (systemically and topically)

of its detrimental effect on body image. Poor nutritional state, infection and oedema all have an adverse effect on a malignant wound. There are a large number of dressings available with different properties suitable for different types of wound (Table 13.6). The aim is not to heal but to keep wounds clean and free of infection, to control pain and to provide maximum comfort. Dressings must be cosmetically acceptable. Antibiotics effective against anaerobes, e.g. metronidazole, given either systemically or topically, can relieve malodour. Tranexamic acid can be applied topically to prevent bleeding. Superficial radiotherapy prevents ulceration of a subcutaneous lesion and can provide local control over limited areas. All dead tissue should be excised. This often needs to be done at regular intervals.

Constipation

Constipation is a common and most distressing symptom in those with advanced breast cancer and, as with pain, treatment should be continuous and anticipatory. Constipation can lead to considerable abdominal discomfort and is a common cause of nausea and vomiting. Unfortunately, almost all strong analgesics cause constipation that is exacerbated by inactivity, poor diet, dehydration and hypercalcaemia.

Table 13.7 • Aperients

Drug	Indication/mechanism of action	Comments
Bulking agents		
Bran Ispaghula husk (Fybogel) Sterculia (Normacol)	Increase stool by absorbing water	Avoid in patients with bowel obstruction Maintain adequate fluid intake
Faecal softeners		
Liquid paraffin	Lubricates and softens impacted faeces	Should not be used in patients with swallowing difficulties (danger of aspiration lipoid pneumonia)
Docusate sodium		Added stimulant properties
Arachis oil enema	For 'per rectum' intervention'	
Osmotic laxatives		
Magnesium sulphate	Retains fluid in bowel	Useful when rapid bowel evacuation is required; use with caution in elderly and debilitated patients
Lactulose	Retains fluid in bowel	Semisynthetic disaccharide, not absorbed from bowel, added antimicrobial effect may take up to 48 hours to act
Movicol	Saline laxative	For constipation resistant to above
Phosphate suppositories	For clearance of rectal impaction	
Bowel stimulants		
Senna Bisacodyl Dantron	Increase colonic motility	May increase colicky pain Avoid in bowel obstruction Colours urine red; skin contact can cause irritation and excoriation
Glycerol suppositories	Rectal stimulant because of irritant action of glycerol	

This condition should be taken seriously and treated aggressively with regular oral laxatives along with enemas and suppositories as indicated (Table 13.7). Opioid-induced constipation is best treated with compound preparations such as Co-danthramer, which contains both a faecal softener (poloxamer) and a stimulant (dantron) or Co-danthrusate (dantron 50 mg, docusate 60 mg). Care must be taken in those patients who are incontinent or catheterised as dantron can cause skin staining, irritation and occasionally excoriation. The combination of bisacodyl or senna and docusate is a logical alternative. Hyperosmotic (e.g. lactulose) or saline laxatives (e.g. Movicol) are recommended second-line therapy for resistant constipation or

for bowel preparation. There is increasing interest in the use of opioid antagonists with low bioavailability for the treatment of morphine-induced constipation. In theory, opioid antagonists that are not well absorbed can counter the effects of morphine on the gut without reversing the central analgesic effect.[31]

Confusion

Common causes of confusion are drug toxicity, infection, hypoxia, hypercalcaemia and direct cancer involvement of the central nervous system. The cause should be actively sought and treated accordingly.

Hypercalcaemia presents with polyuria, polydipsia, dehydration, nausea and vomiting, confusion and somnolence that can progress to coma and death if not treated. Tumour-induced hypercalcaemia (TIH) was a particularly common complication of advanced metastatic bone disease. It is now seen less frequently following the widespread use of bisphosphonates as part of routine therapy. Intravenous bisphosphonates remain the treatment of choice for TIH.[32] They are easy to deliver and relatively devoid of adverse effects. Standard therapy consists of an intravenous infusion of 90 mg pamidronate or 4 mg zoledronic acid following rehydration with normal saline The serum calcium concentration should return to normal within 3–4 days with an improvement in symptoms. The newer bisphosphonates (such as zoledronate) are more potent and result in a more rapid normalisation of serum calcium that is maintained for longer. Hypercalcaemia will almost certainly recur after 2–4 weeks if no further specific systemic anticancer therapy is available. It can be re-treated but will eventually become resistant. TIH is a preterminal event and the median survival after an initial episode of TIH is 2 months, except in those patients in whom further systemic anticancer therapy is available.[33] Although the symptoms associated with hypercalcaemia are distressing and should be treated, the benefit of treating TIH in a patient in whom no further anticancer therapy is possible and who presents with no symptoms must be questioned.

The brain is a common site of metastases, and patients may present with localised weakness, convulsions or personality change as well as confusion. If cerebral secondaries are suspected, the patient should be started on high-dose steroids (e.g. dexamethasone 8 mg b.i.d.) while awaiting confirmation of the diagnosis. An improvement while taking steroids bodes well for subsequent response to radiotherapy. Short courses of radiotherapy (up to five fractions) are as effective as prolonged courses. In one series, the median survival after radiotherapy for cerebral metastases was about 6 months, compared with 1 month for those patients who received symptomatic (corticosteroid) therapy only.[34]

In some patients it will be inappropriate or impossible to treat the underlying cause. This is an indication for sedation. Antipsychotics such as haloperidol, levomepromazine (methotrimeprazine) or olanzapine are recommended first line with the addition of benzodiazepines when added sedation is called for.

Weakness

Weakness, lethargy and fatigue are common but rarely reported symptoms of advanced breast cancer. The incidence of asthenia (defined as physical or mental fatigue/weakness) was reported as 41% in a controlled study of women with advanced breast cancer.[35] Physical (cachexia and weight loss, muscle abnormalities), biochemical, haematological, endocrine and psychological (depression, personality, stress) factors all contribute. Corticosteroids, progestogens, anabolic steroids and psychostimulants have all been tried, but to date no pharmacological treatment has a proven role in this condition.[36]

If a patient suddenly 'goes off her legs', especially if this is associated with bowel or bladder disturbance and sensory loss, malignant cord compression should be considered and investigated immediately. Vertebral bone disease is common in metastatic breast cancer and is often unsuspected until imaged by magnetic resonance[37] (**Fig. 13.5**). Cord compression must be treated with urgency. The success of treatment often depends on early detection.[38] High-dose steroids should be started at first suspicion and continued until treatment is complete. Surgical decompression may be appropriate for single lesions or early in the course of disease, but as this

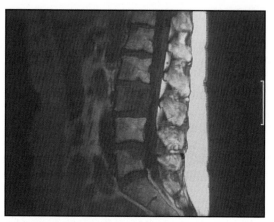

Figure 13.5 • Malignant cord compression as demonstrated by magnetic resonance imaging.

condition is often associated with advanced and widespread metastatic disease, radiotherapy is normally the treatment of choice. The success of treatment is limited and although the prognosis of these patients is generally poor, several patients will survive for a considerable period, which has significant implications for continuing care and local palliative care services.[39]

CARE OF THE DYING

The ability to recognise and acknowledge that a woman with advanced breast cancer is dying is very difficult for many doctors. It requires a change of emphasis of care, with all efforts being directed towards the treatment of symptoms rather than treatment of the disease. All unnecessary investigations and interventions should be discontinued. Essential drugs must be continued and delivered by an appropriate route (see below). Any outstanding ethical issues need addressing, for example resuscitation status, advanced directives and discontinuation of food or fluids.[40]

It is crucial to continue to deliver analgesia to dying patients. Those women who can no longer take oral medications can be given drugs per rectum, transdermally or via a subcutaneous infusion. Diamorphine is the strong opioid of choice in the UK when delivered subcutaneously. It is more soluble than morphine, allowing for large doses to be delivered in a smaller volume. The appropriate dose of subcutaneous diamorphine is one-third the total daily dose of oral morphine, although this will often need to be increased during the terminal phase. Other opioids that can be delivered parenterally include fentanyl, hydromorphone, oxycodone and morphine tartrate.

The ability to deliver drugs subcutaneously has in some ways revolutionised the dying process, although some believe that this has resulted in the institutionalisation of death and a further loss of the ability of a patient to die naturally. Drugs that can be delivered subcutaneously via a syringe driver in this situation are listed in **Table 13.8**. Recommended sites for the placement of subcutaneous needles are shown in **Fig. 13.6** and guidelines for the use of a syringe driver are given in **Box 13.2**.

A common problem encountered when managing the dying patient is terminal restlessness. This state of agitation may be exacerbated by factors such

Table 13.8 • Drugs suitable for subcutaneous administration to the dying patient

Drug	Indication	Comments
Diamorphine*	Analgesia	The 24-hour dose of diamorphine is one-third the 24-hour oral morphine dose
Midazolam	Terminal restlessness and agitation, control of convulsions	Can be mixed with diamorphine in syringe driver Usual dose 20–60 mg 24-hourly
Levomepromazine (methotrimeprazine)	Terminal restlessness plus vomiting	Antipsychotic effect can help terminal confusion, usual starting dose 25 mg 24-hourly
Dexamethasone	Chronic steroid use	Sudden discontinuation can exacerbate terminal distress
Haloperidol	Nausea and vomiting	Commonly used with diamorphine to combat opioid-induced vomiting Sedative at doses >3 mg daily
Cyclizine	Nausea secondary to bowel obstruction	Does not exacerbate colicky pain; may precipitate at concentrations >10 mg/mL
Glycopyrronium	Retained bronchial secretions	No CNS effects; can be used at an earlier stage than hyoscine
Hyoscine hydrobromide	Retained bronchial secretions ('death rattle')	Can result in profound dryness Maximum 24-hour dose 2.4 mg s.c.

*UK only.

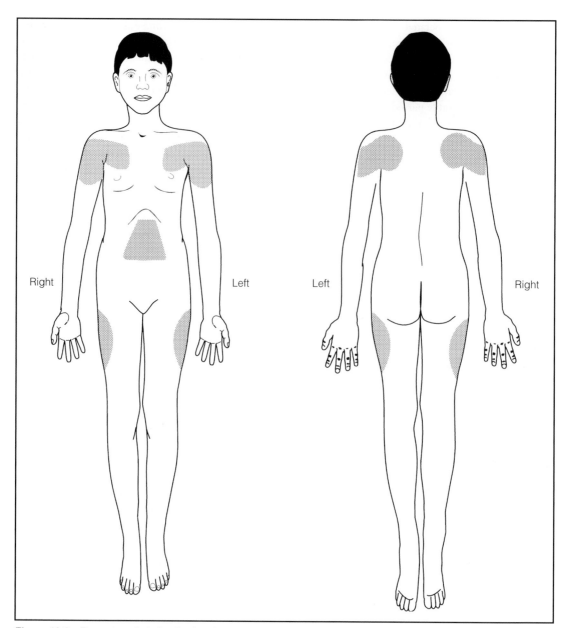

Figure 13.6 • Recommended sites for the placement of subcutaneous needles.

as infection, pain, drug toxicity or withdrawal, the treatment of which are often inappropriate or impossible. Midazolam, a benzodiazepine derivative, is the drug most commonly used to combat terminal restlessness. When nausea and vomiting has been a major problem, a more appropriate agent to use is levomepromazine (methotrimeprazine), which has both antipsychotic, sedative and anti-emetic properties.[26] Both drugs can be delivered subcutaneously. Rectal diazepam provides an alternative choice if the subcutaneous route is not being used.

In terminal dyspnoea the primary aim is to depress respiratory drive, control anxiety and calm the

Box 13.2 • Guidelines for the use of subcutaneous infusions in palliative care

1. Use a simple battery-operated portable syringe driver with a butterfly infusion set to deliver drugs at a predetermined site

2. Place the subcutaneous needle over the shoulder area, abdomen or upper outer thigh (see **Fig. 13.6**)

3. Provided there is evidence of compatibility, selected injections can be mixed in syringe drivers. For example, the following can be used with diamorphine: midazolam, levomepromazine (methotrimeprazine), hyoscine, haloperidol, cyclizine* and dexamethasone*. Avoid more than three drugs in one combination

4. Some medications are *not* suitable for subcutaneous infusion, e.g. chlorpromazine, prochlorperazine and diazepam, all of which cause skin reactions at the injection site

5. Small volumes of water for injection are usually used to dissolve drugs, as normal saline increases the likelihood of precipitation when more than one drug is used

6. The infusion site should be checked regularly; swelling at the site of injection is not an indication for site change whereas pain or obvious inflammation is

7. Cover the infusion site with a semi-occlusive dressing, e.g. Tegaderm, to allow observation of needle site

8. The infusion can be programmed to run over 6, 12 and 24 hours, and drug doses should be reviewed regularly

9. Check syringe driver often to ensure correct administration rate

*May precipitate at higher doses.

patient. This can be achieved pharmacologically with small doses of morphine or diamorphine given regularly in conjunction with benzodiazepines. Retained bronchial secretions can result in alarming sounds of laboured breathing in the dying patient.

This can be distressing to relatives and carers but can be lessened with the judicious use of anti-muscarinic agents, e.g. hyoscine hydrobromide or glycopyrronium bromide, to dry secretions in large airways.

Many relatives and carers find it difficult to cope with the fact that their loved ones are dying and yet not receiving fluid or nourishment when intravenous lines are taken down or removed. Up to 2 L daily of normal saline can be delivered via the subcutaneous route. There is considerable controversy as to the benefits versus possible harm in delivering fluid to dying patients. Every case should be considered individually and the views of the relatives/carers taken into account.[41]

CONCLUSION

Although metastatic breast cancer is an incurable malignancy, it is possible to live with advanced disease for many years. With the provision of good palliative measures it is possible to achieve good quality of life for most women. This encompasses not only the patient but their relatives and carers. Palliative care should be considered early in the course of metastatic disease and should continue throughout the illness trajectory.

Many thousands of women die of breast cancer each year. In the UK, women can usually choose the place of death (hospice, hospital or home) because of the well-developed hospice and palliative care services.[42] Similarly, there are a large number of support services available in the community for patients with breast cancer (e.g. Macmillan nurses, Marie Curie Cancer Care, the Sue Ryder Foundation and the British Association of Cancer United Patients) that provide counselling and general support for women with breast cancer.

Key points

- The provision of good palliative care has the potential to improve the quality of life of women with metastatic breast cancer.
- The pain associated with metastatic breast cancer can be controlled in the majority of cases using relatively simple WHO analgesic guidelines.
- A large number of 'alternative' opioids are now available for those patients with intolerable adverse effects or inadequate pain control on morphine.
- Bisphosphonates have proven efficacy not only in the reduction of skeletal morbidity but also in the control of bone pain.
- Dyspnoea is a subjective phenomenon that can be palliated to some extent with opioids and benzodiazepines.
- Nausea not related to treatment is likely to be multifactorial and therefore best managed with a broad spectrum antiemetic.
- Fatigue is a common and generally underreported symtom in patients with cancer.
- The recognition and acceptance that a patient is dying allows for a change in emphasis in care away from treatment towards symptom control.
- As metastatic breast cancer is an incurable malignancy, palliative care both within the cancer centre and in the community should be mobilised at an early stage.
- Palliative care encompasses the care of the extended family and not just the woman, and occasionally the man, with breast cancer.

REFERENCES

1. Higginson IJ, Findlay IG, Goodwin DM et al. Is there evidence that palliative care teams alter end-of-life experiences of patients and their caregivers? J Pain Symptom Manage 2003; 25:150–68.

   This systematic review is the first to provide evidence that palliative care can affect outcome.

2. World Health Organization. Cancer pain relief, with a guide to opioid availability, 2nd edn. Geneva: WHO, 1996.

   Although criticised in recent years for a lack of proof of efficacy, the WHO analgesic guidelines remain the 'gold standard' for the treatment of pain throughout the world.

3. Jadad AR, Browman GP. The WHO analgesic ladder for cancer pain management. JAMA 1995; 274:1870–3.

4. Eisenberg E, Berkey CS, Carr DB et al. Efficacy and safety of nonsteroidal anti-inflammatory drugs for cancer pain: a meta-analysis. J Clin Oncol 1994; 12:2756–65.

5. McQuay H, Moore A. An evidence-based resource for pain relief, 1998. Oxford: Oxford University Press, 1998.

6. Gajraj NM. Cyclooxygenase-2 inhibitors. Anesth Analg 2003; 96:1720–38.

7. McQuay H. Opioids in pain management. Lancet 1999; 353:2229–32.

8. European Association of Palliative Care. Morphine in cancer pain: modes of administration. Br Med J 1996; 312:823–6.

   International evidence-based guidelines for the use of morphine as published by a working party of the European Association of Palliative Care.

9. Faura CC, Collins SL, Moore RA et al. Systematic review of factors affecting the ratios of morphine and its major metabolites. Pain 1998; 74:43–53.

10. Borgbjerg FM, Nielsen K, Franks J. Experimental pain stimulates respiration and attenuates morphine-induced respiratory depression: a controlled study in human volunteers. Pain 1996; 64:123–8.

11. Cherny N, Ripamonti C, Pereira J et al. Strategies to manage the adverse effects of oral morphine: an evidence-based report. J Clin Oncol 2001; 19:2542–54.

   Fear and uncertainty regarding the adverse effects of opioids is thought to be one of the major reasons why pain is poorly controlled worldwide. This key paper written by the Expert Working Group of the European Association of Palliative Care (EAPC) Network reviews the common opioid adverse effects and their control.

12. Vainio A, Ollila J, Matikainen E et al. Driving ability in cancer patients receiving long term morphine analgesia. Lancet 1995; 346:667–70.

13. Indelico RA, Portenoy RK. Opioid rotation in the management of refratory cancer pain. J Clin Oncol 2002; 20:348–52.

14. Expert Working Group of the EAPC. Morphine and alternative opioids in cancer pain: the EAPC recommendations. Br J Cancer 2001; 84:587–93.

The widespread use of new opioids and opioid formulations over recent years has forced the EAPC to expand its morphine guidelines to include advice on the use of alternative opioids and to review the evidence to support the use of opioids other than morphine.

15. Hardy JR. The use of corticosteroids in palliative care. Eur J Palliat Care 1998; 5:46–50.

16. Sze WM, Shelley MD, Held I et al. Palliation of metastatic bone pain: single fraction versus muti-fraction radiotherapy. A systematic review of randomised trials. Clin Oncol 2003; 15:345–52.

17. Ross JR, Saunders Y, Edmonds P, Patel S, Broadley K, Johnston S. Systematic review of the role of bisphosphonates on skeletal morbidity in metastatic breast cancer. Br Med J 2003; 327:469.

A systematic review that documents the beneficial effect of bisphosphonates on skeletal morbidity in breast cancer.

18. Wong R, Wiffen PJ. Bisphosphonates for the relief of pain secondary to bone metastases (Cochrane review). In: The Cochrane Library, issue 4, 2003. Chichester, UK: John Wiley & Sons.

A Cochrane review, handicapped by a lack of consistency in definitions and endpoints in many of the studies.

19. Mercadante S, Radbruch L, Caraceni A et al. Episodic (breakthrough) pain. Cancer 2002; 94:832–9.

20. British Association of Surgical Oncology. The management of metastatic bone disease in the UK. Eur J Surg Oncol 1999; 25:3–23.

21. McQuay HJ, Moore AR (eds). Antidepressants in neuropathic pain. In: An evidence-based resource for pain relief. Oxford: Oxford Medical, 1998; pp. 231–41.

22. Watson M, Haviland JS, Greer S et al. Influence of psychological response on survival in breast cancer: a population based cohort study. Lancet 1999; 354:1331–6.

23. Antunes G, Neville E, Duffy J et al. BTS guidelines for the management of malignant pleural effusions. Thorax 2003; 58(suppl. ii):29–38.

Evidence-based guidelines published by the British Thoracic Society.

24. Weissberg D, Ben-Zeev I. Talc pleurodesis. Experience with 360 patients. J Thorac Cardiovasc Surg 1993; 106:689–95.

25. Jennings A-L, Davies A, Higgins J et al. Opioids for the palliation of breathlessness in terminal illness (Cochrane review). In: The Cochrane Library, issue 4, 2001. Oxford update software.

Opioids are used widely for the palliation of dyspnoea. This systematic review provides what evidence there is to support the practice.

26. Twycross RG, Barkby GD, Hallwood PM. The use of low dose levomepromazine (methotrimeprazine) in the management of nausea and vomiting. Prog Palliat Care 1997; 5:49–53.

27. Loprinzi CL, Kugler JW, Sloan JA et al. Randomised comparison of megestrol acetate versus dexamethasone versus fluoxymesterone for the treatment of cancer anorexia/cachexia. J Clin Oncol 1999; 17:3299–306.

28. Berenstein EG, Ortiz Z. Megestrol acetate for the treatment of anorexia–cachexia syndrome. Cochrane Database 2005, issue 2, no. CD004310.

29. Davies AN. The management of xerostomia: a review. Eur J Cancer Care 1997; 6:209–14.

30. Foldi E. The treatment of lymphedema. Cancer 1998; 83:2833–4.

31. Kurz A, Sessler DI. Opioid-induced bowel dysfunction. Drugs 2003; 63:649–71.

32. Body JJ, Mancini I. Treatment of tumour-induced hypercalcaemia: a solved problem? Expert Rev Anticancer Ther 2003; 3:241–6.

33. Ling PJ, A'Hern RP, Hardy JR. Analysis of survival following treatment of tumour-induced hypercalcaemia with intravenous pamidronate (APD). Br J Cancer 1995; 72:206–9.

34. Chang EL, Lo S. Diagnosis and management of central nervous system metastases from beast cancer. Oncologist 2003; 8:398–410.

35. Bruera E, Brenneis C, Michaud M et al. Association between asthenia and nutritional status, lean body mass, anaemia, psychological status, and tumor mass in patients with advanced breast cancer. J Pain Symptom Manage 1989; 4:59–63.

36. Stone P, Richards M, Hardy J. Review article: fatigue in patients with cancer. Eur J Cancer 1998; 34:1670–6.

A review of a very common yet underreported complication of cancer and its treatment.

37. Jones AL, Williams MP, Powles TJ et al. Magnetic resonance imaging in the detection of skeletal metastases in patients with breast cancer. Br J Cancer 1990; 62:296–8.

38. Hardy JR, Huddart R. Spinal cord compression: what are the treatment standards? Clin Oncol 2002; 14:132–4.

39. Cowap J, Hardy J, A'Hern R. Outcome of spinal cord compression at a cancer centre: implications for palliative care services. J Pain Sympton Manage 2000; 19:257–64.

40. Stone P, Rees E, Hardy J. End of life care in patients with malignant disease. Eur J Cancer 2001; 37:1070–5.

41. Viola R. The effects of fluid status and fluid therapy on the dying: a systematic review. J Palliat Care 1997; 13:41–52.

42. Higginson IJ, Astin P, Dolan S. Where do cancer patients die? Ten year trend in the place of death of cancer patients in England. Palliat Med 1998; 12:353–63.

Fourteen

Psychosocial issues in breast cancer

Lesley Fallowfield and
Valerie A. Jenkins

INTRODUCTION

In most Western cultures the breasts are viewed as powerful symbols of femininity, inextricably linked to sexual intimacy, feelings of attractiveness, nurture and motherhood. It is therefore of no surprise that a diagnosis of breast cancer has a tremendous psychosocial as well as physical impact on a woman at all stages of her life.

Despite the many advances made in the management of breast cancer over the past 20 years, its diagnosis and treatment remains a source of considerable psychological, social, physical and sexual dysfunction for women, exerting a deleterious impact on the quality of their lives. The number of women who develop psychological problems has barely changed, with a significant minority (25–30%) experiencing affective and adjustment disorders. But what of those who do not merit a diagnosis of clinical depression or anxiety. Are the many changes in diagnostic techniques, service delivery, information and support provision helping women to cope better with their disease? This chapter outlines some of the main sources of psychological, social, physical and sexual problems in breast cancer that impact on quality of life and examines the existing evidence base, assessing the efficacy of interventions aimed at preventing or ameliorating problems.

PSYCHOLOGICAL MORBIDITY

Mastectomy versus breast conservation

For over a century there have been many, largely anecdotal, studies charting the considerable psychological distress associated with breast cancer. Two of the earliest studies reporting psychological morbidity focused predominantly on the postoperative sequelae of mastectomy.[1] At the time, unpleasantly mutilating radical mastectomy was almost the only operative procedure on offer so linking mutilation with anxiety and depression was a reasonable assumption. Surgeons tried hard to reduce some of the mutilation with procedures such as modified radical or simple mastectomy, although women still lost a breast and had an unpleasant scar; moreover, psychological morbidity remained high. Not surprisingly, the development of breast-conserving surgery, followed by radiotherapy, was supported enthusiastically by many. As clinical trial data emerged demonstrating no survival differences between women randomised to mastectomy compared with those randomised to breast conservation,[2,3] surgeons became more confident about offering less mutilating procedures and hopefully preventing unwanted psychosocial sequelae without compromising survival. Unfortunately, a substantial reduction in psychological morbidity has yet to be demonstrated.

One of the first studies to challenge the assumption that breast loss itself promoted most of the psychiatric morbidity observed came from a retrospective assessment of 101 women randomised to either mastectomy or breast conservation.[4] Results were counter-intuitive and disappointing as anxiety and depression were high whatever the surgery performed; 32% of the mastectomy group and 38% of those having breast-conserving surgery experienced clinically significant affective and adjustment disorders. There have been many studies done in many different countries since, demonstrating similar findings and countering the idea that breast loss per se is causal in the psychological morbidity. Whatever the surgery women undergo, all must confront the diagnosis of breast cancer, a potentially life-threatening disease and this often predominates in the thoughts of women initially rather than the fear of breast loss. These findings are not an argument for performing unnecessarily radical surgery. There are undoubted other benefits from less mutilating surgery, in particular some advantages in preserving body image and sparing women the nuisance factor of wearing an external prosthesis. Importantly, many of the studies comparing psychosocial outcomes were performed in the 1980s and early 1990s when many clinicians were less confident about the safety of breast conservation, although trials now show that despite the slightly higher rates of local recurrence, there is no survival disadvantage. It could be possible that this uncertainty was subtly communicated to women.

Choice and decision-making

Some have suggested that psychological morbidity could be prevented if only women were allowed to choose their preferred surgical treatments. Although the proponents of more consumerist approaches strongly assert the putative benefits of active participation by women with breast cancer in treatment decision making, these benefits are rarely supported by firm data. In one study the decision-making preferences of 150 women with newly diagnosed breast cancer were established and compared with those of 200 women with benign breast disease. The majority of women with breast cancer preferred a more passive role, whereas the majority of the benign disease group wished for a more collaborative role.[5] In another study of 269 women treated by surgeons who either favoured one approach (i.e. mastectomy or breast-conserving surgery) or who offered choice between options whenever possible, psychological morbidity was lowest for the women treated by surgeons who offered the choice. However, benefits to those treated by 'choice' doctors were observed irrespective of whether the choice could in fact be offered.[6] What helped women adapt and adjust to their disease and treatment had less to do with choice than satisfaction with the communication they had with their doctors about the rationale for one treatment rather than another. Those satisfied with the communication at the time that diagnosis was given and the treatment options discussed experienced less psychological morbidity at 12, 24 and 36 months follow-up compared with those who felt that communication had been inadequate.[7]

A more recent meta-analysis summarising the findings of 40 publications suggests that better techniques and improved specialist medical and nursing care for women are starting to show some benefits. The mean weighted effect sizes calculated for psychosocial outcomes, which included psychological morbidity, partnership/sexual and social adjustment, body/self-image and cancer fears, demonstrated modest advantages for women who had breast-conserving surgery.[8]

Impact of axillary surgery on quality of life

Management of the axilla in breast cancer surgery is a controversial area. Arm morbidity following both clearance and sampling is well documented. Extensive surgery aimed at clearing the axilla of positive nodes might well reduce recurrence and improve survival but comes at considerable cost to the patient in terms of arm morbidity. Complications such as muscle weakness, numbness, pain and lymphoedema are common and can have a deleterious impact on a woman's quality of life even if she is cured of her breast cancer.[9,10] Research has shown that up to 83% women will experience at least one arm problem following surgery.[11] Assessment of arm morbidity using traditional objective methods rather than patient self-report has often proved inconsistent and may fail to capture the extent of patients' problems. More recently, a robust and validated patient self-report measure (FACT-B+4) has been developed that may prove useful in monitoring the presence and longevity of arm morbidity in trials of new techniques aimed at minimising problems.[12] This instrument has been used in the UK-based Axillary Lymphatic Mapping Against Nodal Axillary Clearance (ALMANAC) trial, a multicentre randomised clinical trial comparing sentinel node biopsy with conventional axillary surgical techniques in women presenting with clinically node-negative breast cancer. ALMANAC showed that the benefits of sentinel node biopsy are not only reduction of unnecessary resection of the axilla but also a marked reduction in unwanted sequelae such as arm morbidity, thus permitting a better quality of life, without sacrificing any staging accuracy.

Interventions to reduce psychological morbidity

The large numbers of women who still experience considerable psychological morbidity, despite improvements in service provision, a greater awareness of women's likely problems and concerted efforts to ameliorate these through better information and communication, counselling and support groups, is puzzling and needs some explanation. The almost obsessional, often sensational and excessive preoccupation with breast cancer by the media surely has some responsibility for this. Women are bombarded by mixed messages about things such as the risks and benefits of screening, the value of self-examination and breast awareness. They are also surrounded by misleading and often inaccurate claims about the causes of breast cancer, ranging from dietary factors to the use of deodorants. Campaigns to promote breast awareness often use young women, perpetuating unreasonable fears among the very age groups least at risk of developing the disease. Not surprisingly, women overestimate their risk of getting breast cancer, especially when figures such as 1 in 10 or 12 are bandied about, failing to convey the fact that this is a woman's lifetime risk of developing breast cancer.[13] So at a time when there has never been quite so much information available or so many resources directed at trying to prevent or ameliorate

psychological stress, we appear to have created as much if not more anxiety than was discernible previously. The key is to help guide women through reliable information sources and to ensure that verbal communication and support provided by health-care professionals is congruent with information accessed through other media. As a group, the needs of women with breast cancer are probably better served than many other cancers. Charities such as CancerBACUP, Breakthrough Breast Cancer, Breast Cancer Care, and Cancer Care, to name but a few, provide some excellent websites and materials.

Counselling/specialist nurses

Despite its prevalence, patients with cancer experience psychological dysfunction that is rarely documented during routine clinic visits.[14] This is unfortunate as evidence is growing that if psychological morbidity is recognised, then a number of different psychosocial interventions of proven efficacy can be offered.[15,16] In busy clinics some surgeons feel that they do not have time, even if they possess the skills needed, to enquire into the psychological functioning of patients. Responsibility for this often falls on specialist breast cancer nurses.

One of the first studies to demonstrate the potential value of specialist nurses was a controlled trial evaluating their ability to prevent the psychiatric morbidity associated with mastectomy.[17] The psychological morbidity of 75 women who received counselling before and after surgery, with home visits and assessment at follow-up clinics, was compared with that of 77 women receiving normal surgical unit care. Counselling failed to prevent morbidity but regular monitoring by the nurse specialist meant that problems were recognised and 76% of those needing more specialised help from a psychiatrist gained early referral. In contrast only 15% of the control group had their problems recognised and as a result received help. Another small study of 40 consecutive patients randomised to either counselling or routine care reported a transiently favourable outcome to the counselled group in terms of less depression and a greater sense of control at 3 months postoperatively, although this difference had disappeared by 12 months.[18] Despite the equivocal evidence of efficacy, the high prevalence of psychological and sexual dysfunction associated with breast cancer has led to the creation of many posts for specialist nurses with counselling skills. Their role is now firmly established in breast cancer clinics; indeed, it seems difficult to recall a time when clinics were organised without them. Initially, the specialist nurse doubled up as a stoma nurse, as one of her primary roles was to offer advice about breast prostheses. However, the modern specialist nurse now has to undergo considerable training in the skills required to recognise and treat some of the psychological problems found in women with breast cancer. Although there is not a substantial methodologically sound research base demonstrating the efficacy of specialist nurse counsellors, many women and clinicians attest to the benefits of their work. A recently published Australian study examined the implementation of an evidence-based model of care using specialist breast cancer nurses and reported improvements in many areas of care, in particular information and support for women and more appropriate referrals.[19]

Support groups

Another source of help for women with breast cancer comes from support groups and there are many different types available. There is a large body of research suggesting strong associations between emotional distress and immunological and neuro-endocrine responses in women with breast cancer. This link has been responsible for a burgeoning interest in support groups that putatively lead to improved psychological and physiological outcomes, and is an area full of controversy.[20] In 1989, the *Lancet* published an important paper by Spiegel et al.[21] reporting the results from the 10-year follow-up of a prospective randomised trial of supportive–expressive group therapy in women with metastatic breast cancer. An earlier report by this group had shown that this intervention, which included professionally led peer group support encouraging emotional expression, relaxation therapy and autohypnosis, produced significant psychological benefits. Those women randomised to group support compared with the control group reported better mood states, fewer maladaptive coping responses and fewer phobic reactions.[22] Although the study was designed to establish the

potential benefits on psychological well-being, Spiegel at al. examined post hoc the death records to determine the impact of the intervention on disease progression and mortality. This showed a statistically significant difference in mean survival that favoured the intervention group (36.6 months vs. 18.9 months for the control). This work has been criticised by many[23,24] and others have failed to replicate Spiegel's findings of an effect on survival,[24,25] but it did stimulate an interesting and important body of research aimed at establishing plausible psychoendocrine and psychoneuroimmunological explanations for improved survival.[26] Spiegel's original research was never designed to test the impact support groups would have on survival but rather its overall impact on quality of life and he always cautioned against over-interpretation of the research. However, more recent work evaluating quality of life in women with metastatic breast cancer, who were randomised to supportive–expressive group therapy or a control arm, failed to show any benefits of the intervention.[27] In studies that have shown a modest impact on survival, advantages are probably due to psychotherapeutic benefits improving such things as compliance, better nutrition and physical activity.[28] It could be argued that one of the most important aspects of supportive–expressive group therapy is to help patients to face the fact of their breast cancer and to confront the reality of death, with a strong focus on living better, not necessarily longer.

The supportive–expressive group approach is in marked contrast to those who try to encourage patients to fight their cancer and thereby assume responsibility for outcomes including poor ones. The 'fighting spirit' approach stemmed from research originally reported by Greer et al.[29] This longitudinal prospective study examined the relationship of the psychological response of 69 women with early-stage breast cancer to their diagnosis and treatment and the ultimate effect of this on survival. Using results from standardised psychological tests of depression and personality together with an open-ended interview, the authors grouped women's responses into four mutually exclusive categories: denial, fighting spirit, stoic acceptance and help-lessness/hopelessness. The authors reported a statistically significant association between the initial psychological responses at 3 months with outcomes at 5 years,[29] 10 years[30] and then 15 years.[31] Recurrence-free survival was more apparent in women who had an initial response of fighting spirit than in those exhibiting stoic acceptance or helplessness/hopelessness. The study did suffer from many weaknesses, including a small sample size with considerable attrition over time and thus had low statistical power. Furthermore, no adjustment was made for one of the most important prognostic factors, namely lymph node status, as this was not routinely assessed at commencement of the study. Despite these limitations, it was a landmark study as many had recognised that a reductionist biomedical model of breast cancer does not satisfactorily explain the behaviour of the disease. It helped to stimulate a renewed interest in psychoneuroimmunology among psychologists, clinicians and other scientists.

Unfortunately, the results were also embraced enthusiastically by the lay press and alternative therapists, all of whom extrapolated far beyond the data presented and offered a variety of psychological programmes and exercises, together with dietary regimens aimed at helping patients to cure their cancer through adoption of a fighting spirit. (Interestingly enough, the response of denial had also been associated with improved survival but this fact was conveniently ignored.) A later, much sounder prospective study of 578 women with early breast cancer and 5-year follow-up showed the fallacy of encouraging a fighting spirit.[32] The authors failed to find any significant effect of fighting spirit on survival but did detect a modest detrimental effect of helplessness/hopelessness and high depression scores on survival. It is precisely these responses to breast cancer that can potentially be helped through cognitive-behaviour therapy or counselling delivered by a specialist nurse.[33]

PSYCHOSEXUAL MORBIDITY

Although much has been written about the effects that treatments have on body image and self-esteem, one quality-of-life issue that has received rather less attention is the effect that diagnosis and treatment for breast cancer has on a woman's psychosexual functioning. Often it is towards the end of cancer treatment that most sexual dysfunction caused by therapy occurs, when a woman has completed her main hospital treatments and the initial threat of death and dying is slowly replaced with trying to get back to a normal life. In a recent review of sexual dysfunction, Schover et al.[34] note that although sexuality in breast cancer patients was studied as an aspect of quality of life over 40 years ago, little progress has been made since then. Early research focused on the initial impact of mastectomy versus breast-conserving surgery and the benefits of reconstruction, but less was known about the effects of chemotherapy and different hormone therapies on sexuality. There is still relatively little systematic research into the effect that different treatments have on a woman's feelings of altered body image and loss of sexual desire, and even fewer interventions in place to help these women. Much of the available data on sexuality following breast cancer treatment is too general, and it is rare for women to be assessed before, during and after treatment in order to determine when problems begin and how long they last, let alone develop and examine ameliorative interventions.

Different treatments undoubtedly affect a woman's psychosexual well-being. Surgery can leave a woman with feelings of mutilation, and a loss of sense of femininity. The introduction of better surgical techniques, including immediate reconstructive surgery, may help patients retain a more intact sense of body image and self-esteem and thus adjust more easily. An early study by Schain et al.[35] reported that those patients who had immediate reconstructive surgery had significantly less recalled distress about their mastectomy at 1 year than those who had delayed reconstruction, although initial differences in adjustment disappeared over time. However, another report assessing psychosocial morbidity in 254 patients who had undergone breast-conserving surgery for primary breast cancer showed that the final cosmetic result had a marked bearing on the subsequent psychological outcome. Al-Ghazal et al.[36] reported significant correlations between cosmesis and levels of anxiety and depression and between cosmesis and body image, sexuality and self-esteem. In a more recent study of patients receiving either immediate reconstructive surgery or breast-conserving treatment, no differences were found between the groups in self-reported quality of life or changes in body image.

Interestingly, significant differences were found in cosmetic outcomes favouring immediate reconstruction over breast-conserving surgery as rated by the surgical team.[37] However, objective assessment of cosmesis does not always correlate with patients' perceptions about body image.

Harcourt et al.[38] showed in a prospective study that breast reconstruction is not a universal panacea for the emotional and psychological consequences of mastectomy. Women in this study chose whether to have reconstructive surgery (immediate or delayed) and completed self-assessments of anxiety, depression, body image and quality of life preoperatively and postoperatively at 6 and 12 months. Psychological distress decreased following surgery in all groups, but women still reported feeling conscious of altered body image 12 months later regardless of whether or not they had breast reconstruction. This finding should alert health-care professionals not to assume that breast reconstructive surgery necessarily confers psychological benefits compared with mastectomy alone.

Surgery for women at high genetic risk

Another group of women with issues about eventual cosmesis and its impact on sexuality are those at high genetic risk who are contemplating prophylactic surgery in order to reduce their chance of developing breast cancer later in life. Hatcher et al.[39] assessed the psychosocial impact of either accepting or declining bilateral prophylactic surgery in 143 women with increased risk of breast cancer. Quality of life, psychiatric morbidity, body image and sexual activity was measured at baseline and at 6 and 18 months. Results showed a significant decrease in psychological morbidity in those women who chose surgery, whereas those who opted for regular surveillance and declined surgery experienced anxiety and depression that did not decrease significantly over an 18-month period. There was no significant difference between the groups in the degree of sexual pleasure experienced over time. Women who opted for surgery (most of whom had immediate reconstruction) maintained a positive body image. There were some interesting personality differences between women who pursued prophylactic surgery and those who declined. The decliners had significantly higher anxiety personality traits than those who had surgery and tended to use detachment as a coping strategy rather than the problem-focused approach used more frequently by those who had surgery. Thus regular surveillance for an at-risk woman who had a predisposition to worry and who usually coped with anxiety by trying to ignore it only made these women more anxious. Women clearly need careful preoperative counselling and assessment prior to embarking on any prophylactic management policy.[40]

Psychosexual impact of adjuvant therapies

Increasing numbers of women are receiving neoadjuvant or adjuvant hormonal and chemotherapy treatments for breast cancer, yet the impact of these on psychosocial and sexual well-being is less well explored. Chemotherapy can produce overtly disfiguring side effects, for example alopecia and weight gain, and other debilitating problems such as nausea and fatigue. On top of this, most premenopausal women will experience a premature menopause, with all its associated adverse effects including hot flushes, cold sweats, vaginal dryness or discharge, and dyspareunia.

A research group in the Netherlands evaluated the impact of tamoxifen on subjective and psychosexual well-being in 98 breast cancer patients in relation to their menopausal status and any prior chemotherapy;[41] 44% of women reported a decreased interest in sexual activity during tamoxifen therapy that was unrelated to the type of chemotherapy they had received or menopausal status. However, after tamoxifen was stopped, patients who had received high-dose chemotherapy reported sexual dysfunction more often than patients who received the standard dose. Berglund et al.[42] examined the effects of different adjuvant treatments on sexuality in a prospective study. The women were all premenopausal and taking part in a European clinical trial in which they were randomised to tamoxifen or goserelin, a combination of tamoxifen and goserelin or no adjuvant endocrine therapy. Results indicated that women who received chemotherapy had a higher level of sexual dysfunction than patients who had not. The addition of endocrine treatment did not alter this result; however, in those women who did not receive chemotherapy, goserelin alone and combined with tamoxifen produced a significantly higher level of sexual dysfunction from 1 to 2 years compared with those who received tamoxifen alone or no endocrine therapy.

The effect that tamoxifen has on psychological and sexual functioning has been studied closely in chemoprevention studies for women at high risk of developing breast cancer.[43] Almost 500 women have participated in these double-blind trials, 254 randomised to the tamoxifen arm and 234 to the placebo arm. Psychological morbidity was assessed using standardised anxiety and depression tools and sexual functioning was measured using Fallowfield's Sexual Activity Questionnaire,[44] a self-report questionnaire that describes sexual functioning in terms of activity, pleasure and discomfort. Changes in anxiety, mood state and sexual functioning were not associated with treatment group. Nor were there differences in the proportions of women experiencing vaginal dryness, pain or discomfort during penetration.[43] However, the women taking tamoxifen were more likely to report vaginal discharge. This may be a reason why sexual activity was not impaired. The preliminary 2-year quality-of-life data from the Arimidex or Tamoxifen, Alone, Combined (ATAC) trial shows that at 3 months after treatment, patients receiving an aromatase inhibitor experienced significantly more vaginal dryness, pain on intercourse and loss of sexual interest than those women receiving tamoxifen.[10]

Although it is evident that most treatments for breast cancer impact in some way on a woman's psychosexual functioning, few are informed that these problems can occur and how to ameliorate adverse effects before they become a problem. One reason may be that health professionals feel embarrassed or inadequate about dealing with such issues. However, sexuality and intimacy are important concerns particularly for patients with breast cancer and need to be addressed.

Interventions to help psychosexual morbidity

Although much literature exists on the need for intervention for sexual dysfunction in patients with cancer, few results are available from randomised controlled clinical trials.[45] A very early study looked at psychosexual counselling for couples where the woman had had a mastectomy.[46] Couples who attended a four-session sex therapy group within 3 months following mastectomy did show increased sexual satisfaction but no differences in marital and psychological adjustment. A study from the USA evaluated a nurse-led intervention for postmenopausal women with breast cancer that aimed to provide relief of menopausal symptoms, improvement in sexual functioning and quality of life.[47] The intervention took place over a 4-month period and focused on symptom assessment, education, counselling, and specific pharmacological and behavioural interventions; 72 women completed the study, half receiving the usual care and half the intervention. Results revealed a significant improvement in sexual functioning and menopausal symptoms but no difference in quality of life between the groups.

Although there are guidelines available for health professionals on assessment and treatment of sexual dysfunction in breast cancer patients, encouragement and support to attend educational programmes is required. Too few recognise that counselling patients about sexual issues is an important aspect of patient care.

PSYCHOLOGICAL ASPECTS OF SERVICE DELIVERY

Delay in presentation with breast cancer

Anxiety about the disease and fears about treatment can lead women to delay seeking advice. Delay can be described in terms of patient or provider delay. Patient delay refers to the interval between first detection of symptoms and first medical consultation. The period that most authors accept as prolonged delay is 12 weeks or more,[48] although Nosarti et al.[49] regard patient delay as 4 weeks or more. Provider or system delay is defined as the interval between first presentation to the GP and initial treatment and is not easy to define. Although guidelines in the UK now suggest no longer than 2 weeks should elapse between first presentation to the GP with a suspicious lump and referral to a specialist, surgical treatment can be delayed for a wide variety of reasons. Delayed presentation of symptomatic breast cancer is associated with lower survival, particularly delays of 3–6 months or longer.[50] Therefore it is important to identify which factors influence patient delay and also whether provider delay contributes to poorer outcomes that may affect survival.

A retrospective analysis was performed on 36 222 patients with breast cancer registered with the Yorkshire Cancer Registry between 1976 and 1995 in order to examine whether provider delay adversely affected outcomes. Results found no evidence that provider delays of longer than 90 days adversely influenced survival.[51] However, there were some differences in that 48% of younger patients had their first treatment within 30 days compared with 64% of those over 50 years of age. The authors concluded that delays of longer than 60 days do not significantly impair survival and that even delays of more than 90 days are unlikely to have an impact on survival.

A systematic review of risk and delay in presentation by Ramirez et al.[48] found 86 studies in patients and 28 in providers. Only 23 studies were of adequate quality to include in the assessment. The authors generated hypotheses about the relationship between putative risk factors for patient and provider delay and assigned strength of evidence according to a combination of the number and size of studies that supported, failed to support or refuted their hypotheses. The risk factors for patient delay were grouped under the following headings: sociodemographic, clinical, psychological and social. The results showed strong evidence for an association between older age and delay and strong evidence that marital status was unrelated to delay by patients. Provider delay was associated with younger age and presentation with a breast symptom other than a lump.

Ramirez's group and others have examined delay from a number of perspectives, involving both quantitative and qualitative research. In one study they interviewed 185 women with breast cancer 2 months after their diagnosis in order to examine the incidence and effects of patient and provider delay;[52] 19% of women delayed 12 weeks or more and a number of factors predicted delay, including initial breast symptoms other than a lump, and not disclosing discovery of the breast lump immediately to somebody close. Patient delay was also related to a clinical tumour size of 4 cm or more and a higher incidence of metastatic disease.

Of these women, 46 (15 non-delayers and 31 delayers) were also interviewed to determine any differences between the groups.[53] Results suggested that those who recognised the seriousness of their symptoms presented promptly to the GP. The perceived seriousness was influenced by the nature of the symptom and how far it matched the individual's expectations of breast cancer as a painless lump. Other factors that influenced the seeking of help included beliefs about the consequences of treatment for breast cancer and attitudes to GP attendance. These results showed that women's knowledge about the symptoms and treatments of breast cancer was very limited despite the fact that it is a high-profile topic.

To this end, an additional survey by the group investigated healthy women's knowledge and beliefs regarding breast cancer.[54] Participants were randomly selected through the Postal Address File and data collected through the Office of National Statistics. Trained interviewers elicited each participant's knowledge of (i) any woman's and her own lifetime risk of developing breast cancer, (ii) risk factors for developing breast cancer, (iii) knowledge of breast cancer symptoms and (iv) perceptions of the management of breast cancer. Responses from 996 participants showed that despite breast cancer receiving a great deal of media attention, the majority of women in the UK had limited familiarity of their relative risk of developing breast cancer, of associated factors and of the diversity of potential breast cancer-related symptoms. Only 23% of women rated their own lifetime risk of developing breast cancer correctly, 35% thought it was 1 in 100 and 31% thought it was 1 in 1000. In addition, older women (mean age 75 years) identified fewer types of symptoms than younger women and thought themselves too old to develop breast cancer. The authors suggest this may explain the strong association between older age and delay in seeking help. However, women's knowledge of treatments was more on target, with 87% mentioning surgery, 66% chemotherapy and 49% radiotherapy. Only 5% spontaneously mentioned hormone treatment. Despite this, 80% of women believed treatments to be long-lasting and arduous.

Although one might expect to see strong cultural variations, similar reasons for delay are found across the continents. A cross-sectional study conducted in Tehran examined the extent of patient delay in a group of 190 newly diagnosed breast cancer patients;[55] 75% presented to the doctor within 3 months, while 25% delayed more than 3 months. Multivariate analysis showed a risk of delay in widowed or divorced women, women with a positive family history of breast cancer and in less educated patients. Again, delay in presentation was associated with late-stage disease and larger tumours. In Pakistan, the frequency and reasons for delay in seeking medical advice was examined in 138 women recently diagnosed with breast cancer at a national cancer centre in Karachi.[56] Delay was defined as greater than 1 month between initial perception of the lump and seeking medical advice. On average women took 8.7 weeks to inform the family and 17.2 weeks until they visited a physician. In total, 53% delayed seeking medical advice. Common reasons were use of alternative therapies (34%), fear of surgery (22%), lack of significance attached to the problem (23%) and fear of cancer (5%). Complementary and alternative medicine was used by 29% before visiting the doctor; the majority of this comprised homoeopathy, spiritual therapy (15%) and Ayurvedic medicine (13%). Complementary and alternative medicine was associated with delay at presentation and presentation at an advanced stage. In Nigeria, fear of mastectomy is the most common factor responsible for late presentation of carcinoma of the breast.[57] These women also sought help from prayers and spiritual healing (13.5%), and had a preference for herbalists and native doctors (23.1%). Health-care professionals may be unaware of the extent to which women with breast cancer utilise complementary and alternative medicine. Although some may be of value, or merely benign, others may have serious consequences that delay presentation and treatment of breast lumps.

One-stop clinics

Since the early 1990s there have been many patient demands for a comprehensive cancer service and an increasing professional requirement on the part of clinicians for improved health-care delivery in breast cancer through published guidelines such as BASO, SIGN and the Patient's Charter. The guidelines have suggested the establishment of organised specialist breast clinics with the aim of providing rapid diagnosis for patients with malignant disease and reassurance for symptomatic patients who do not have breast cancer. Requests for fast results, quicker throughput of patients and a decrease in unnecessary outpatient follow-up has led to the introduction of one-stop clinics within these centres. Alongside this came the 2-week referral rule for a woman reporting a breast lump to her GP. These were seen as potentially helpful developments, as 'waiting for results' is perceived by many women as one of the most traumatic periods during the whole breast cancer experience. However, there are increasing concerns that all these changes might not be providing the beneficial outcomes that were expected. In particular, the increase in demand for immediate referral reinforces the idea that breast cancer is a dire medical emergency, which it is not; rather it is an emotional emergency.

One-stop clinics have become a double-edged sword. The primary health-care sector is referring more and more women and does not always follow published guidelines, leading to a huge increase in patient numbers but not the staff to deal with them. In one prospective audit of 321 referrals to a Glasgow one-stop clinic,[58] 10% of women had breast cancer and 90% had benign disease or no pathology. The authors highlighted the fact that over one-third of referrals from the primary health-care sector were inappropriate and inevitably reduced the efficiency of the service provided for patients. Another audit in London[59] examined whether the service to women had improved since the original audit 5 years previously. This was a prospective audit of four consecutive clinics and a total of 300 patients were seen. Forty women had one-stop investigations and 86% of these had benign disease, demonstrating yet again that the majority of women referred to a breast clinic and those attending post-screening assessment have benign breast disease.

What does attendance at one-stop clinics do to a woman's psychological condition, be it a benign or malignant result? Most patients with benign disease will be in a state of heightened anxiety until they have undergone specialist assessment, the necessary investigations and eventual reassurance. In contrast, women who receive a diagnosis of breast cancer will still have heightened anxiety for many months during and following their treatment.[6]

One study[60] examined the costs and benefits of a one-stop clinic compared with a dedicated breast clinic. As part of the assessment, anxiety was measured at baseline, 24 hours, 3 weeks and 3 months in the 478 women who participated (267 at the one-stop clinic and 211 at the standard clinic). Results showed that in both groups mean anxiety scores at all time points were lower than at baseline. Reduction in mean anxiety was significantly greater for one-stop clinic patients at 24 hours but not for other time points. Harcourt et al.[61] showed a similar initial reduction in anxiety in one-stop clinic patients. Another study[62] reported the psychological distress associated with waiting for results in a delayed-results breast clinic. The findings from 126 women showed that the waiting sustained but did not exacerbate psychological distress. The qualitative aspect of this study also suggested that the structure of the delayed-results clinic might facilitate psychological preparation for test results.

Psychological aspects of mammographic screening

The National Mammographic Breast Screening Programme was initiated in response to the recommendations of a working group chaired by Sir Patrick Forrest.[63] Research has been published suggesting that the screening programme has lowered mortality rates in breast cancer.[64] Similarly, in 2002 the World Health Organisation concluded that trials have provided sufficient evidence to show that mammographic screening reduces deaths from breast cancer in women aged 55–69 years. However, there have been some vociferous debates about the true value of screening and even whether breast screening is associated with health benefits; it also has financial, physical and emotional costs for patients. Women who attend for screening have to offset potential health gains against such things as work time lost, fears of radiation, pain of the mammographic procedure, and the physical and psychological consequences of recall for further examinations where the initial mammogram was interpreted as indeterminate or abnormal.

The existing literature is inconsistent in its conclusions as to whether recall has short- or long-term psychological consequences. Some researchers have reported that women who receive false-positive results experience elevated anxiety after receiving a letter recalling them for further mammography,[65]

and that increased levels of anxiety and concern can last from 1 month[66] up to 6 months.[67] The effect can last even longer, as shown in a UK study of women who had initially been recalled with false-positive results.[68] Three years later, just before being invited for their next routine breast screening despite having received a final clear result 3 years previously, women who had undergone fine-needle aspiration, surgical biopsy or had been placed on early recall had significantly greater adverse psychological consequences at 1 month before their next screening appointment than women who had received a clear result after their initial mammogram at their last routine breast screening. In contrast, others have shown that although recalled women are more likely to have borderline or clinically significant anxiety than at baseline or screening, this effect lasts less than 5 weeks.[69] Similar findings of moderate negative short-term distress have been reported in other studies.[70,71] However, one of these, a large Finnish study[71] of 1718 patients noted that women who received false-positive findings experienced intrusive thoughts and worry about breast cancer at 2 months which still prevailed at 12 months. Similarly, Sandin et al.[72] examined differences between 597 women attending a second-stage breast cancer screening and 598 women attending routine screening with regard to affective cognitive distress and psychopathology and whether the psychological impact was temporary or longer-lasting. Results showed that women recalled for further assessment had higher levels of affective cognitive impact, specifically worry, fear and thinking about getting breast cancer. However, this distress did not persist following notification of the benign result.

Since a proportion of recalled women experience undesirable psychological consequences, there have been calls for interventions that offer support and counselling for these women.[66,71,73] Many breast assessment centres offer counselling by telephone or in the screening centre when women receive notification that they need further assessments. However, staff in Australia noted that some women continue to contact breast screening centres for support and reassurance despite receiving the all-clear. Undoubtedly, a number of factors influences the behaviour of such patients, including a person's coping style, level of social support and personality type. These factors were considered in a randomised trial of counselling interventions for women who were recalled for further investigations at breast screening centres in Melbourne, Australia.[73] Women were randomised to face-to-face counselling ($N = 66$), telephone counselling ($N = 68$) or usual care ($N = 71$). Usual care referred to women who received no further contact after being told they did not have cancer. Each woman completed a psychological consequences questionnaire, a social support questionnaire, a measure of dispositional optimism, and a coping strategy questionnaire following the all-clear and following the counselling intervention. There were no main effects for the intervention; in fact 32% (23) of the women randomised to receive face-to-face counselling refused the offer and 15 of them ended up participating in the telephone session instead. The researchers noted that women who tended to expect the worst were those who experienced the most disruption and represented an 'at-risk' group who would probably find counselling most useful, but the study was not powered to test this. More research is needed to characterise optimal support services for women who undergo screening, but good communication is a key requirement throughout the entire mammography process.

NEWER RESEARCH ISSUES ASSOCIATED WITH TREATMENTS

Cognition and chemotherapy/ endocrine therapy

The increased and widespread use of adjuvant treatments for breast cancer has produced a new aspect of research, namely the possible harmful effects that these treatments have on memory and attention. Complaints of slight forgetfulness or difficulty in concentration have been cited along with reports of patients experiencing poor quality of life because of the severity of the symptoms. Interest in this area has grown as evidence from both animal and clinical research has shown that estrogen has a very important role in memory and cognition. Estrogen receptors are found in key areas of the brain important for cognitive performance,

for example the amygdala, cerebral cortex and hippocampus. Separate studies have shown that removal of the ovaries in rats results in learning impairments and that the deficits are ameliorated by giving estrogen.[74,75] Similarly, both chemotherapy and hormone treatments for breast cancer disrupt the bioavailability of estrogen, which may contribute to the cognitive problems experienced by some but not all patients. There are other ways that chemotherapy treatments could affect cognition, including direct toxicity to the brain, metabolic changes, increased levels of cytokines, and microinfarcts. In addition, there are factors that are known to affect memory and must always be accounted for when an assessment is made, including a person's age, level of intelligence, and mood.

In recent years there have been several reviews on neuropsychological functioning in women treated for breast cancer.[76–78] The most recent reports the main findings from eight studies, six of which suggest impaired neuropsychological functioning.[76] However, the pattern of impairments found in the studies is not consistent, with some studies reporting deficits in both verbal and visual recall[79,80] and others deficits in verbal memory and psychomotor functioning.[81,82] As mentioned earlier, chemotherapy may have a direct toxic effect on the brain, and if so one would predict that those women who receive high-dose therapy might experience worse problems. Van Dam's early work concurs with this, in that substantial cognitive deficits were found in 32% of patients treated with high-dose marrow ablative chemotherapy and autologous stem cell support compared with 17% of women treated with standard therapy and 9% of control patients.[83] These impairments were observed 2 years after treatment was completed. Unfortunately, most of the studies suffer from poor methodology, are cross-sectional and have relatively small numbers, making it difficult to generalise and interpret what aspects of cognition are the most impaired, what impact this has on a patient's life and who will experience the problems. Preliminary studies suggest that there may be a genetic predisposition; in particular the e4 allele of apolipoprotein E (ApoE) has been associated with reduced neuropsychological performance.[84] Carriers of the e4 allele with breast cancer or lymphoma who were treated with chemotherapy tended to score lower on tests of visual memory, spatial ability and psychomotor functioning than survivors with other alleles of APOE.[84]

Making sense of the results from any of these studies is compounded by many other factors associated with cancer diagnosis and treatment. These include the stress, anxiety and depression that can negatively affect a patient's ability to focus, concentrate and organise, together with the effect that fatigue and pain has on multitasking and processing speed.[85] Finally, emerging studies using neuroimaging tools and techniques such as functional magnetic resonance imaging and positron emission tomography will hopefully illuminate the mechanisms for chemotherapy-related changes in brain function.

SUMMARY

Despite the many advances made in treating breast cancer, improvements in the delivery of care and provision of support services, the diagnosis of breast cancer still causes considerable distress. Women cope in many different ways with the knowledge that they have a potentially life-threatening disease requiring unpleasant treatments. For some it is a major emotional and social catastrophe, whereas others approach it with a degree of equanimity or stoicism. It is sometimes difficult to predict how women will react, adapt and adjust to what lies ahead. Greater awareness of some of the psychosocial, sexual and cognitive dysfunction associated with different treatments should enable us to design interventions to prevent or ameliorate their problems, but the importance of good clear information delivered in a supportive, honest and empathic manner should not be overlooked. The communication skills of a surgeon can exert a surprisingly useful psychotherapeutic impact on a woman and her ability to cope with the disease and its treatment.

REFERENCES

1. Renneker RE, Cutler R, Hora J et al. Psychoanalytical explorations of emotional correlates of cancer of the breast. Psychosom Med 1963; 25:106–23.

2. Veronesi U, Saccozzi R, Del Vecchio M et al. Comparing radical mastectomy with quadrantectomy, axillary dissection, and radiotherapy in patients with small cancers of the breast. N Engl J Med 1981; 305:6–11.

3. Fisher B, Bauer M, Margolese R et al. Five-year results of a randomized clinical trial comparing total mastectomy and segmental mastectomy with or without radiation in the treatment of breast cancer. N Engl J Med 1985; 312:665–73.

4. Fallowfield LJ, Baum M, Maguire GP. Effects of breast conservation on psychological morbidity associated with diagnosis and treatment of early breast cancer. Br Med J 1986; 293:1331–4.

5. Beaver K, Luker KA, Owens RG et al. Treatment decision making in women newly diagnosed with breast cancer. Cancer Nurs 1996; 19:8–19.

6. Fallowfield LJ, Hall A, Maguire P et al. Psychological effects of being offered choice of surgery for breast cancer. Br Med J 1994; 309:448.

7. Fallowfield L. Offering choice of surgical treatment to women with breast cancer. Patient Educ Couns 1997; 30:209–14.

8. Moyer A. Psychosocial outcomes of breast-conserving surgery versus mastectomy: a meta-analytic review. Health Psychol 1997; 16:284–98.

Meta-analysis of 40 studies examing the psychological sequelae of breast-conserving surgery versus mastectomy for early-stage disease. Modest advantages for breast-conserving surgery for psychological, marital–sexual and social adjustment, body image and cancer-related fears.

9. Hack TF, Cohen L, Katz J et al. Physical and psychological morbidity after axillary lymph node dissection for breast cancer. J Clin Oncol 1999; 17:143–9.

10. Poole K, Fallowfield LJ. The psychological impact of post-operative arm morbidity following axillary surgery for breast cancer: a critical review. Breast 2002; 11:81–7.

11. Liljegren G, Holmberg L. Arm morbidity after sector resection and axillary dissection with or without postoperative radiotherapy in breast cancer stage I. Results from a randomised trial. Uppsala-Orebro Breast Cancer Study Group. Eur J Cancer 1997; 33:193–9.

12. Coster S, Poole K, Fallowfield LJ. The validation of a quality of life scale to assess the impact of arm morbidity in breast cancer patients post-operatively. Breast Cancer Res Treat 2001; 68:273–82.

Validation paper of the FACT-B+4 quality of life scale. Scale demonstrated good internal consistency and stability, is psychometrically robust and sensitive to patient rehabilitation, making it suitable for use in longitudinal surgical trials.

13. Baum M. Epidemiology versus scare mongering: the case for the humane interpretation of statistics and breast cancer. Breast J 2000; 6:331–4.

14. Fallowfield L, Ratcliffe D, Jenkins V, Saul J. Psychiatric morbidity and its recognition by doctors in patients with cancer. Br J Cancer 2001; 84:1011–15.

15. Fallowfield L. Psychosocial interventions in cancer. Br Med J 1995; 311:1316–17.

16. Meyer BJ, Russo C, Talbot A. Discourse comprehension and problem solving: decisions about the treatment of breast cancer by women across the life span. Psychol Aging 1995; 10:84–103.

17. Maguire P, Tait A, Brooke M et al. Effect of counselling on the psychiatric morbidity associated with mastectomy. Br Med J 1980; 281:1454–6.

18. Watson MD, Denton S, Baum M et al. Counselling breast cancer patients: a specialist nurse service. Counselling Psychol Q 1988; 1:25–34.

19. Liebert B, Parle M, Roberts C et al. An evidence-based specialist breast nurse role in practice: a multicentre implementation study. Eur J Cancer Care (Engl) 2003; 12:91–7.

20. Luecken LJ, Compas BE. Stress, coping, and immune function in breast cancer. Ann Behav Med 2002; 24:336–44.

21. Spiegel D, Bloom JR, Kraemer HC, Gottheil E. Effect of psychosocial treatment on survival of patients with metastatic breast cancer. Lancet 1989; ii:888–91.

22. Spiegel D, Bloom JR, Yalom I. Group support for patients with metastatic cancer. A randomized outcome study. Arch Gen Psychiatry 1981; 38:527–33.

23. Fox BH. A hypothesis about Spiegel et al.'s 1989 paper on psychosocial intervention and breast cancer survival. Psychooncology 1998; 7:361–70.

24. Cunningham AJ, Edmonds CV, Jenkins GP et al. A randomized controlled trial of the effects of group psychological therapy on survival in women with metastatic breast cancer. Psychooncology 1998; 7:508–17.

25. Goodwin PJ, Leszcz M, Ennis M et al. The effect of group psychosocial support on survival in metastatic breast cancer. N Engl J Med 2001; 345:1719–26.

In this multicentre trial, 235 women with metastatic breast cancer were randomly assigned to either an intervention group that participated in weekly supportive expressive group therapy (158) or a control group that received no intervention (77). The primary outcome was survival. Women assigned to supportive–expressive therapy had greater improvement in psychological symptoms and reported less pain (P = 0.04) than women in the control group. A significant interaction of treatment-group assignment with baseline psychological score was found (P ≤0.003 for the comparison of mood variables; P = 0.04 for the comparison of pain); women who were more distressed benefited, whereas those who were less distressed did not. The psychological intervention did not prolong survival, median survival being 17.9 months in the intervention group and 17.6 months in the control group (hazard ratio for death according to the univariate analysis 1.06, 95% CI 0.78–1.45; hazard ratio according to the multivariate analysis 1.23, 95% CI 0.88–1.72).

26. Temoshok LR, Wald RL. Change is complex: rethinking research on psychosocial interventions and cancer. Integr Cancer Ther 2002; 1:135–45.

27. Bordeleau L, Szalai JP, Ennis M et al. Quality of life in a randomized trial of group psychosocial support in metastatic breast cancer: overall effects of the intervention and an exploration of missing data. J Clin Oncol 2003; 21:1944–51.

28. Kogon MM, Biswas A, Pearl D et al. Effects of medical and psycho-therapeutic treatment on the survival of women with metastatic breast carcinoma. Cancer 1997; 80:225–30.

29. Greer S, Morris T, Pettingale KW. Psychological response to breast cancer: effect on outcome. Lancet 1979; ii:785–7.

30. Pettingale KW, Morris T, Greer S, Haybittle JL. Mental attitudes to cancer: an additional prognostic factor. Lancet 1985; i:750.

31. Greer S, Morris T, Pettingale KW, Haybittle JL. Psychological response to breast cancer and 15-year outcome. Lancet 1990; 335:49–50.

32. Watson M, Haviland JS, Greer S et al. Influence of psychological response on survival in breast cancer: a population-based cohort study. Lancet 1999; 354: 1331–6.

This study investigated the effect of psychological response on disease outcome in 578 women with early-stage breast cancer. The women were followed up for 5 years. Cox's proportional-hazards regression was used to obtain the hazard ratios for the measures of psychological response, with adjustment for known clinical factors associated with survival. At 5 years, 395 women were alive and without relapse, 50 were alive with relapse, and 133 had died. There was a significantly increased risk of death from all causes by 5 years in women with a high score on the HAD scale category of depression (hazard ratio 3.59, 95% CI 1.39–9.24). There was a significantly increased risk of relapse or death at 5 years in women with high scores on the helplessness and hopelessness category of the MAC scale compared with those with a low score in this category (hazard ratio 1.55, 95% CI 1.07–2.25). There were no significant results found for the category of 'fighting spirit'.

33. McArdle JM, George WD, McArdle CS et al. Psychological support for patients undergoing breast cancer surgery: a randomised study. Br Med J 1996; 312:813–16.

34. Schover LR, Yetman RJ, Tuason LJ et al. Partial mastectomy and breast reconstruction. A comparison

of their effects on psychosocial adjustment, body image, and sexuality. Cancer 1995; 75:54–64.

35. Schain WS, Wellisch DK, Pasnau RO, Landsverk J. The sooner the better: a study of psychological factors in women undergoing immediate versus delayed breast reconstruction. Am J Psychiatry 1985; 142:40–6.

36. Al-Ghazal SK, Fallowfield L, Blamey RW. Does cosmetic outcome from treatment of primary breast cancer influence psychosocial morbidity? Eur J Surg Oncol 1999; 25:571–3.

37. Cocquyt VF, Blondeel PN, Depypere HT et al. Better cosmetic results and comparable quality of life after skin-sparing mastectomy and immediate autologous breast reconstruction compared to breast conservative treatment. Br J Plast Surg 2003; 56:462–70.

38. Harcourt DM, Rumsey NJ, Ambler NR et al. The psychological effect of mastectomy with or without breast reconstruction: a prospective, multicenter study. Plast Reconstr Surg 2003; 111:1060–8.

This prospective multicentre trial examined the psychological implications of women's decisions for or against breast reconstruction. Psychological assessments were made preoperatively and at 6 and 12 months postoperatively. There was a reduction in psychological distress over the year in patients whether or not they received reconstructive surgery but women in all groups (mastectomy, early or delayed reconstruction) also reported concerns over altered body image 1 year postoperatively.

39. Hatcher MB, Fallowfield L, A'Hern R. The psychosocial impact of bilateral prophylactic mastectomy: prospective study using questionnaires and semi-structured interviews. Br Med J 2001; 322:76.

This study investigated the psychosocial impact of bilateral prophylactic mastectomy in 143 women who had high genetic risk of developing breast cancer; 79 women chose to receive surgery and 66 declined. Psychological morbidity was assessed over a 2-year period. Psychological morbidity decreased significantly over time for the 79 women who chose to have surgery but not in those who declined. The decliners had significantly higher anxiety personality traits than those who had surgery and tended to use detachment as a coping strategy rather than the problem-focused approach used more frequently by those who had surgery.

40. McAllister M, O'Malley K, Hopwood P et al. Management of women with a family history of breast cancer in the North West Region of England: training for implementing a vision of the future. J Med Genet 2002; 39:531–5.

41. Mourits MJ, Bockermann I, de Vries EG et al. Tamoxifen effects on subjective and psychosexual well-being, in a randomised breast cancer study comparing high-dose and standard-dose chemotherapy. Br J Cancer 2002; 86:1546–50.

42. Berglund G, Nystedt M, Bolund C et al. Effect of endocrine treatment on sexuality in premenopausal breast cancer patients: a prospective randomized study. J Clin Oncol 2001; 19:2788–96.

43. Fallowfield L, Fleissig A, Edwards R et al. Tamoxifen for the prevention of breast cancer: psychosocial impact on women participating in two randomized controlled trials. J Clin Oncol 2001; 19:1885–92.

44. Thirlaway K, Fallowfield L, Cuzick J. The Sexual Activity Questionnaire: a measure of women's sexual functioning. Qual Life Res 1996; 5:81–90.

45. Shell JA. Evidence-based practice for symptom management in adults with cancer: sexual dysfunction. Oncol Nurs Forum 2002; 29:53–66; quiz 67–9.

46. Christensen DN. Postmastectomy couple counseling: an outcome study of a structured treatment protocol. J Sex Marital Ther 1983; 9:266–75.

47. Ganz PA, Greendale GA, Petersen L et al. Managing menopausal symptoms in breast cancer survivors: results of a randomized controlled trial. J Natl Cancer Inst 2000; 92:1054–64.

48. 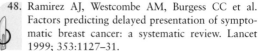 Ramirez AJ, Westcombe AM, Burgess CC et al. Factors predicting delayed presentation of symptomatic breast cancer: a systematic review. Lancet 1999; 353:1127–31.

This review reported strong evidence for an association between older age and delay by patients, and strong evidence that marital status was unrelated to delays by patients. Younger age and presentation with a breast symptom other than a lump were strong risk factors for delays by providers.

49. Nosarti C, Crayford T, Roberts J et al. Delay in diagnosis in breast cancer. Lancet 1999; 353:2154; author reply 2155.

50. Richards MA, Smith P, Ramirez AJ et al. The influence on survival of delay in the presentation and treatment of symptomatic breast cancer. Br J Cancer 1999; 79:858–64.

51. Sainsbury R, Johnston C, Haward B. Effect on survival of delays in referral of patients with breast-cancer symptoms: a retrospective analysis. Lancet 1999; 353:1132–5.

52. Burgess CC, Ramirez AJ, Richards MA, Love SB. Who and what influences delayed presentation in breast cancer? Br J Cancer 1998; 77:1343–8.

53. Burgess C, Hunter MS, Ramirez AJ. A qualitative study of delay among women reporting symptoms of breast cancer. Br J Gen Pract 2001; 51:967–71.

54. Grunfeld EA, Ramirez AJ, Hunter MS, Richards MA. Women's knowledge and beliefs regarding breast cancer. Br J Cancer 2002; 86:1373–8.

This survey of 996 women revealed that women had limited knowledge of their relative risk of developing breast cancer, of associated risk factors and of the diversity of potential breast cancer-related symptoms. Older women were particularly poor at identifying symptoms of breast cancer, risk factors associated with breast cancer and their personal risk of developing the disease. Poorer knowledge of symptoms and risks among older women may help to explain the strong association between older age and delay in seeking help.

55. Montazeri A, Ebrahimi M, Mehrdad N et al. Delayed presentation in breast cancer: a study in Iranian women. BioMed Central Women's Health 2003; 3:1–6.

56. Malik IA, Gopalan S. Use of CAM results in delay in seeking medical advice for breast cancer. Eur J Epidemiol 2003; 18:817–22.

57. Ajekigbe AT. Fear of mastectomy: the most common factor responsible for late presentation of carcinoma of the breast in Nigeria. Clin Oncol (R Coll Radiol) 1991; 3:78–80.

58. Patel RS, Smith DC, Reid I. One stop breast clinics: victims of their own success? A prospective audit of referrals to a specialist breast clinic. Eur J Surg Oncol 2000; 26:452–4.

59. Chan SY, Berry MG, Engledow AH et al. Audit of a one-stop breast clinic: revisited. Breast Cancer 2000; 7:191–4.

60. Dey P, Bundred N, Gibbs A et al. Costs and benefits of a one stop clinic compared with a dedicated breast clinic: randomised controlled trial. Br Med J 2002; 324:507.

61. Harcourt D, Ambler N, Rumsey N, Cawthorn S. Evaluation of a one stop breast clinic: a randomised controlled trial. Breast 1998; 7:314–19.

62. Poole K, Hood K, Davis BD et al. Psychological distress associated with waiting for results of diagnostic investigations for breast disease. Breast 1999; 8:334–8.

63. Forrest A. Breast cancer screening: report to the health ministers of England, Wales, Scotland and Northern Ireland. London: HMSO, 1986.

64. Blanks RG, Moss SM, McGahan CE et al. Effect of NHS breast screening programme on mortality from breast cancer in England and Wales, 1990–8: comparison of observed with predicted mortality. Br Med J 2000; 321:665–9.

65. Sutton S, Saidi G, Bickler G, Hunter J. Does routine screening for breast cancer raise anxiety? Results from a three wave prospective study in England. J Epidemiol Community Health 1995; 49:413–18.

66. Lowe JB, Balanda KP, Del Mar C, Hawes E. Psychologic distress in women with abnormal findings in mass mammography screening. Cancer 1999; 85:1114–18.

67. Olsson P, Armelius K, Nordahl G et al. Women with false positive screening mammograms: how do they cope? J Med Screen 1999; 6:89–93.

68. Brett J, Austoker J. Women who are recalled for further investigation for breast screening: psychological consequences 3 years after recall and factors affecting re-attendance. J Public Health Med 2001; 23:292–300.

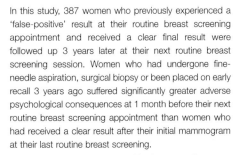

In this study, 387 women who previously experienced a 'false-positive' result at their routine breast screening appointment and received a clear final result were followed up 3 years later at their next routine breast screening session. Women who had undergone fine-needle aspiration, surgical biopsy or been placed on early recall 3 years ago suffered significantly greater adverse psychological consequences at 1 month before their next routine breast screening appointment than women who had received a clear result after their initial mammogram at their last routine breast screening.

69. Gilbert FJ, Cordiner CM, Affleck IR et al. Breast screening: the psychological sequelae of false-positive recall in women with and without a family history of breast cancer. Eur J Cancer 1998; 34:2010–14.

70. Ellman R, Angeli N, Christians A et al. Psychiatric morbidity associated with screening for breast cancer. Br J Cancer 1989; 60:781–4.

71. Aro AR, Pilvikki Absetz S, van Elderen TM et al. False-positive findings in mammography screening induces short-term distress: breast cancer-specific concern prevails longer. Eur J Cancer 2000; 36:1089–97.

72. Sandin B, Chorot P, Valiente RM, et al. Adverse psychological effects in women attending a second-stage breast cancer screening. J Psychosom Res 2002; 52:303–9.

73. Bowland L, Cockburn J, Cawson J et al. Counselling interventions to address the psychological consequences of screening mammography: a randomised trial. Patient Educ Couns 2003; 49:189–98.

74. Singh M, Meyer EM, Millard WJ, Simpkins JW. Ovarian steroid deprivation results in a reversible learning impairment and compromised cholinergic function in female Sprague-Dawley rats. Brain Res 1994; 644:305–12.

75. O'Neal MF, Means LW, Poole MC, Hamm RJ. Estrogen affects performance of ovariectomized rats in a two-choice water-escape working memory task. Psychoneuroendocrinology 1996; 21:51–65.

76. Morse R, Rodgers J, Verrill M, Kendell K. Neuropsychological functioning following systemic treatment in women treated for breast cancer: a review. Eur J Cancer 2003; 39:2288–97.

This review evaluated the effect of treatment and illness-related factors on neuropsychological functioning in women treated for breast cancer. Six of the eight studies reviewed suggest that neuropsychological functioning may be impaired following chemotherapy treatment but the authors highlight a number of important methodological issues that limit interpretation of these results. Therefore, it is unclear whether neuropsychological outcome differs according to a range of treatment, biomedical and psychological factors.

77. Rugo HS, Ahles T. The impact of adjuvant therapy for breast cancer on cognitive function: current evidence and directions for research. Semin Oncol 2003; 30:749–62.

78. Phillips KA, Bernhard J. Adjuvant breast cancer treatment and cognitive function: current knowledge and research directions. J Natl Cancer Inst 2003; 95:190–7.

79. Wieneke M, Dienst, ER. Neuropsychological assessment of cognitive functioning following chemotherapy for breast cancer. Psychooncology 1995; 4:61–6.

80. Schagen SB, Hamburger HL, Muller MJ et al. Neurophysiological evaluation of late effects of adjuvant high-dose chemotherapy on cognitive function. J Neurooncol 2001; 51:159–65.

81. Ahles TA, Saykin AJ, Furstenberg CT et al. Neuropsychologic impact of standard-dose systemic chemotherapy in long-term survivors of breast cancer and lymphoma. J Clin Oncol 2002; 20:485–93.

82. Jenkins V, Shilling V, Fallowfield LJ et al. Does hormone therapy for the treatment of breast cancer have a detrimental effect on memory and cognition? Psychooncology 2004; 13:61–6.

83. van Dam FS, Schagen SB, Muller MJ et al. Impairment of cognitive function in women receiving adjuvant treatment for high-risk breast cancer: high-dose versus standard-dose chemotherapy. J Natl Cancer Inst 1998; 90:210–18.

84. Ahles TA, Saykin AJ, Noll WW et al. The relationship of APOE genotype to neuropsychological performance in long-term cancer survivors treated with standard dose chemotherapy. Psychooncology 2003; 12:612–19.

85. Meyers CA. Neurocognitive dysfunction in cancer patients. Oncology 2000; 14:75–9; discussion 79, 81–2, 85.

Fifteen

Benign breast disease

Steven Thrush and
J. Michael Dixon

INTRODUCTION

The majority (>90%) of patients presenting to a
breast clinic suffer from benign breast disease.[1]
An understanding of the aetiology, symptoms and
management will ensure correct treatment and
satisfied patients. The expectation that the breast
surgeons' role is simply to diagnose or exclude
breast cancer has long disappeared. Benign breast
disease causes considerable morbidity and anxiety.
Effective treatment includes accurate diagnosis
followed by adequate explanation of the condition
and how it is best managed. With increasing
specialisation and patient awareness, the number of
benign patients seen is likely to increase, as are
expectations of care. Diagnosis and management of
benign breast disease is a rewarding part of a breast
specialist's workload.

Benign breast disease can be divided into congenital abnormalities, aberrations of normal breast
development and involution (ANDI) and conditions
secondary to some extrinsic precipitatory factors
(non-ANDI).

CONGENITAL ABNORMALITIES

Although not diseases as such, developmental
abnormalities of the breast can cause considerable
concern and are not uncommon reasons for referral
to a breast clinic.

Supernumerary nipples and accessory breast tissue

Accessory breast tissue is usually found in the axilla
and supernumerary or accessory nipples are usually
below the breast and above the umbilicus. Accessory
nipples can be excised if causing irritation.
Accessory breast tissue can become more prominent
or obvious during pregnancy (**Fig. 15.1**). As with
normal breast tissue, both benign and malignant
conditions can develop within the accessory breast
tissue. Reassurance and an explanation of the cause

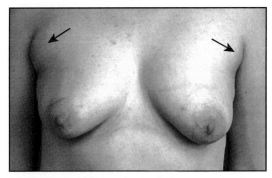

Figure 15.1 • Accessory breast tissue.

of the 'lump' is usually all that is required. Surgical excision should be reserved for those truly symptomatic as they are difficult to excise cosmetically and surgery is associated with significant morbidity.[2]

Breast hypoplasia

This is failure of a breast to develop fully. It is usually unilateral but can be bilateral. Poland's syndrome is a group of conditions in which amastia develops with associated degrees of pectoralis absence and syndactyly.[3] It is extremely rare and usually only partial in nature. An ipsilateral latissimus dorsi pedicled flap, with or without an implant, can be used to reconstruct the muscle defect and produce symmetry.

Asymmetry is a much commoner problem which usually only necessitates reassurance. If marked, augmentation of the smaller breast with or without reduction of the opposite breast may be required. Expandable implants can be overinflated and then reduced in size to try to improve contour in such cases.

Hypoplasia can also be associated with tubular breasts. This deformity can affect one or both breasts and is caused by a constricting ring at the base of the breast, limiting vertical and horizontal growth. The surgical management of this group of conditions is challenging and often unsatisfactory. Tissue expansion combined with radial incisions on the deep aspect of the breast to divide the constricting ring usually improves contour.

ABERRATIONS OF NORMAL BREAST DEVELOPMENT AND INVOLUTION

Defining what represents breast disease and what is normal is not a new problem. The ANDI classification[4] was developed to provide a framework to help understanding of the pathogenesis and subsequent management of benign breast disease. Most benign diseases arise from normal physiological processes and range from normality to mild abnormality (aberration) to severe abnormality (disease). The breast passes through three phases related to the levels of circulating hormones and their effects on the ducts, lobule and stroma. The three phases

Table 15.1 • Aberrations of normal breast development and involution

Age (years)	Normal process	Aberration
<25	Breast development Stromal	Juvenile hypertrophy
25–40	Lobular Cyclical activity	Fibroadenoma Cyclical mastalgia Cyclical nodularity (diffuse or focal)
35–55	Involution Lobular Stromal Ductal	Macrocysts Sclerosing lesions Duct ectasia

are development, cyclical change and involution (**Table 15.1**).

Fibroadenomas

A fibroadenoma is classified as an aberration of normal breast development and is made up of a combination of connective tissue and proliferatory epithelium.[5] Fibroadenomas arise from the hormone-dependent lobule of the terminal duct lobular unit. The stromal element of these tumours defines its classification and behaviour. A 'simple' fibroadenoma contains stroma of low cellularity and regular cytology. Phyllodes tumours probably arise from fibroadenomas and contain stroma with marked cellularity and atypia. They cannot always be differentiated on core biopsy.

SIMPLE FIBROADENOMAS

These are benign, extremely mobile, discrete, rubbery masses that present symptomatically in young women or are an incidental finding during breast imaging. They are a 'frequent' condition and are seen most commonly at the time of greatest lobular development in the late teens and early twenties. They are highly mobile due to encapsulation and pliability of the breast tissue. This can make them appear to be much more superficial on examination than their true position, important when embarking on removal under local anaesthetic. When observed for 2 years in women under 40 years of age, the majority do not change in size

(55%), some get smaller or resolve (37%) and a small number increase in size (8%).[6]

In older women the picture is less classical; differentiating breast cancer from a fibroadenoma is essential. Rapid growth of a fibroadenoma is rare but can occur in either adolescence (juvenile fibroadenoma) or the perimenopausal age group. Tumours over 5 cm are termed 'giant fibroadenoma' and are more commonly seen in African countries.[7] On macroscopic appearance fibroadenomas are discrete, bosselated, whitish tumours that appear to bulge when cut through. Only rarely does cancer develop within a fibroadenoma but when it does it tends to be non-invasive and lobular in nature.[8]

Management

The management of fibroadenomas depends on the patients' age and preference as well as the results of the triple assessment. Patients aged less than 30 years with cytological confirmation of the diagnosis of fibroadenoma can be managed conservatively,[6] with repeat imaging being recommended in 6 months to check that the lesion is not increasing in size. Older patients should have a core biopsy and if a diagnosis of fibroadenoma is made, the patient can be reassured and discharged. Excision is recommended if a fibroadenoma increases significantly in size, where the tumour results in distortion of the breast profile or where the lesion is over 4 cm in size, if there is any histological concern about stromal activity, or if the patient wishes excision. It is important to take account of the wishes of the patient; these are influenced by the manner in which the facts are presented.

Excision should ideally be undertaken through cosmetically placed incisions. Another option is to remove fibroadenomas with an 8G mammotome.[9] With larger tumours (>5 cm where histology has shown no suggestion that it could be a phyllodes tumour), it is safe to section the tumour in situ and remove it through a small incision to improve cosmetic outcome. Large lesions can be removed cosmetically through an inframammary incision. Removal of excess skin is rarely required in young women, particularly when removing a large juvenile fibroadenoma. Recurrence can occasionally occur but is rare. When it does so, it may be due to undiagnosed adjacent lesions rather than incomplete excision.

PHYLLODES TUMOUR AND SARCOMA

The aetiology of phyllodes (leaf-like) tumours is unknown. They are less common than fibroadenomas (ratio of presentation 1:40[10]) and constitute about 2.5% of all fibroepithelial tumours. The age of onset is 15–20 years later than fibroadenomas. They tend to grow rapidly, producing marked distortion and cutaneous venous engorgement, which can lead to ulceration. The majority are benign in nature and so they are rarely fixed to skin or muscle. When cut during removal they are more brownish in colour than fibroadenomas and can have areas of necrosis within. If a diagnosis of phyllodes tumour is made before operation, then the aim should be to remove it with a 1-cm macroscopic margin.

Differentiating benign from malignant phyllodes can be difficult and involves assessment of the size, ratio of stroma and epithelium, the border of the lesion, stromal cellularity and the number of stromal mitoses, and the presence or absence of necrosis.

Overall, phyllodes tumours recur locally in approximately 20% of patients. Most locally recurrent tumours are histologically similar to the original lesions. Malignant phyllodes tumours recur earlier on average than benign lesions. Regional lymph node metastases very rarely develop from malignant phyllodes tumours, with nodes being affected in approximately 5%. Metastatic lesions, when they occur, resemble sarcomas. Fewer than 5% of all phyllodes tumours metastasise and approximately 25% of those classified as malignant metastasise depending on the exact criteria used for classification. Treatment of metastatic disease has been discouraging, with no sustained remissions from radiation, hormonal treatment or chemotherapy.

Nipple discharge

Nipple discharge accounts for 5% of referrals to a breast clinic,[11] with 5% of these caused by in situ or malignant disease.[12] The important features to assess are whether the discharge is from one duct or many, is induced or spontaneous and is affecting one or both breasts. The frequency, colour and consistency of the discharge should also be noted. The aim is to differentiate between physiological causes and ductal pathology. Discharge can be elicited by squeezing around the nipple in 20% of women[13] and is often noted following mammography. If discharge is associated with a lump, then management is directed to the diagnosis of the lump.

Galactorrhoea should only be diagnosed if the discharge is bilateral, copious, off-white in colour and from multiple ducts. Some women continue to produce milk for many months after they have stopped breast-feeding but galactorrhoea usually develops long after cessation of breast-feeding. Prolactin levels should be checked and if raised (>1000 mIU/L) the cause can be secondary to medication or a pituitary tumour. If the serum prolactin is normal, then reassurance and a full explanation of the aetiology are often all that is required. If there are persistent symptoms, the ducts underneath the nipple can be ligated.

Coloured opalescent discharge, from multiple ducts, is common. It may be physiological discharge or it can be from duct ectasia. Serosanguineous and/or bloody discharge from a single duct is more likely to be associated with papillomas, epithelial hyperplasia or carcinoma.

INVESTIGATION

Assessment includes a careful breast examination to identify the presence or absence of a breast mass. Firm pressure applied around the areola can help to identify the site of any dilated duct (pressure over a dilated duct will produce the discharge); this is helpful in defining where an incision should be made for any subsequent surgery. The nipple is squeezed with firm digital pressure and if fluid is expressed, the site and character of the discharge are recorded. Testing of the discharge for haemoglobin determines whether blood is present. Fewer than 10% of patients who have a blood-stained discharge or who have a discharge containing moderate or large amounts of blood have an underlying malignancy. The absence of blood in nipple discharge is not an absolute indication that the discharge is unrelated to an underlying malignancy, as demonstrated in a recent series of 108 patients where the sensitivity of Haemoccult testing was only 50%.[14] Nipple discharge cytology is of little use due to its poor sensitivity.[15,16]

Two techniques have evolved to determine the aetiology and avoid unnecessary surgery. Ductoscopy, using a microendoscope passed into the offending duct, allows direct visualisation and has the potential for biopsy. There are encouraging reports of its use (see Chapter 3), especially in directing duct excision at surgery[17] and detecting deeper lesions often missed by blind central excision.[18] Ductal lavage is a technique in which the duct is cannulated, irrigated with saline and the subsequent discharge (encouraged with massage) examined cytologically. This technique increases cell yield by 100 times that of simple discharge cytology.[19] At present, the role of ductoscopy appears to be as an adjunct to surgery; by using simple transillumination of the skin overlying the lesion during ductoscopy, limited duct excision is possible. The role of ductal lavage has been questioned due to large variations in its sensitivity and specificity.[20] During ductoscopy, visualised lesions can be biopsied and in one report 38 of 46 women with biopsy-proven papillomas were observed for 2 years with no reported missed cancers.[18] The role of ductoscopy in the assessment of nipple discharge is set to increase as the quality of equipment improves and it becomes more widely available.

A mammogram should be performed as part of the assessment of patients over 35 years of age with a discharge. The sensitivity in this group of patients is low at 57%.[15] Ultrasound can sometimes identify papillomas and malignant lesions in the ducts close to the nipple.[21]

If no abnormality is found on clinical or mammographic examination, patients are managed according to whether the discharge is from a single duct or multiple ducts (**Fig. 15.2**). Any patient with spontaneous single-duct discharge should undergo surgery if it is:

- bloodstained or contains moderate to large amounts of blood on testing;
- persistent (at least twice per week);
- associated with a mass;
- a new serosanguineous discharge in a postmenopausal woman.

AETIOLOGY

Duct ectasia

This is benign dilatation and shortening of the terminal ducts within 3 cm of the nipple. It is a common condition and increases in incidence with age. It should not be confused with periductal

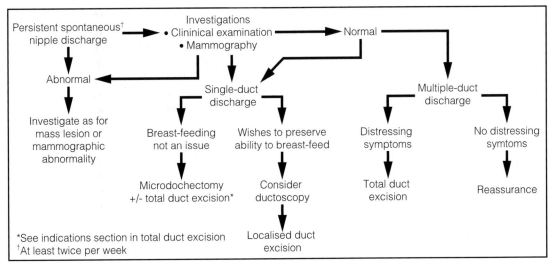

Figure 15.2 • Investigation of nipple discharge. *See indications in section Total duct excision or division.

mastitis, which occurs in younger women and is secondary to cigarette smoking. Duct ectasia can present as nipple discharge, nipple retraction (giving a slit-like appearance) or a palpable mass. It is usually asymptomatic. The discharge is usually creamy and cheesy in nature.

Ductal papillomas

There are three main forms: a solitary-duct discrete papilloma, multiple papillomas or a juvenile papilloma. The commonest is a single papilloma, which occurs in a large duct (within 5 cm of the nipple) and presents with either bloody or serous single-duct discharge. As papillomas have a thin stalk, they have the potential to tort and necrose. Half of women with papillomas have bloody discharge while the other half have a serous discharge.[22]

Multiple intraductal papillomas describes a condition where a woman has many peripheral duct papillomas. These tend not to present as nipple discharge but as a palpable lump. They are only associated with an increased risk of malignancy if they contain areas of severe atypical hyperplasia. Juvenile papilloma is a very rare condition occurring in young women and usually presents as a mass (similar to fibroadenoma).

Ductal carcinoma in situ

One-third of symptomatic in situ cancers present as nipple discharge.[23] Only rarely does an invasive cancer cause nipple discharge in the absence of a clinical mass. In most series, ductal carcinoma in situ (DCIS) is responsible for up to 10% of unilateral nipple discharge.[13] The diagnosis is usually made only following surgical excision of the affected duct.

Bloody nipple discharge in pregnancy

A bloody nipple discharge detected either visibly or on testing during pregnancy or lactation is common. In 20% of women who develop nipple discharge during pregnancy, blood is evident on testing. The likely cause is hypervascularity of developing breast tissue; it is benign and requires no specific treatment.[24]

SURGERY

Microdochectomy

A single duct can be removed using microdochectomy. This is performed via a circumareolar incision. Expression of the nipple discharge should not be performed until the patient is in theatre and fully draped in order to provide the best chance of identifying the offending duct. This duct is canulated with a lacrimal probe and the incision made. The probe aids identification of the relevant duct and dissection of this from surrounding ducts/breast tissue. A length of at least 2–3 cm should be removed. The excised duct should be opened to ensure a cause for the discharge is present and the distal remnant inspected to ensure that all the dilated duct has been excised. If the duct is still dilated, then it should be split, opened and inspected. Microdochectomy should not damage surrounding normal ducts and allows subsequent breast-feeding.

Total duct excision or division

In women of non-childbearing age, total duct excision is an option for a single-duct discharge. Total duct excision can also be used for multiple-duct discharge if the discharge is copious and affecting quality of life, and is often performed for periductal mastitis. The operation involves dividing all the ducts from the underside of the nipple and removing surrounding breast tissue to a depth of 2 cm behind the nipple–areola complex.[25] A circumareolar incision is used. Patients should be warned that there is a small risk of nipple tip necrosis, reduced sensation and nipple inversion associated with this operation. Patients undergoing surgery for periductal mastitis require total removal of all ducts from behind the nipple; leaving remnants of ducts predisposes to recurrence.

For patients having cosmetic nipple eversion, the procedure can be performed through a limited incision and the ducts divided sufficiently to ensure the nipple everts naturally without the need for sutures.

Mastalgia

Most women at some point during their lives will suffer from breast pain. The aim for clinicians is to differentiate between true mastalgia (pain originating within the breast) and referred pain. Women with referred pain will describe the pain as unilateral, associated with activity and reproduced by pressure on the chest wall. Non-steroidal anti-inflammatory drugs, either taken orally or applied topically, can relieve such symptoms. True mastalgia is associated with swelling and nodularity of the breasts. It resolves spontaneously in 20–40% of women but can recur.

Due to the hormonal aetiology, the pain is often worse before and relieved after menstruation. Differentiating cyclical and non-cyclical mastalgia is of little clinical importance as treatment is identical. Exacerbating factors include the perimenopausal state (where hormone levels fluctuate) and the use of exogenous hormones (hormone replacement therapy or the oral contraceptive pill).

The cause of mastalgia is unknown but suggestions include excess production of prolactin,[26] excess estrogen,[27] insufficient progesterone,[28] or increased receptor sensitivity in breast tissue caused by a raised ratio of saturated fatty acids to essential fatty acids.[29]

ASSESSMENT

A full history and examination should be performed. In women over 35 years of age, mammography should be performed to exclude an occult malignancy (approximately 5% of women with breast cancer complain of pain,[10] while 2.7% of women presenting with pain as their main problem are diagnosed with breast cancer[30]). If a lump is palpable, then this will dictate further management. An ill-fitting bra is an easily rectified cause of breast pain.

The use of a pain chart allows interpretation of the pattern of the pain, gives objective evaluation of treatment and indicates the effect it is having on the patients' life. (Patients with minimal pain are unlikely to fully complete a 3-month chart!)

TREATMENT

Reassurance that the symptoms are not related to an underlying malignancy is probably the most effective treatment for mastalgia.[31] Following this, the majority will require no further treatment.

Evening primrose oil (EPO) has recently been withdrawn from prescription by the Medicines Control Agency, as there was no clinical evidence to support its use. Two recent double-blind, randomised, controlled trials using EPO versus placebo in a cross-over pattern have shown no benefit for EPO.[32,33] The original work that advocated its use has never been published other than in abstract form.[34] Other agents that have been shown to have benefit include phytoestrogens (e.g. soya milk)[35] and Agnus castus (a fruit extract).[36]

Reducing fat intake to less than 15% of dietary calories has been shown to improve symptoms in cyclical mastalgia.[37] The patients who responded showed changes in their serum lipid profiles but the study was not blinded so placebo effects cannot be excluded.

In severe pain, prescribed medication can be used but complications need to be explained. Second-line treatment should be either tamoxifen (10 mg daily) or danazol. Tamoxifen 20 mg daily was found to be superior to placebo in a double-blind, randomised, controlled trial and pain relief was maintained in 72% of women 1 year after use.[38] Tamoxifen given in the luteal phase of the menstrual cycle abolished pain in 85% of women. Recurrent pain at 1 year was 25%, and the rate of adverse effects was 21%.[39] Tamoxifen 10 mg daily has been compared with danazol 200 mg daily.[40] Tamoxifen was found to be superior to danazol, with fewer adverse effects: 53% of patients receiving tamoxifen were pain-free at 1 year compared with 37% of patients receiving danazol. Tamoxifen (10 mg daily) or danazol can be given during the luteal phase of the cycle with similar improvements in symptoms but with a marked reduction in adverse effects.[39,41] Tamoxifen is not licensed for use in mastalgia.

Bromocriptine use has diminished due to its high rate of adverse effects (80%).[42] Selective serotonin reuptake inhibitors have shown some benefit in mastalgia as part of premenstrual syndrome;[43] they also have effects on fatty acid profiles.

Breast cysts

Palpable breast cysts are a common presentation to a breast clinic and affect 7% of women.[10] Cysts can be as either macrocysts or microcysts. Microcysts have no significance except their potential to grow. Macrocysts present typically in the fifth decade and are usually multiple in nature. Cysts can be divided into apocrine and non-apocrine depending on the consistency of the fluid found within the cyst. The relevance of this is that apocrine cysts have a higher tendency to recur.[44]

IMAGING

Mammographically, breast cysts have characteristic halos but ultrasound is essential to the management of cystic disease. Not only does it distinguish between solid and cystic lesions but also provides information on the cyst lining and fluid consistency. It is also an adjunct in ensuring accurate differentiation of simple from complex cysts, as well as allowing complete aspiration. A simple cyst shows a smooth outline with no internal echoes and posterior enhancement. If the cyst wall shows any projections, this may indicate the presence of an intracystic papilloma or carcinoma.

MANAGEMENT

Asymptomatic cysts should be left alone. Large or painful cysts should be aspirated to dryness. If the fluid is blood-stained, it should be sent for cytology; otherwise it should be discarded. If a palpable mass is still present after aspiration, further imaging and biopsy are indicated. If the cyst recurs, then repeat aspiration can be performed. There is a slightly increased relative risk of developing breast cancer in women with cysts but not significant enough to warrant surveillance.

Sclerotic/fibrotic lesions

Stromal involution can produce areas of fibrosis. Three different groups of such lesions are described: sclerosing adenosis, radial scars and complex sclerosing lesions (CSL). Sclerosing adenosis can present with a palpable mass and breast pain. Mammographically, it can be associated with microcalcificaton. It differs histologically from radial scars and CSL in the degree of excessive myoepithelial proliferation seen in addition to the fibrosis. Radial scars and CSL are usually asymptomatic and discovered as part of mammographic screening but can present as a palpable mass. They are considered to be the same process but are differentiated on size (radial scar, ≤1 cm; CSL, >1 cm). All these lesions, though benign in nature, are difficult to distinguish from malignant conditions mammographically, macroscopically and histologically. Biopsy or excision of such lesions (open excision) is usually required.

A form of sclerosis can occur in patients who usually have type 1 diabetes, diagnosed histologically as sclerosing lymphocytic lobulitis or 'diabetic mastopathy'. It does not seem to predispose to breast carcinoma or lymphoma and in patients without diabetes has an unknown aetiology.[45]

NON-ANDI CONDITIONS

Breast infections

Infection is a common problem affecting the breast,[46] and can be divided into lactational, non-lactational and postsurgical. The skin overlying the breast can also become infected either primarily or secondarily because of infection developing in an existing lesion such as a sebaceous cyst or as a consequence of a generalised condition such as hidradenitis suppurativa.

LACTATIONAL INFECTIONS

Mastitis secondary to breast-feeding occurs in approximately 5% of puerperal women and is most common during the first month or during weaning as the baby's teeth develop. *Staphylococcus aureus* is the usual organism and it enters the duct system through the nipple. There is usually a history of a cracked nipple and/or problems with milk flow. Patients initially present with pain, localised erythema and swelling. If this progresses, the inflammation can affect the whole of the breast and the patient can become toxic. Promoting milk flow by continuing to breast-feed and the early use of appropriate antibiotics markedly reduces the rate of subsequent abscess formation. Infections developing within the first few weeks are often from organisms transmitted in hospital and may be resistant to commonly used antibiotics. Over half of organisms that cause breast infection produce penicillinase.[47] Co-amoxiclav or flucloxacillin and erythromycin are the antibiotics of preference. Tetracycline, ciprofloxacin, and chloramphenicol should not be used to treat infection in breast-feeding women because these drugs enter breast milk and may harm the child.

NON-LACTATIONAL INFECTIONS

Non-lactational infections are grouped into peripheral or periareolar. Those infections in the periareolar area are seen in young women and are often secondary to periductal mastitis (associated with heavy cigarette smoking).[48] How cigarette smoking causes periductal mastitis is unclear. Substances in cigarette smoke may directly or indirectly damage the wall of subareolar ducts. Accumulation of toxic metabolites, such as lipid peroxidase, epoxides, nicotine and cotinine, in the breast ducts has been demonstrated to occur in smokers within 15 minutes of a woman starting to breast-feed.[49] Smoking has also been shown to inhibit growth of Gram-positive bacteria, leading to an overgrowth of Gram-negative bacteria.[50] This may affect the normal bacterial flora and allow overgrowth of pathogenic aerobic and anaerobic gram-negative bacteria, and would explain the presence of these organisms in the lesions of periductal mastitis. Microvascular changes have also been recorded and may cause local ischaemia. The combination of damage due to toxins, microvascular damage by lipid peroxidases, and altered bacterial flora are almost certainly responsible for the clinical manifestations of periductal mastitis.

Patients present with periareolar inflammation associated with a mass or abscess. The organisms are usually mixed, including anaerobes. Very rarely an infection is related to underlying comedo necrosis in DCIS. For this reason a mammogram should be performed in those patients over 35 years of age after resolution of the inflammation. Periareolar sepsis has a high rate of recurrence.

Peripheral non-lactational breast abscesses are three times more common in premenopausal women than in menopausal or postmenopausal women. The aetiology of these infections is unclear but some are associated with diabetes, rheumatoid arthritis, steroid treatment and trauma.[51] The usual organism responsible is *S. aureus*.

POSTSURGICAL INFECTION

Infections can present in the acute postsurgical period or after the wound has healed. There is conflicting evidence for the use of prophylactic antibiotics during clean breast surgery.[52] The most common organisms causing infection in the acute period include normal skin flora or organisms derived from the terminal ducts.[53] Studies have shown that a single dose of antibiotics given to patients undergoing more complicated breast and/or axillary surgery reduces the rate of postoperative infection. Most surgeons give antibiotics routinely to patients having implants inserted. Patients having surgery for periductal mastitis are at increased risk of postoperative infection and all these patients should have intraoperative and postoperative antibiotics that cover the range of organisms isolated from this condition. 'Seromas' are frequent and can become infected either during aspiration or as a result of reduced resistance to infection during chemotherapy. Radiotherapy interferes with both the blood and lymphatic flow to the breast and its effect is to reduce resistance to infection in the treated area; when infection occurs, prolonged and high-dose antibiotic therapy is usually required. Delayed infections after breast-conserving surgery or mastectomy are not uncommon (especially after radiotherapy). It is important not to confuse this with so-called 'delayed cellulitis', where the breast becomes painful, red and oedematous. It is unresponsive to antibiotics and has an incidence of 3–5% in patients following radiotherapy for breast-conserving surgery.[54]

If an implant becomes infected, intensive antibiotic therapy is occasionally effective but usually the prosthesis has to be removed. Replacing an infected implant following thorough lavage has been reported to be effective but is rarely performed.[55] It is not uncommon for implants to become infected after a minor surgical intervention (such as dental work) or during chemotherapy given as adjuvant therapy or as treatment for metastatic disease. Prophylactic antibiotics should be considered for patients with implants undergoing major dental work.

TREATMENT

The basis of treatment for all breast infections is use of a broad-spectrum antibiotic and draining any collections of pus. Due to the difficulty of predicting the presence of pus within an inflamed breast, ultrasound with or without aspiration should be performed.[56] The need for open drainage in breast abscesses has been superseded by the use of aspiration.[57–59] This has allowed management to become outpatient based. Protocols validated within the Edinburgh Breast Unit have demonstrated that few if any breast abscesses require incision and drainage under general anaesthesia.[60] All abscesses should be assessed by ultrasound and if pus is present the surgeon or radiologist aspirates this, usually under ultrasound guidance (**Fig. 15.3**).

Patients are reviewed regularly every 2–3 days and any further collections aspirated until no further pus forms. Drainage under local anaesthesia is performed in patients where the overlying skin is thinned or necrotic (**Fig. 15.4**; see Plate 13, facing p. 116). The incision to drain any breast abscess should be just large enough to allow the pus to drain (usually 1 cm or less), while minimising later scarring. Ultrasound provides a simple method of differentiating an abscess from cellulitis and allows assessment of loculation and permits complete aspiration of all pus. Experience in the Edinburgh Breast Unit of using ultrasound to assist aspiration of breast abscesses is that it is quick and simple to learn and use. When used with local anaesthetic injected into the breast and irrigated into the abscess, aspiration is relatively painless and the local anaesthetic dilutes the pus to allow aspiration. Periareolar non-lactational abscesses can be treated and cured by repeated aspiration. Due to the recurrent nature of this condition, persistent abscess formation is common and in such patients careful surgical excision of any residual abscess and affected ducts is often required.[26] A mammary duct fistula (an abnormal connection between the infected duct and the skin around the areola) develops in up to one-third of patients after incision and drainage of a periareolar abscess.[61] These require definitive surgical management, with complete excision of the tract (plus the affected ducts under the nipple) and ideally primary closure with antibiotic cover (**Fig. 15.5**). Laying open the fistula and allowing it to heal by secondary intention is effective but leaves an ugly scar across the nipple.

(a)

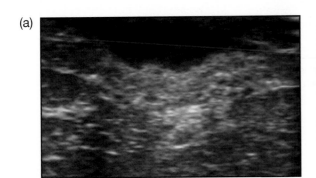

(b)

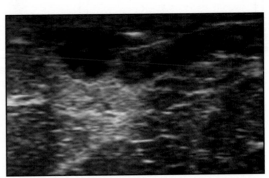

Figure 15.3 • Aspiration of abscess under ultrasound guidance: **(a)** ultrasound view of a breast abscess; **(b)** the needle can be seen entering the abscess and aspiration performed.

(a)

(b)

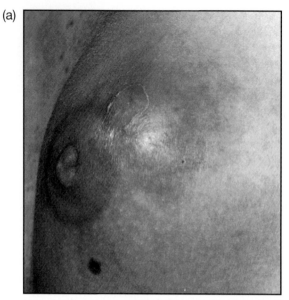
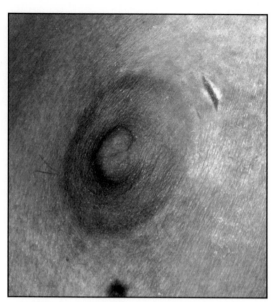

Figure 15.4 • Abscess of the left breast with thinned overlying skin **(a)** before and **(b)** after incision and drainage through a small stab incision.

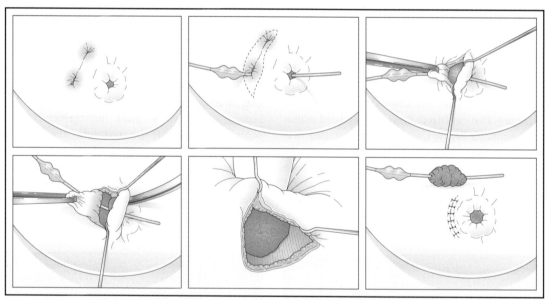

Figure 15.5 • Diagrammatic illustration of the steps involved in excision of a mammary duct fistula performed through a circumareolar incision with primary wound closure under antibiotic cover.

An important aspect of the management of puerperal breast infections is the continued expression of milk, with the most efficient breast pump being the baby's mouth. Emptying the breast increases the rate of a good outcome in infective mastitis[62] and although bacteria and the antibiotic are present in the milk, this does not appear to harm the child.[63] It is rarely necessary to suppress lactation but in severe unremitting or repeated infections, agents such as cabergoline are effective at stopping milk flow.

It is essential to remember that inflammatory carcinoma can be difficult to differentiate from breast infection. If the breast does not settle on appropriate management, then fine-needle aspiration and/or core biopsy of the abnormal area should be considered.

Other infections

HIV ASSOCIATED

Immunocompromised patients are susceptible to breast infection. This is true of both male and female sufferers.

GRANULOMATOUS MASTITIS

This is a rare condition, characterised by non-caseating granulomas and microabcesses confined to a breast lobule.[64] Patients present with a hard mass (which is often indistinguishable from a carcinoma) or multiple or recurrent abscesses. The mass can be extremely tender. Young parous women are most frequently affected. The role of organisms in the aetiology of this condition is unclear but a recent study isolated corynebacteria from 9 of 12 women with granulomatous lobular mastitis.[65] The most common species isolated was the newly described *Corynebacterium kroppenstedtii*, followed by *Corynebacterium amycolatum* and *Coryne-acterium tuberculostearicum*. Confirmation of these findings is required but if these organisms are the cause of this condition, then specific antibiotic therapy to eradicate corynbecacteria should be effective. These organisms are usually sensitive to penicillin and tetracycline, but treatment should be based on sensitivities as reported by the local bacteriological service. In patients presenting with a breast mass diagnosed on core biopsy as granulomatous lobular mastitis, excision of the mass should be avoided, as it is often followed by persistent wound discharge and failure of the wound to heal. Steroids have been used with varying reports of their efficacy; we do not use them.[66]

HIDRADENITIS SUPPURATIVA

Hidradenitis is infection associated with the apocrine glands, affecting axillae, perineum and/or breast areas. It is commoner in smokers and the organisms responsible are similar to those present in periareolar sepsis. Treatment in the acute phase comprises management of any infection/abscesses. Excision of the affected area with skin grafting is

effective in approximately 50% of patients and may be the only long-term option for some patients.

Montgomery's glands

Throughout the areola are blind-ending ducts that produce fluid to lubricate the areola during breast-feeding. These glands can block, forming hard nodules on the periphery of the areola. Occasionally these can become infected. Unless symptomatic, the management of these prominent Montgomery's glands is reassurance.

Lipomas

Due to the fatty nature of the breast it is not surprising that lipomas develop. They tend to present in the fifth decade[10] and have to be distinguished from any sinister cause. Imaging shows a radiolucent lobulated mass. Needle aspiration is often reported inadequate (C1) due to fat only being aspirated. A pseudolipoma is a mass that clinically appears to be a simple lipoma but is actually caused by a small cancer that produces compressed fat lobules as the suspensory ligaments of the breast shorten. Liposarcomas occur only very rarely in the breast.[67]

Fat necrosis

Following trauma to the breast, fat necrosis can occur. Fat necrosis can produce either a mass similar on palpation and imaging to breast carcinoma or a cystic oily collection. Usually, but not always with fat necrosis, patients give a history of direct trauma to the affected breast and examination may reveal bruising. It is important to assess such patients with imaging and not dismiss dimpling and bruising as fat necrosis. Some of these patients have underlying carcinomas that have only been noticed following (usually trivial) trauma.

Mondor's disease

Mondor's disease is spontaneous superficial thrombophlebitis of a breast vein. It is often initially painful and occasionally there may be a history of trauma or surgery to the breast. Clinically, there may be a thickened palpable cord with associated erythema. Its aetiology in the absence of surgery, trauma or infection is unknown but is not thought to be of any significance. It is a self-limiting condition that normally resolves within a couple of weeks. Non-steroidal anti-inflammatory agents rubbed over the area of tenderness improve pain.

Gynaecomastia

True gynaecomastia is caused by hyperplasia of the stromal and ductal tissue of the male breast. It is responsible for considerable embarrassment and worry and is the commonest condition affecting the male breast. Pseudogynaecomastia gives a similar appearance but is due to excess adipose tissue with no increase in stromal or ductal tissue. Both types can present together.[68]

Gynaecomastia can occur from any age, is usually unilateral and presents as a concentric painful swelling. It is a common condition, occurring in at least 35% of men at some time. It is benign and usually reversible. An important differential diagnosis is a primary breast cancer.

The aetiology of gynaecomastia is due to a relative hyperestrogenism.[69] This is caused by decreased androgen production, increased estrogen production or an increase in peripheral aromatisation. In those cases where no endocrine abnormality or drug is found, the cause may be a reduction in androgen receptors and/or a local increase in aromatase activity.[70] Causes can be divided into physiological, pathological, drug induced (medicinal and recreational) and idiopathic.

1. Physiological, or primary, gynaecomastia shows a trimodal pattern, with peaks in the neonatal period, puberty and senescence. It is often self-limiting but will occasionally require treatment.
2. Pathological causes are listed in **Box 15.1**.
3. Common drugs that produce gynaecomastia include spironolactone (antiandrogen); histamine H_2 antagonists, antipsychotics and methyldopa (gonadotrophin disturbance); digoxin, cannabis and griseofulvin (estrogen receptor competitors); and anabolic steroids (**Box 15.2**).

The degree of gynaecomastia is classified using appearance (**Box 15.3**). A thorough history will usually elicit the underlying cause. Examination

Box 15.1 • Pathological causes of gynaecomastia

DECREASED ANDROGENS

Reduced production

- Chromosomal abnormalities, e.g. Klinefelter's syndrome
- Bilateral cyptorchidism
- Hyperprolactinaemia
- Bilateral torsion
- Viral orchitis
- Renal failure

Androgen resistance

- Testicular feminisation

INCREASED ESTROGENS

Increased secretion

- Testicular tumours
- Carcinoma of the lung

Increased peripheral aromatisation

- Liver disease
- Adrenal disease
- Thyrotoxicosis

of breast, axilla, testes and abdomen should be performed.

Investigations of gynaecomastia are directed to excluding a primary breast carcinoma or a secondary pathological cause. Biochemical assessment (liver and renal function tests, gamma-glutamyltransferase, prolactin, alpha-fetoprotein, beta-human chorionic gonadotrophin and total testosterone) is only required in rapidly growing gynaecomastia. Imaging (with mammography and/or ultrasound) plus biopsy (fine-needle aspiration cytology and/or core biopsy) can be performed if the cause of the gynaecomastia is indeterminate or cancer is suspected.

TREATMENT

Reassurance of the transient and benign nature is often all that is required in the management of physiological gynaecomastia. In drug-related gynaecomastia, the withdrawal of the drug or change to an alternative should be considered. For pathological gynaecomastia, the underlying cause needs to be addressed.

Box 15.2 • Drugs associated with gynaecomastia

Hormones

- Anabolic steroids (body-builders)
- Estrogenic agonists
- Antiandrogens (treatment of prostate cancer), e.g. cyproterone acetate, goserelin

Recreational drugs

- Alcohol
- Cannabis
- Heroin

Cardiovascular drugs

- Digoxin
- Spironolactone
- Captopril
- Enalapril
- Amiodarone
- Nefedipine
- Verapamil

Antiulcer drugs

- Cimetidine
- Ranitidine
- Omeprazole

Antibiotics

- Ketoconazole
- Metronidazole
- Minocycline

Psychoactive agents

- Tricylic antidepressants
- Diazepam
- Phenothiazines

Others

- Domperidone
- Metoclopramide
- Penicillamine
- Phenytoin
- Theophylline

Box 15.3 • Classification of gynaecomastia[71]

Grade	Clinical appearance
I	Small but visible breast development with little redundant skin
IIa	Moderate breast development with no redundant skin
IIb	Moderate breast development with redundant skin
III	Marked breast development with much redundant skin

From Simon BE, Hoffman S, Kahn S. Classification and surgical correction of gynecomastia. Plast Reconstr Surg 1973; 51:48–52.

For those cases requiring treatment there are two options: medical treatment and surgical excision. Medical management benefits from a high success rate and avoidance of an operation. The evidence for the three commonly prescribed drugs (danazol,[72] tamoxifen[73] and clomifene[74]) is based on small non-randomised trials and does not include recurrence rates, optimum dose, length of treatment or associated long-term risks. In the UK, only danazol is licensed for the treatment of gynaecomastia. A short 6-week course is recommended, with 100 mg b.d. for the first week followed by 100 mg t.d.s. for the second to sixth weeks, response being assessed at the eighth week. Imaging and clinical photography can be used to evaluate success of treatment. Repeat courses may be required. Tamoxifen at a daily dose of 10 mg produces excellent response rates and is favoured in our practice.

Due to the high risk of poor cosmesis associated with gynaecomastia surgery and subsequent risk of litigation, surgery should only be undertaken after medical failure or where the stage of the problem is too large (class IIa/III). Marking the extent of the gynaecomastia prior to surgery is essential. The procedure should be performed via a periareolar incision to reduce scarring. The use of lighted retractors and diathermy aid surgery. A disc of breast tissue should be left behind the nipple combined with an intact pectoral fascia and overlying fat to prevent retraction and fixation to the muscle (saucer deformity). Skin flaps are kept thick to prevent deformity and skin necrosis.

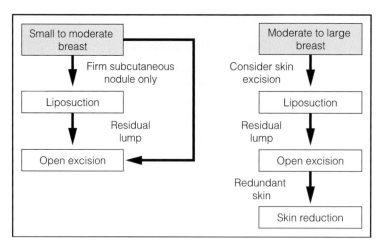

Figure 15.5 • Algorithm for management of gynaecomastia.

Patients should be warned about nipple necrosis, sensory changes and recurrence as well as cosmetic problems. In extreme cases excess skin is removed, requiring repositioning of the nipple and even free nipple grafts.[75] In young patients, the excess skin will correct itself without need for excision. The use of liposuction alone or combined with limited surgery has been reported to improve cosmetic outcomes. Ultrasound-assisted liposuction allows treatment of more fibrous areas and increases the number of patients suitable for this technique.[76] An approach to management including liposuction is outlined in **Fig. 15.6**.[77]

ASSESSMENT OF PATIENTS WITH BENIGN BREAST DISEASE

Commonly encountered questions include the following.

- Is a one-stop clinic the best method of diagnosing breast disease?
- Fine-needle aspiration cytology, core biopsy or both?
- Should benign breast disease become the remit of nurse specialists?

One-stop clinics

The aim of the one-stop clinic is to provide the patient with all the relevant investigations and diagnosis at the initial visit. This requires the availability of a breast specialist, cytopathologist and breast radiologist to provide immediate interpretation of the examination and investigations. Even with all these available, a definitive diagnosis is not always possible.[78] There are benefits in reducing anxiety in such a service (especially with benign disease) but this benefit is only in the short term.[79] Patients like these clinics and they reduce the number of clinic visits and letters, improving administration efficiency. The increased cost of such a service, concerns that immediate reporting may affect accuracy and the possible detrimental psychological aspect for those with cancer[80] need to be considered. It is well recognised that at the time when a patient is given bad news, little else of the consultation is remembered. By concentrating on establishing and delivering a diagnosis at the first visit, it is then possible to have a more useful and constructive second visit when management can be considered. One-stop clinics are likely to continue as patients prefer them but they may only be feasible in larger units where they are cost-efficient.

Fine-needle aspiration cytology, core biopsy or both?

Fine-needle aspiration cytology has been the mainstay of diagnosis of symptomatic breast lumps for the last 30 years. Its introduction allowed preoperative diagnosis and avoided a large number of open excision biopsies. It has the benefit of being easy to perform, causes little patient discomfort and has a high sensitivity and specificity (in experienced hands[81]). The result can be interpreted quickly, allowing rapid diagnosis. Its major disadvantage is that it does not provide architectural information on the area examined and therefore cannot differentiate in situ and invasive disease. It is also possible to grade tumours[82] and provide estrogen receptor status[83] from cytology. Core biopsy is increasingly the preoperative technique of choice for diagnosing palpable breast lumps and areas of nodularity.[84] The use of local anaesthesia is required and the risk of haematoma is higher than in fine-needle aspiration cytology. However, the improved sensitivity and specificity and greater information available (architecture, estrogen receptor and HER-2 status, grade, presence of vascular invasion or calcification) with core biopsy is the reason for this change. The use of roll cytology, from cores, allows rapid initial diagnosis and adds the benefit of a subsequent histological assessment.[85]

Performing both a core biopsy and fine-needle aspiration cytology has been shown to provide the greatest sensitivity and does prevent potential de-skilling of cytologists. It is especially indicated in the hands of those with limited experience, due to the improvement in sensitivity of the combination compared with each test alone.[86] The cost–benefit of such a protocol needs assessment.

There is increasing evidence that symptomatic lumps should be biopsied under ultrasound guidance.[87] This ensures that the actual lump is visualised with the biopsy needle within it, improving sensitivity. Suitably trained surgeons or breast physicians can undertake these biopsies, thus ensuring that radiologists are not inundated with further work.[88]

FUTURE MANAGEMENT OF BENIGN BREAST DISEASE

The last few years has seen the expansion of breast physicians, nurse specialists and the formation of nurse consultants. Their roles have expanded to help with the increasing breast workload, 2-week rule and lack of breast specialists. There is evidence that such professionals can help in symptomatic clinics, perform follow-up clinics and run symptom-specific clinics (e.g. mastalgia clinics) as long as there is specialist back-up.[89,90] The future roles of both these individuals and breast surgeons are likely to continue to evolve. The breast surgeons of the future may be less involved in diagnosis, and more active surgically.

REFERENCES

1. Thrush S, Sayer G, Scott-Coombes D, Roberts JV. Is the grading of referrals to a specialist breast unit appropriate or effective? Br Med J 2002; 324:1279.
2. Down S, Barr L, Baildam AD, Bundred N. Management of accessory breast tissue in the axilla. Br J Surg 2003; 90:1213–14.
3. Nerakha GJ. In: Gallager HS, Leis HP, Synderman RK et al. (eds) The Breast. St Louis, MI: Mosby, 1978; pp. 442–51.
4. Hughes LE, Mansel RE, Webster DJ. Aberrations of normal development and involution (ANDI): a new perspective on pathogenesis and nomenclature of benign breast disorders. Lancet 1987; ii:1316–19.
5. World Health Organisation. Histological typing of breast tumours, 2nd edn. Geneva: WHO, 1981.
6. Dixon JM, Dobie V, Lamb J et al. Assessment of the acceptability of conservative management of fibroadenoma of the breast. Br J Surg 1996; 83:264–5.
7. Hughes LE, Mansel RE, Webster DJT. Benign disorders of the breast. London: Baillière Tindal, 2001.
8. Ozzello L, Gump FE. The management of patients with carcinomas in fibroadenomatous tumors of the breast. Surg Gynecol Obstet 1985; 116:99–104.
9. Sperber F, Blank A, Metser U et al. Diagnosis and treatment of breast fibroadenomas by ultrasound guided vacuum-assisted biopsy. Arch Surg 2003; 138:796–800.
10. Haagenson CD. Diseases of the breast, 3rd edn. Philidelphia: WB Saunders, 1986.
11. Dixon JM, Mansel RE. ABC of breast diseases: symptoms, assessment and guidelines for referral. Br Med J 1994; 309:722.
12. King EB, Chew KC, Petrakis NL, Ernster VL. Nipple aspiration cytology for the study of pre-cancer precursors. J Natl Cancer Inst 1983; 71:1115–21.
13. Ambrogetti D, Berni D, Catarzi S et al. The role of ductal galactography in the differential diagnosis of breast carcinoma. Radiologia Medica 1996; 91:198–201.
14. Sandison AT. An autopsy of the human breast. National Cancer Institute Monograph No. 8. US Dept of Health, Education and Welfare, 1962, pp. 1–145.

15. Simmons R, Adamovich T, Brennan M et al. Non-surgical evaluation of pathologic nipple discharge. Ann Surg Oncol 2003; 10:113–16.

16. Groves AM, Carr M, Wadhera V, Lennard TWJ. An audit of cytology in the evaluation of nipple discharge: a retrospective study of 10 years' experience. Breast 1996; 5:96.

17. Dooley WS. Routine operative breast endoscopy for bloody nipple dicharge. Ann Surg Oncol 2002; 9:920–3.

18. Matsunaga T, Ohta D, Misaka T et al. A utility of ductography and fibreoptic ductoscopy for patients with nipple discharge. Breast Cancer Res Treat 2001; 70:103–8.

19. Shen KW, Wu J, Lu JS et al. Fiberoptic ductoscopy for breast cancer patients with nipple discharge. Surg Endosc 2001; 15:1340–5.

20. Khan SA, Baird C, Staradub VL, Morrow M. Ductal lavage and ductoscopy: the opportunities and the limitations. Clin Breast Cancer 2002; 3:185–95.

21. Cabioglu N, Hunt KK, Singletary SE et al. Surgical decision making and factors determining a diagnosis of breast cancer in women presenting with nipple discharge. J Am Coll Surg 2003; 196:354–64.

22. Van Zee KJ, Ortega Perez G, Minnard E et al. Preoperative galactography increases the diagnostic yield of major duct excision for nipple discharge. Cancer 1998; 82:1874–80.

23. Rosen PP, Cantrell B, Mullen DL, DePalo A. Juvenile papillomatosis (Swiss cheese disease) of the breast. Am J Surg Pathol 1980; 4:3–12.

24. Lafreniere R. Bloody nipple discharge during pregnancy: a rationale for conservative treatment. J Surg Oncol 1990; 43:228–30.

25. Dixon JM, Kohlhardt SR, Dillon P. Total duct excision. Breast 1998; 7:216–19.

26. Peters F, Pickardt CR, Zimmerman G, Breckwoldt PRL, TSH and thyroid hormones in benign breast disease. Klin Wochenschr 1981; 59:403–7.

27. England PC, Skinner LG, Cotterell KM, Sellwood RA. Serum oestradiol-17β in women with benign and malignant breast disease. Br J Cancer 1974; 30:571–6.

28. Sitruk-Ware R, Sterkers N, Mauvais-Jarvis P. Benign breast disease. 1. Hormonal investigation. Obstet Gynecol 1979; 53:457–60.

29. Gateley CA, Maddox PR, Pritchard GA et al. Plasma fatty acid profiles in benign breast disorders. Br J Surg 1992; 79:407–9.

30. Mansel RE. ABC of breast diseases: breast pain. Br Med J 1994; 309:866–8.

31. Barros AC, Mottola J, Ruiz CA et al. Reassurance in the treatment of mastalgia. Breast J 1999; 5:162–5.

32. Khoo SK, Munro C, Battistutta D. Evening primrose oil and treatment of premenstrual syndrome. Med J Aust 1990; 153:189–92.

33. Blommers J, de Lange-De Klerk ES, Kuik DJ et al. Evening primrose oil and fish oil for severe chronic mastalgia: a randomised, double blind controlled trial. Am J Obstet Gynecol 2002 187:1389–94.

34. Pashby NH, Mansel RE, Hughes LE et al. A clinical trial of evening primrose oil in mastalgia. Br J Surg 1981; 68:801–24.

35. McFayden IJ, Chetty U, Setchell KDR et al. A randomized double blind cross over trial of soya protein for the treatment of cyclical breast pain. Breast 2000; 9:271–6.

36. Halaska M, Raus K, Beles P et al. Treatment of cyclical mastodynia using an extract of Vitex agnus castus: results of a double blind comparison with a placebo. Ceska Gynecol 1998; 63:388–92.

37. Boyd NF, McGuire V, Shannon P et al. Effect of a low-fat high-carbohydrate diet on symptoms of clinical mastopathy. Lancet 1988; ii:128–32.

38. Fentiman IS, Caleffi M, Brame K et al. Double blind controlled trial of tamoxifen therapy for mastalgia. Lancet 1986; i:287–8.

39. GEMB Group Argentine. Tamoxifen therapy for cyclical mastalgia: dose randomised trial. Breast 1997; 5:212–13.

40. Kontostolis E, Stefanidis K, Navrozoglou I, Lolis D. Comparison of tamoxifen with danazol for treatment of cyclical mastalgia. Gynecol Endocrinol 1997; 11:393–7.

41. O'Brien PM, Abukhalil IE. Randomised controlled trial of the management of premenstrual syndrome and premenstrual mastalgia using luteal phase-only danazol. Am J Obstet Gynecol 1999; 180:18–23.

42. Blichert-Toft M, Anderson AN, Henrikson D, Mygind T. Treatment of mastalgia with bromocriptine: a double blind crossover study. Br Med J 1979; 1:273.

43. Eriksson E. Serotonin reuptake inhibitors for the treatment of premenstrual dysphoria. Int Clin Psychopharmacol 1999; 14(suppl. 2):S27–S33.

44. Dixon JM, McDonald C, Elton RA, Miller WR. Risk of breast cancer in women with palpable breast cysts. Lancet 1999; 353:1742–5.

45. Kudva YC, Reynolds CA, O'Brien T, Crotty TB. Mastopathy and diabetes. Curr Diabetes Rep 2003; 3:56–9.

46. Thrush S, Banergee S, Sayer G, et al. Breast sepsis: a unit's experience. Br J Surg 2002; 89(suppl. 1): 75–6.

47. Goodman MA, Benson EA. An evaluation of the current trends in the management of breast abscesses. Med J Aust 1970; 1:1034–9.

48. Schafer P, Furrer C, Merillod B. An association between smoking with recurrent subareolar breast abscess. Int J Epidemiol 1988; 17:810–13.

49. Petrakis NL, Maack CA, Lee RE et al. Mutagenic activity of nipple aspirates of breast fluid. Cancer Res 1980; 40:188–9.

50. Ertel A, Eng R, Smith SM. The differential effect of cigarette smoke on the growth of bacteria found in humans. Chest 1991; 100:628–30.

51. Rogers K. Breast abscess and problems with lactation. In: Smallwood JA, Talor I (eds) Benign breast disease. London: Edward Arnold, 1990; p. 96.

52. Gupta R, Sinnett D, Carpenter R et al. Antibiotic prophylaxis for post-operative wound infection in elective breast surgery. Eur J Surg Oncol 2000; 26:363–6.

53. Collis N, Mirza S, Stanley PR et al. Reduction of potential contamination of breast implants by the use of 'nipple shields'. Br J Plast Surg 1999; 52:445–7.

54. Zippel D, Siegelmann-Danieli N, Ayalon S et al. Delayed breast cellulitis following breast conservation operations. Eur J Surg Oncol 2003; 29:327–30.

55. Nahabedian MY, Tsangaris T, Momen B et al. Infectious complications following breast reconstruction with expanders and implants. Plast Reconstr Surg 2003; 112:467–76.

56. Hayes R, Mitchell M, Nunnerley HB. Acute inflammation of the breast: the role of breast ultrasound in diagnosis and management. Clin Radiol 1991; 44:253–6.

57. Dixon JM. Repeated aspiration of breast abscesses in lactating women. Br Med J 1988; 297:1517–18.

58. O'Hara RJ, Dexter SPL, Fox JN. Conservative management of infective mastitis and breast abscesses after ultrasonographic assessment. Br J Surg 1996; 83:1413–14.

59. Dixon JM. Outpatient treatment of non-lactational breast abscesses. Br J Surg 1992; 79:56–7.

60. Dixon JM (ed.). ABC of Breast. London: BMJ Publications, 2000.

61. Bundred NJ, Dixon JM, Chetty U, Forrest AM. Mammary fistula. Br J Surg 1991; 78:1185.

62. Thomsen AC, Espersen T, Maigaard S. Course and treatment of milk stasis, non-infectious inflammation of the breast and infectious mastitis in nursing women. Am J Obstet Gynecol 1984: 149:492–5.

63. Anonymous. Puerperal mastitis. Br Med J 1991; 302:1367–71.

64. Howell JD, Barker F, Gazet J-C. Granulomatous lobular mastitis: report of further two cases and comprehensive literature review. Breast 1994; 3:119–23.

65. Paviour S, Musaad S, Roberts S et al. *Corynebacterium* species isolated from patients with mastitis. Clin Infect Dis 2002; 35:1434–40.

66. Taylor GB, Paviour SD, Musaad S et al. A clinicopathological review of 34 cases of inflammatory breast disease showing an association between corynebacteria infection and granulomatous mastitis. Pathology 2003; 35:109–19.

67. Blanchard DK, Reynolds CA, Grant CS, Donohue JH. Primary nonphylloides breast sarcomas. Am J Surg 2003; 186:359–61.

68. Daniels IR, Layer GT. How should gynaecomastia be managed? Aust NZ J Surg 2003; 73:213–16.

69. Carlson HE. Gynecomastia. N Engl J Med 1980; 303:795–9.

70. Ismail AA, Barth JH. Endocrinology of gynaecomastia. Ann Clin Biochem 2001; 38:596–607.

71. Simon BE, Hoffman S, Kahn S. Classification and surgical correction of gynecomastia. Plast Reconstr Surg 1973; 51:48–52.

72. Jones DJ, Holt SD, Surtees P et al. A comparison of danazol and placebo in the treatment of adult idiopathic gynecomastia: results of a prospective study in 55 patients. Ann R Coll Surg Engl 1990; 72:296–8.

73. Khan HN, Blamey RW. Endocrine treatment of physiological gynaecomastia. Br Med J 2003; 327:301–2.

74. Plourde PV, Kulin HE, Santner SJ. Clomiphene in the treatment of adolescent gynecomastia. Clinical and endocrine studies. Am J Dis Child 1983; 137:1080–2.

75. Wray RC Jr, Hoopes JE, Davis GM. Correction of extreme gynaecomastia. Br J Plast Surg 1974; 27:39–41.

76. Samdal F, Kleppe G, Amland PF, Abyholm F. Surgical treatment of gynaecomastia. Five years' experience with liposuction. Scand J Plast Reconstr Surg Hand Surg 1994; 28:123–30.

77. Fruhstorfer BH, Malata CM. A systematic approach to the surgical treatment of gynaecomastia. Br J Plastic Surg 2003; 56:237–46.

78. Eltahir A, Jibril JA, Squair J et al. The accuracy of 'one stop' diagnosis for 1110 patients presenting to a symptomatic breast clinic. J R Coll Surg Edinb 1999; 44:226–30.

79. Dey P, Bundred N, Gibbs A et al. Costs and benefits of a one stop clinic compared with a dedicated breast clinic: randomised controlled trial. Br Med J 2002; 324:507–10.

80. Harcourt D, Ambler N, Rumsey N, Cawthorn S. Evaluation of a one-stop breast clinic: a randomised controlled trial. Breast 1998; 7: 314–19.

81. Dixon JM, Lamb J, Anderson TJ. Fine needle aspiration of the breast: importance of the operator. Lancet 1983; ii:564.

82. Robinson IA, McKee G, Nicholson A et al. Prognostic value of cytological grading of fine-needle aspirates from breast carcinomas. Lancet 1994; 343:947–9.

83. Zoppi JA, Rotundo AV, Sundblad AS. Correlation of immunocytochemical and immunohistochemical determination of estrogen and progesterone receptors in breast cancer. Acta Cytol 2002; 46:337–40.

84. Britton PD. Fine needle aspiration or core biopsy? Breast 1999; 8:1–4.

85. Albert US, Duda V, Hadji P et al. Imprint cytology of core needle biopsy specimens of breast lesions. A rapid approach to detecting malignancies, with comparison of cytologic and histopathologic analyses of 173 cases. Acta Cytol 2000; 44:57–62.

86. Thrush S, Kunasingam K, Russell G, Bentley P. Needle biopsy in the breast clinic: core biopsy, fine-needle aspiration cytology or both? Eur J Cancer 2003; 1(suppl. 4).

87. Hatada T, Ishii H, Ichii S et al. Diagnostic value of ultrasound-guided fine needle aspiration biopsy, core needle biopsy, and evaluation of combined use in the diagnosis of breast lumps. J Am Coll Surg 2000; 190:299–303.

88. Whitehouse PA, Baber Y, Brown G et al. The use of ultrasound by breast surgeons in outpatients: an accurate extension of clinical diagnosis. Eur J Surg Oncol 2001; 27:611–16.

89. Garvican L, Grimsey E, Littlejohns P et al. Satisfaction with clinical nurse specialists in a breast care clinic: questionnaire survey. Br Med J 1998; 316:976–7.

90. Earnshaw JJ, Stephenson Y. First two years of a follow-up breast clinic led by a nurse practitioner. J R Soc Med 1997; 90:258–9.

Sixteen

What we can expect from trials in the next 5 years?

J. Richard C. Sainsbury

INTRODUCTION

The management of patients with breast cancer has evolved continuously over the last 100 years. These advances have occurred because of new techniques (e.g. sentinel node biopsy, partial breast radio-therapy), better understanding of the biology of the disease (estrogen receptors, growth factor receptors, etc.) and newer pharmacological agents (tamoxifen, aromatase inhibitors, etc.). Fundamental to the introduction of these technologies has been the demonstration of benefit using clinical trials rather than allow a technological development or a new drug be an end in itself. Breast cancer has led the way in the field of cancer medicine in organising well-run clinical trials and this trend continues. The first randomised trial was probably conducted at sea, where the benefit of citrus fruits in preventing scurvy was overwhelmingly proven, only to be ignored by the Admiralty.

There are major concerns over the new European legislation and it may be that the clinical trial, as we currently know it, is no longer viable. There are vexed questions about who will sponsor some trials and the associated paperwork means fewer small pilot studies will be possible. In the UK, the Cancer Research UK trial units (with funding of approved studies by the National Cancer Research Institute)

are helping raise trial entry but there is still much to be done.

Running a trial is no longer the easy pastime it once was. One cannot run studies without ethical approval and they require investment of much time, financial support, statistical support, data management and pairs of hands to collect the data. If a trial is going to be used for regulatory purposes (e.g. for a new drug), then standards have to be commensurately higher and it is only with pharmaceutical industry support that such trials can be undertaken successfully. Increasingly, clinicians involved with the management of patients (or their managers) require payment for study entry. There is an increasing reluctance to allow tissue blocks or sections to leave pathology departments for subsequent biological studies without payment. Once a trial is complete there are problems if the result is negative in that publication is harder. Publication itself brings many tribulations, particularly when considering authorship, with a balance required between recognition for those who originated the study and those at the 'coal face' who contributed the patients. Nonetheless, there have been many worthwhile studies and there will continue to be so (European legislation permitting).

The major subspecialities of breast disease management (surgery, radiotherapy and chemo-endocrine therapy) are considered separately in this chapter; in addition, there is a miscellaneous group of trial activities. Trials likely to report within the next few years are considered, as are areas where forthcoming trials would be of value.

PREVENTION TRIALS

Following the result from the IBIS-1 study[1] (tamoxifen vs. placebo for women at 1.5–2 times risk), combined with the results from the underpowered Italian and Royal Marsden studies and the adequately powered but prematurely terminated American P-1 study, it is clear than tamoxifen does reduce the incidence of breast cancer by about 40%. The duration of benefit persists after cessation of therapy but the extent of this is unknown. The effect is seen in estrogen receptor-positive tumours. The long-term adverse effects are difficult to interpret (**Table 16.1** and **Fig. 16.1**).

In the study Multiple Outcomes of Raloxifene Evaluation (MORE) study, the incidence of breast cancer was reduced by about 60%. Raloxifene is a selective estrogen receptor modulator like tamoxifen that was developed for the prevention and treatment of osteoporosis. It suffers, like tamoxifen, from an excess of thromboembolic events. Following the

Table 16.1 • Trials of prevention therapy

Trial (entry dates)	Population	Number randomised	Agent (vs. placebo) and daily dose	Intended duration of treatment
Royal Marsden (1986–96)	High risk Family history	2471	Tamoxifen 20 mg	5–8 years
NSABP-P1 (1992–97)	>1.6% 5-year risk	13 388	Tamoxifen 20 mg	5 years
Italian (1992–97)	Normal risk Hysterectomy	5408	Tamoxifen 20 mg	5 years
IBIS-I (1992–2001)	More than twofold relative risk	7139	Tamoxifen 20 mg	5 years
Adjuvant overview (1976–95)	Women with ER+ operable breast cancer in 11 trials	~15 000	Tamoxifen 20–40 mg with or without chemotherapy in both arms	3 years or more (average ~5 years)

ER+, estrogen receptor positive.

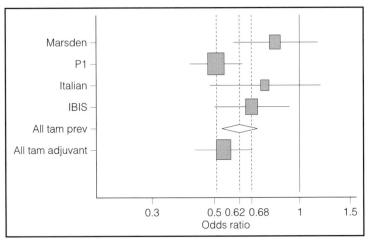

Figure 16.1 • Summary of effects of four randomised prevention trials of tamoxifen. DCIS, ductal carcinoma in situ.

MORE findings,[2] the Study of Tamoxifen and Raloxifene (STAR) study was launched in the USA. The trial entry of 7000 patients has nearly been achieved and a result is expected in 2008. The ongoing evaluation of MORE, known as CORE, has continued to show a 50–60% reduction in the incidence of breast cancer. This figure is consistently higher than that achieved with tamoxifen. It is interesting that no trials of raloxifene as therapy have reported; if it is an effective preventative, might not it have therapeutic potential?

Other prevention trials using the retinoid compounds have ceased recruiting, proven inconclusive or disappeared.

SURGICAL TRIALS

Ongoing trials: sentinel node biopsy

Sentinel node biopsy is moving from a research tool to routine use. It was the first surgical technique to be adopted in the UK after a prospective audited phase of competence. The Axillary Lymph Node Mapping and Nodal Clearance (ALMANAC) trial was a two-phase study. Initially, surgeons were required to carry out 40 procedures, some of which were mentored by an external surgeon. A less than 5% false-negative rate was permitted before individuals were judged as competent. Sentinel node were identified by both radioisotope and blue dye localisation in order to find the relevant node reliably.

The second phase of the ALMANAC trial was a randomisation between sentinel node and routine axillary surgery (be it clearance or sampling). If the nodes were found to be positive, either axillary clearance was performed as a secondary procedure or axillary radiotherapy was given. The outcomes evaluated were, in the short term, quality of life, length of stay and a health economic evaluation. Axillary recurrence rates are a secondary endpoint. Analysis of the quality of life showed a marked difference between the two arms. Sentinel node biopsy was superior for all outcome measures in the quality-of-life analysis, although a formal health economic analysis has yet to be reported. A large European (EORTC) trial (AMAROS) has currently

recruited about 1000 patients. This trial is expected to report in 2008. In the USA, there are two randomised studies run by the American College of Surgeons. Z10 is examining the management of the positive axilla following sentinel node staging, asking whether radiotherapy is sufficient to achieve local control or whether complete axillary surgery is necessary. Z11 is examining patients found to have micrometastatic disease on nodal sectioning.

Other surgical trials

Trials have demonstrated the benefit of prophylactic mastectomy for *BRCA1/2* gene carriers in reducing breast cancer incidence and mortality.[3] The BASO-II trial of radiotherapy and tamoxifen in women with small good-prognosis tumours was to have been updated at the San Antonio Breast Cancer Symposium in December 2004, but these important results were presented at Nottingham in September 2005. There is a suggestion that radiotherapy may not be necessary for older women with completely resected good-prognosis tumours. These results are important for guiding the next generation of trials on partial breast radiotherapy.

TRIALS IN RADIOLOGY AND BREAST SCREENING

The Comparative Effectiveness in MR Imaging in Breast Cancer (COMICE) study aims to compare repeat operation and mastectomy rates in patients evaluated either by standard triple assessment or by magnetic resonance imaging (MRI) as well as triple assessment. There is an economic evaluation to this study. A total of 1840 women are needed; recruitment has been slow but additional centres have now become involved.

The FH01 study is a single-arm study of annual mammography in women aged 40–49 years at enhanced familial risk of breast cancer. Its aims are to estimate the difference in breast cancer mortality in women under the age of 50 with a significant family history (defined as a 1.5 times risk) in those screened and those not screened and to estimate the cost-effectiveness of this strategy; 10 000 patients are required and 1400 have been recruited to date. There is an associated psychosocial study (PIMMS) assessing the psychological impact of mammographic surveillance; 3000 women will be sampled by questionnaire prior to mammography, at 2 weeks after their final result and 6 months later. An additional face-to-face interview will take place on a subset of women and those in whom an interval cancer is detected or if recalled for assessment and then reassured.

The MARIBS study is a comparison of MRI and conventional mammography in high-risk women and is complete. It has shown that MRI is a valuable screening tool in high-risk young women.

TRIALS OF ENDOCRINE THERAPY

It is clear that endocrine therapy should only be offered to those women whose tumours are hormonally responsive as assessed by estimation of estrogen and progesterone receptors. Increasingly, c-erbB-2 (HER-2) is being measured as this may modify choice of agent.

Tamoxifen has been the mainstay of endocrine therapy for the last 30 years but its place is being challenged by the aromatase inhibitors.

Premenopausal breast cancer

The role of ovarian suppression as part of adjuvant management remains controversial. While oophorectomy (by surgery, radiation or luteinising hormone releasing hormone agonists) prolongs survival in the absence of chemotherapy, the situation is less

clear with modern treatments. Many women become amenorrhoeic during chemotherapy and progress to an early menopause. Current practice is to offer ovarian ablation to those with hormone receptor-positive tumours who continue menstruation or restart their periods.

The trials of ovarian suppression using goserelin (Zoladex) are shown in **Table 16.2**. The populations studied differ in nodal positivity rates and completeness of determination of estrogen receptor status at entry.[4-7] It is unfortunate that the ZIPP collaboration is only reported in abstract form[8] and a full paper is overdue.

The ABC study (see later) failed to show a benefit for ovarian suppression in addition to chemotherapy in patients also treated with tamoxifen, although there is a suggestion that these may be beneficial in women under 40. There are two new trials opening to study this question further: Suppression of Ovarian Function and Tamoxifen (SOFT) and Premenopausal Endocrine Responsive Chemotherapy (PERCHE).

Postmenopausal breast cancer

Tamoxifen has been the treatment for postmenopausal patients with hormone receptor-positive breast cancer for the last two decades and has saved many lives. It is beneficial in both node-positive and node-negative patients and remains the most commonly prescribed adjuvant hormonal agent worldwide. It has adverse effects, which have become more important as newer agents emerge. Currently, the recommendation is for 5 years use. Two trials,

Table 16.2 • Trials of adjuvant endocrine ablation using goserelin (Zoladex). For trial details see text

Trial	Agents	Population	Result
ZEBRA[4] ($N = 1640$)	Z vs. CMF	Node positive, 74% ER positive	Z equivalent to CMF
ACO[5] ($N = 1045$)	Z + T vs. CMF	Node positive/negative, ER positive	Z + T >> CMF
GROCTA[6] ($N = 244$)	T + OS vs. CMF	Node positive/negative, ER positive	NS
INT 0101[7] ($N = 1504$)	CAF vs. CAFZ vs. CAFZT	Node positive, ER positive	CAFZ > CAF CAFZT > CAFZ
ZIPP[8] ($N = 2710$)	Std vs. Std + Z	Node positive/negative, 70% ER positive	Std + Z >> Std

CAF, cyclophosphamide, Adriamycin and 5-fluorouracil; CMF, cyclophosphamide, methotrexate and fluorouracil; ER, estrogen receptor; OS, overall survival; Std, standard therapy; T, tamoxifen; Z, Zoladex.

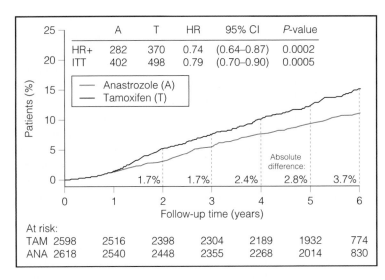

Figure 16.2 • ATAC trial: time to recurrence curves for the hormone receptor-positive (HR+) patients. The absolute differences in recurrence rate are shown. ITT, intention to treat.

ATLAS and AttOM, are examining whether continuing therapy longer than this is indicated. AttOM has recruited 8000 patients and the international ATLAS aims for 15 000 and is still open for recruitment. The plan is to ensure that all patients are estrogen receptor positive, so further recruitment in the AttOM trial is required as only 6599 patients fall into this group.

The third-generation aromatase inhibitors (anastrozole, letrozole and exemestane) are potent suppressors of the enzyme aromatase, which is responsible for the generation of most postmenopasual estrogen. Anastrozole and letrozole are non-steroidal competitive inhibitors, whereas exemestane is a steroidal molecule that binds irreversibly to the aromatase enzyme (suicidal effect). After trials demonstrating benefit in postmenopausal, hormone-responsive, advanced disease, these drugs have been studied in the adjuvant setting. There are randomised trials assessing their use at three different time points: as primary de novo agents in patients completing surgery, in patients switching at 2 years from tamoxifen (or vice versa), and after 5 years of tamoxifen therapy.

Trials of de novo adjuvant therapy include the ATAC study and BIG I-98 trial. They differ in that ATAC (Arimidex, Tamoxifen Alone and in Combination) randomised patients to one of three arms for 5 years (anastrozole or tamoxifen or the combination), whereas the BIG (Breast International Group) I-98 study is a four-arm study. Two arms received either tamoxifen or letrozole for 5 years,

whereas the other two arms crossed over with patients receiving 2 years of tamoxifen followed by 3 years of letrozole or vice versa.

The ATAC study was the largest breast cancer adjuvant trial, recruiting 9300 patients from 23 countries (**Fig. 16.2**; this also appears as Fig. 11.3 and is reproduced here for the reader's convenience). It showed no difference between the combination and tamoxifen alone and analysis of the combination arm was dropped. There was a significant difference in disease-free survival in favour of anastrozole at the time of first and second protocol analysis, with an absolute benefit of 1.2 and 2.3% respectively.[9] An overall survival benefit was recently presented. There was a 42% reduction in contralateral breast cancer, lending support to the IBIS-II study. The BIG I-98 study also showed a significant improvement in disease-free and distant disease-free survival, with a 48% reduction in contralateral disease (**Fig. 16.3**; this also appears as Fig. 11.4 and is reproduced here for the reader's convenience).

There was a very different side-effect profile between the aromatase inhibitors and tamoxifen, with significantly fewer endometrial, thromboembolic and other vascular events in favour of anastrozole and letrozole. The most common adverse effect of all aromatase inhibitors is musculoskeletal pain and bone loss. This may be a limiting toxicity for some and bone density measurement is now considered necessary for this group. The musculoskeletal disorder is often helped by cyclooxygenase (COX)-2

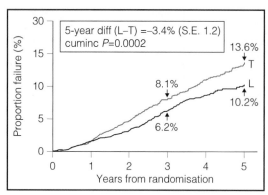

Figure 16.3 • First results from BIG I-98 trial: relapse-free survival in patients in the monotherapy arms.

inhibitors. There appeared to be a slight excess of cardiac events in the BIG I-98 study.

Switching

Three studies have reported. The largest report, the International Exemestane Study (IES),[10] used exemestane after 2–3 years of tamoxifen and demonstrated a significant prolongation in disease-free survival for those switching treatments (**Fig. 16.4**; this also appears as Fig. 11.6 and is reproduced here for the reader's convenience). Given this result the trial was stopped early, so the long-term adverse effects of exemestane will not be identifiable. There was increased bone resorption in the group receiving exemestane. It must be remembered that

tamoxifen has bone-sparing properties (as a partial agonist) so comparison between the two agents is difficult. A smaller study, the Italian Tamoxifen Anastrozole (ITA) trial,[11] also showed a reduction in recurrence rates for the aromatase inhibitor. The third trial (ARNO) also used anastrozole as the comparator.[12] This has shown a benefit for switching from tamoxifen to anastrozole at 2 years.

One observation that emerged from the ATAC trial was that there was an additional benefit for patients taking anastrozole when their tumours were estrogen receptor positive but progesterone receptor negative. This was not seen in the exemestane study (although patients received 2 years of tamoxifen before exposure to aromatase inhibitor) but was seen in the ARNO study. A treatment algorithm might be that estrogen receptor-positive, progesterone receptor-positive cancers could be treated with tamoxifen, whereas estrogen receptor-positive, progesterone receptor-negative tumours should receive an aromatase inhibitor up front, and tumours that lose progesterone receptor sensitivity with time should benefit from switching. All patients in the BIG I-98 study were estrogen receptor positive and no effect of progesterone receptor status was seen at the first analysis.

Continuation after 5 years

The only trial randomising patients at 5 years is the MA17 trial of letrozole versus continuing tamoxifen.

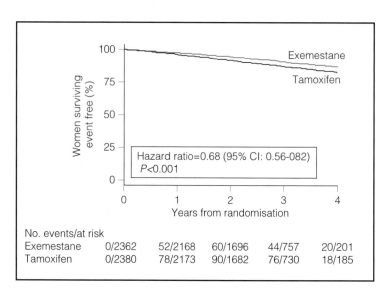

Figure 16.4 • Results from International Exemestane Study: patients were randomised to switch to exemestane or continue tamoxifen after 2–3 years of tamoxifen. © 2004, Massachusetts Medical Society.

This showed a relapse-free benefit for the group taking letrozole after about 2 years of additional therapy. The trial was stopped early and the long-term adverse effects are not known. This trial will not be repeated as earlier introduction of aromatase inhibitors or switching may well become common-place. There was a survival benefit in node-positive patients who switched to letrozole.

It must be remembered that each of these trials involved different populations of women and direct comparisons and extrapolations should be treated with care. The ATAC study recruited de novo patients whereas IES, ARNO and ITA recruited patients who had not relapsed at 2 years of tamoxifen. Similarly, MA17 recruited those who remained relapse free after 5 years of tamoxifen. The bone toxicities in these studies may well be different given the exposure to tamoxifen prior to the aromatase inhibitor, although the data from IES shows bone loss is detectable within 6 months of switching therapy.

One trial of endocrine therapy was recently relaunched and modified: the TEAM study started life as a randomisation of 5 years of exemestane or 5 years of tamoxifen. After the results of the IES sequential exemestane study were published, the TEAM trial was relaunched as 2 years of tamoxifen changing to 3 years of exemestane versus 5 years of exemestane. Its design has thus changed from an ATAC-type comparison to one-half of the BIG trial. A group of higher-risk patients was deliberately chosen in order to see an early difference in event rate. (Patients had to have positive nodes or larger node-negative lesions in addition to being estrogen receptor positive.) Quality of life, bone markers and pathology tissue collection were all included in this study. By 2003, 600 patients were recruited, with 100 in the bone subprotocol out of 6000 world-wide. The revised protocol requires 8740 patients and will complete recruitment by the end of 2005.

BONE TRIALS

A trial from the Royal Marsden Hospital showed that oral clodronate, an early bisphosphonate drug, reduced the incidence of bone metastases and hinted at an overall survival benefit.[13] There are now bisphosphonates available that are many hundreds of times more potent and larger studies are under way. The AZURE study randomises patients to a 6-monthly injection of zoledronic acid (after an initial loading course) in addition to standard chemotherapy in patients with stage II/III breast cancer; 3300 patients are required, with the primary endpoint being disease-free survival.

CHEMOTHERAPY TRIALS

Chemotherapy trials are divided into those that have finished recruiting and will hopefully report in the next few years and those open for recruitment. Each trial and its aims are described, with a comment at the end of each section.

Recently closed trials

TACT

The Taxotere as Adjuvant Chemotherapy (TACT) trial randomised standard anthracycline-based chemotherapy with either 5-fluorouracil, epirubicin and cyclophosphamide (FEC) or epirubicin, cyclo-phosphamide, methotrexate and 5-fluorouracil (Epi-CMF) (eight cycles) as the control arms versus four cycles of FEC followed by four cycles of sequential docetaxel. This was followed by tamoxifen for 5 years if the patient was estrogen receptor positive. From February 2001 to June 2003, 4162 patients were recruited. The original intention had been to recruit 3340 patients but the study was kept open when it became clear that the control arms were more effective than had been assumed when the power calculations for the study were first performed.

The aim was to compare eight cycles of standard chemotherapy with four cycles of anthracycline chemotherapy followed by four cycles of a taxane. Overexpression of HER-2 was not an entry require-ment. It may well be that only with analysis of HER-2 status will results be interpretable. Another criticism is that eight cycles of chemotherapy was not the routine used at that time and thus the trial may not be relevant to the general population of women receiving six cycles of chemotherapy or may encourage a creep from six to eight cycles as standard practice, which is not evidence based.

Tissue from all tumour blocks has been tested for HER-2 in three reference centres and tissue micro-arrays made for future study of putative biomarkers.

A subset of patients also contributed to a study where peripheral blood has been assayed for DNA markers of response.

TOPIC 2

This is a small study comparing vinorelbine/epirubicin with Adriamycin/cyclophoshamide (AC) as preoperative (neoadjuvant) treatment for patients with breast cancers larger than 3 cm. This trial followed on from TOPIC, which compared response rates for ECF with infusional SFU and AC, where similar clinical response rates were seen. The aims were to assess response rates as well as disease-free and overall survival. In addition, the proportion receiving conservation surgery as opposed to mastectomy was studied. The trial opened in 1998 and closed in 2002, with 499 patients entered. Originally, there had been a third arm of vinorelbine/mitozantrone (mitoxantrone) that ceased recruitment in 2000. This arm will make the trial difficult to analyse and it may be that there are insufficient numbers for statistical probity.

HERCEPTIN TRIALS

Herceptin or trastuzumab is a humanised monoclonal antibody that has activity against the 20% of cancers that overexpress the oncogene *HER2* or *CERBB2*.

Studies in the metastatic setting have shown activity of Herceptin as a single agent or in combination with anthracyclines and taxanes. Cardiotoxicity appears a particular problem when combined with Adriamycin. Recently combinations of Herceptin and chemotherapy given as a neoadjuvant therapy to patients with large operable or locally advanced breast cancer resulted in a significant increase in the pathological clinical response rate compared with chemotherapy alone. The most dramatic results have come in the adjuvant setting. At ASCO in 2005 combined results of two large trials involving 1679 women randomised to AC followed by paclitaxel and 1672 patients randomised to AC followed by paclitaxel combined with Herceptin showed a greater than 50% reduction in disease-free survival (HR = 0.48, $P = 3 \times 10^{-12}$), a similar reduction in time to first distant recurrence (HR = 0.47, $P = 8 \times 10^{-10}$), a significant improvement in overall survival (HR = 0.67, $P = 0.015$) – despite a median follow-up period of over 2 years. These are enormously impressive results and were confirmed by the results of a European adjuvant Herceptin study which reported a significant 46% reduction in events in women receiving herceptin. HER-2 testing is now being introduced as routine practice and, although costly, Herceptin is likely to become an integral part of the adjuvant therapy of women whose tumours overexpress HER-2. New studies are ongoing to assess how Herceptin works and what is the optimal way to give it – weekly vs. 3-weekly, 1 year vs. 2 years.

Open trials

The Adjuvant Cytotoxic Chemotherapy in Older Women (ACTION) trial aims to test the benefit of adjuvant chemotherapy, either AC or epirubicin/cyclophosphamide (EC), in women over 70 years old. The primary endpoint is relapse-free survival in a group where there is uncertainty over the value of chemotherapy. This study will also look at accelerated therapy using granulocyte colony-stimulating factor (G-CSF) in terms of toxicity and acceptability. A total of 1000 patients will be randomised, firstly to chemotherapy versus no chemotherapy and then, within the chemotherapy group, to either 3-weekly or 2-weekly injections with G-CSF. A review after 200 patients will be performed to assess feasibility.

ICCG C/14/96 DEVA is an International Collaborative Cancer Group study examining sequential chemotherapy using epirubicin followed by docetaxel compared with epirubicin alone in postmenopausal patients also receiving prolonged tamoxifen. It will allow examination of whether concurrent or sequential administration of tamoxifen is better. The design is a 2 × 2 factorial with patients randomised between sequential chemotherapy or epirubicin alone, and in some centres to sequential or concurrent tamoxifen if estrogen receptor positive. This trial will add to the data on the benefit of taxanes but also help understand the results seen in a SWOG trial of an 18% better disease-free survival in patients whose tamoxifen was delayed until after chemotherapy.[14] Another study (GEICAM; Spanish Breast Cancer Research Group) proved inconclusive.[15] Overall 800 patients will be needed, of whom 722 are currently randomised in five countries and 35 units. Even 800 patients may not be enough to answer the question clearly.

HERA is a three-arm study of 1 year of Herceptin versus 2 years of Herceptin versus no Herceptin in women with HER-2-positive breast cancer; 4818 patients have been recruited worldwide, the UK contributing 492. There was initially some confusion over what constituted positive HER-2 status but the majority used the accepted criteria of 3+ on immuno-staining with the Herceptest or 2+ on fluorescence in situ hybridisation. This study is important as it will allow assessment of the value of Herceptin as an adjuvant agent and if effective the optimal duration. There is an associated important biological study, Trans HERA, which aims to collect, store and analyse breast tumour tissue and serum from patients in the HERA trial in order to investigate whether any biological markers correlate with out-come. This part of the study is funded by Roche, who also sponsor the main trial, but the company is not involved in the storage or analysis of the samples. Consenting of patients has begun but no tissue has yet been collected.

The Trial of Accelerated Chemotherapy (TACT-2) is a 2×2 randomisation assessing whether acceler-ated administration of epirubicin, when given before CMF or capecitabine, will improve its efficacy, and will evaluate whether the use of oral capecitabine instead of CMF (after epirubicin) is as effective as CMF and less toxic. A total of 4400 women will be recruited into this complicated trial. Additional quality-of-life and health economic studies, as well as tumour collection, will be performed. No details on recruitment are available nor is it clear whether adjuvant endocrine therapy is allowed. The ran-domisation is shown in **Box 16.1**.

TANGO has finished recruiting. It is a ran-domisation of adding gemcitabine to paclitaxel given after four cycles of epirubicin and cyclo-phosphamide. It is based on the demonstration that addition of sequential paclitaxel to standard AC prolongs survival (CALGB 9344 and NSABP B28 trials). The addition of gemcitabine to paclitaxel has shown good response in a trial of metastatic disease where patients were heavily pretreated with anthracyclines, hence this arm. A total of 3000 patients were recruited, with 783 also taking part in the quality-of-life substudy. One reason the trial recruited well was that it was the only trial open at this time where free taxane was available. The oncology community in some countries continues to struggle with funding of newer drugs.

NeoTANGO is a neoadjuvant study of sequential EC and paclitaxel with or without gemcitabine (as above) in high-risk patients with large operable or locally advanced breast cancer. There are four arms looking at different schedules (see below), with 800 patients needed. In addition, there are two subtrials: NeoTANGO Science is concerned with prospective molecular profiling and candidate gene analysis on paraffin-embedded tumour samples along with serum proteomics, while CTCR-BR01 is per-forming molecular profiling and gene analysis on fresh tissue before, during and after chemotherapy and will also include serum proteomics. The science side is as yet poorly defined but should start to bring clinical trials and bench science closer.

The taxanes do not appear to be as efficacious in either the adjuvant or neoadjuvant setting as was first thought. At the 2004 San Antonio Breast Cancer Congress there were mixed results over the additional benefit of taxanes to conventional chemotherapy. Preliminary results of NSABP27 showed no signifi-cant differences in disease-free or overall survival with the addition of a taxane, although there was a trend towards a better local relapse-free survival. A similar lack of difference in disease-free and overall survival was seen in the French PACS O1 trial where docetaxel was added to standard FEC.

Anglo-Celtic IV Will Weekly Win is a smaller study comparing weekly paclitaxel treatment with a 3-weekly schedule in patients with advanced/metastatic breast cancer using time to disease progression as the endpoint. Gene polymorphisms responsible for paclitaxel metabolism will be analysed and linked to response rates. The arms of this study will receive different amounts of drug over different time periods (12 doses of 90 mg/m^2

Box 16.1 • TACT-2 randomisation options

Epirubicin for four cycles (every 3 weeks) followed by four cycles of 'classic' CMF

Epirubicin for four cycles (every 3 weeks) followed by four cycles of oral capecitabine

Epirubicin for four cycles (every 2 weeks) followed by four cycles of 'classic' CMF

Epirubicin for four cycles (every 2 weeks) followed by four cycles of oral capecitabine

CMF, cyclophosphamide, methotrexate and fluorouracil.

on a weekly basis vs. six doses of 175 mg/m^2 every 3 weeks). So far, 345 of the necessary 600 patients have been recruited.

Anglo-Celtic III Sprog is a randomised comparison of G-CSF secondary prophylaxis versus conservative management of chemotherapy-induced neutropenia to maintain dose intensity in chemotherapy for breast cancer. A total of 816 patients are required for this study, which is available as an add-on for any chemotherapy where G-CSF is not routinely administered; 171 patients have been recruited to date.

SOFT evaluates the benefit of ovarian suppression plus tamoxifen compared with tamoxifen alone in premenopausal women with hormone receptor-positive breast cancer after surgery with or without chemotherapy. A third group will examine the role of exemestane in addition to ovarian suppression. Surgery, radiation or 5 years of gonadotrophin-releasing hormone (GnRH) analogue are all acceptable as a method of achieving ovarian suppression. A total of 3000 patients worldwide are being sought and the trial is being coordinated by the Breast International Group. This study is one of several examining whether there are any additional benefits of aromatase inhibitors in women who are premenopausal at the start of treatment but who will be rendered postmenopausal by the treatment.

Anglo-Celtic V OPTION examines ovarian protection in premenopausal women receiving chemotherapy. The GnRH agent goserelin is used to suppress menstruation prior to and during chemotherapy in order to examine whether ovarian function is preserved after cessation of chemotherapy. This will be performed in patients with estrogen receptor-negative disease who will not receive endocrine therapy postoperatively. To date, only two of the necessary 400 patients have been recruited. This is an interesting trial as many oncologists empirically offer goserelin to younger women in an attempt to protect fertility without any large database to support this.

SEQUENCING TRIALS

SECRAB, which has recently closed, has randomised 2298 patients in order to address the question of the optimal sequence of adjuvant chemotherapy and radiotherapy. There were five permitted radiotherapy schedules and four permitted chemotherapy regimens. Patients were randomised to a sequential schedule or a synchronous schedule. There was an associated quality-of-life study and a cosmesis study.

RADIOTHERAPY TRIALS

START

This trial, which closed recently, followed on from a national survey by the Royal College of Radiologists. This revealed that a large number of different radiotherapy fractionation schedules were in use at the time for the treatment of women with breast cancer. Centres were allowed to take part in either trial A or trial B. Trial A entered 2236 patients and trial B 2215 (**Box 16.2**). Quality-of-life studies, photographic assessments and blood sampling with family history questionnaires were completed in some patients.

HOT

This is a randomised phase II trial of hyperbaric oxygen therapy for patients with chronic arm lymphoedema after radiotherapy for early breast cancer. The primary aim is to test the efficacy of hyperbaric oxygen therapy in reducing arm lymphoedema in patients suffering long-term adverse effects of high-dose radiotherapy for early breast cancer. A secondary aim is to test mechanisms of tissue reperfusion and healing in response to hyperbaric oxygen. Patients will be compressed to 242 kPa and will receive a total of 30 pressure exposures (5 days per week for 6 weeks). The pressure chamber is at the Royal Hospital Haslar in Gosport and requires the patient to be resident locally, which might reduce trial entry.

Box 16.2 • START trial randomisation options

Trial A
50 Gy in 25 fractions every 5 weeks vs. 41.6 Gy in 13 fractions every 5 weeks vs. 39 Gy in 13 fractions every 5 weeks

Trial B
50 Gy in 25 fractions every 5 weeks vs. 40 Gy in 15 fractions every 3 weeks

FAST

This is a radiation fractionation trial with randomisation to 5.7 and 6 Gy given in five fractions versus 25 fractions of 2.0 Gy; 300 patients will be required in each arm. This follows on from the START trial of standardisation of radiotherapy. The primary endpoint is change in breast appearance measured by photographs taken at baseline, year 2 and year 5. The secondary endpoint is tumour recurrence in the breast. The implication is that larger fractions sizes have no disadvantages, and perhaps some significant advantages, for women with early breast cancer. If this trial does demonstrate equivalence, it will mean that women can be treated more quickly. Currently up to 40% of the workload of a radiotherapy unit is related to breast cancer treatment; freeing time would reduce costs and increase efficiency.

RACE

This is a translational research project looking at DNA sequence variations associated with late radiotherapy complications in women treated for early breast cancer. The endpoint is examination of a single blood test for single nucleotide polymorphisms within/close to candidate genes.

PRIME

This is a randomised phase III trial assessing the need for breast radiotherapy in 'low-risk', older, node-negative patients treated by breast-conserving surgery and adjuvant endocrine therapy. Endpoints are local recurrence rates and overall survival. The recruitment target is 1000 patients, with a projected closure date of December 2007. Postoperative breast irradiation has been standard following breast-conserving surgery and adjuvant endocrine therapy irrespective of age. However, the differences between older and younger patients in response to treatment are poorly defined, since patients over 70 are frequently excluded from trials on the basis of their age. There is no doubt that elderly women as a group are undertreated and the results of this trial will add to the information as to whether radiotherapy can be safely omitted in this age group. The results from a Dutch trial show that boost can safely be omitted at this age.

Cambridge Breast Intensity-modulated Radiotherapy Trial

The primary aim of this study is to examine whether correction of dose homogeneity using forward-planned intensity-modulated radiotherapy improves the cosmetic outcome. Again, photographic assessments will be used. A total of 312 patients have been recruited, off whom 231 have been randomised. Blood samples are again being collected to look at single nucleotide polymorphisms. This trial is only available for patients having radiotherapy in Cambridge.

SUPREMO

This trial has just been funded and examines the role of postmastectomy chest wall radiotherapy in a group of patients at moderate risk. Data from two trials of chest wall radiotherapy have shown improved survival with this modality but have been criticised for their use of what is now considered inappropriate chemotherapy and suboptimal treatment of axillary disease. This trial may have difficulty in recruiting as the mastectomy rate continues to fall, but will be important for defining the role of postmastectomy radiotherapy in the modern era.

Trials of partial breast radiotherapy

The adverse effects of whole-breast radiotherapy include cardiac irradiation (if the tumour is left-sided), lung damage and irradiation of local muscles and the shoulder joint. All these can cause morbidity and so the question of whether partial breast radiotherapy alone is sufficient is a valid one. This is being tackled in a number of centres by different techniques. These include single fractions of radiotherapy given perioperatively (TARGIT and Milan trials) and the use of balloon devices with afterloading of radioactive source, with treatments given over typically 5 days. Some radiation biologists feel that a one-off dose of low-energy radioactivity will be insufficient to achieve local control and that the 5-day treatment may be better. Unfortunately, no direct head-to-head comparisons are being made and there is likely to be confusion on the issue of local radiotherapy for some time to come. The TARGIT trial randomises patients to intraoperative radiotherapy using a low-energy X-ray source. The additional time taken is of the order of 40–60 minutes. If resection margins are found to be positive, the patient undergoes a further resection and standard external beam radiotherapy. This study is recruiting well, with centres in the UK, Italy, Germany and Australia contributing. The equipment needed is relatively straightforward and operating theatres require no modification, unlike the Milan trial where one operating theatre has been converted to accept a linear accelerator. This somewhat limits its general use. Patients receive a much higher dose of radiation in Milan than in the TARGIT trial. Both these treatments have the advantage that if they are shown to be as effective as standard external beam radiotherapy, they will save many radiotherapy visits thus freeing up the machines for other patients. The balloon studies are being coordinated by the American College of Surgeons and preliminary data presented at San Antonio showed good cosmesis. Trials are not yet mature enough to provide any results on local control.

OTHER TRIALS

Ductal carcinoma in situ

Within the IBIS II trial there is a subtrial for patients with estrogen receptor-positive ductal carcinoma in situ (DCIS). These patients will be randomised to placebo or anastrozole but may be given radiotherapy as part of their primary treatment. This trial is obviously for a postmenopausal population and 4000 patients are needed. There is another trial (ERISAC) looking at the antiproliferative effect of exemestane and COX-2 inhibitors, either in isolation or together, in patients with estrogen receptor-positive DCIS. Patients take 14 days of treatment prior to definitive surgery. The numbers needed for this study are not given but to date 40 patients have been recruited.

Hormone replacement therapy

A randomised trial of hormone replacement therapy in women with a history of early breast cancer was launched in March 2002 but closed in July 2004 because of slow recruitment; 197 patients

had been recruited at this date. One problem for this trial was the publication of the Women's Health Initiative and Million Women Study results.[16] The HABITS[17] and Stockholm studies were the first of the randomised trials looking at breast cancer patients to be published. Over 800 patients were available for analysis, in whom 56 breast cancer recurrences had been diagnosed (hazard ratio 1.79). The debate about hormone replacement therapy continues but the current recommendation is that it should be used in the short term only for the normal population (up to 5 years). There are no current recommendations for breast cancer survivors. Many physicians will use it in patients whose tumours are estrogen receptor negative. LIBERATE is evaluating the gonadomimetic agent tibolone in patients on tamoxifen.

FOLLOW-UP

A randomised controlled trial aiming to demonstrate equivalence between standard hospital outpatient follow-up and telephone intervention administered by specialist breast nurses is underway. A total of 350 patients will be randomised using the following outcome measures: meeting information needs, psychological morbidity, clinical outcomes and an economic evaluation. Recruitment commenced in March 2003 and 258 patients have been randomised. There is an interesting Finnish trial that examined both intensity of follow-up and the use of tests such as radiography and liver function tests. Patients were randomised to one of four arms, either intensive follow-up with intensive tests, intensive follow-up with no tests, limited hospital contact with no tests, and limited hospital contact with intensive tests. The results of this study are currently being submitted for publication and will influence further studies in this area.

TIMING OF SURGERY

This Yorkshire-based intervention timing and survival study recruited 612 patients and assessed their menstrual cycle status at the time of first tumour handling and subsequent surgery. The date of the last period as recalled by the patient, as well as biochemical measurement of estrogen, progesterone, follicle-stimulating hormone and luteinising hormone, were recorded. This study was set up after publication of data demonstrating a survival benefit for women operated on in the luteal phase of their cycle. A first analysis of the subgroup who had normal menstrual cycles and had not taken the contraceptive pill within the last 6 months showed no difference between follicular and luteal timing of surgery.[18] This was based on patient recall of their last menstrual period and further reports using biochemical estimation of the cycle are awaited. A similar study from the Mayo Clinic also showed no difference in survival with prospectively collected data.[19] The Yorkshire study used the Nottingham Prognostic Index to calculate the likely event rate but found that actual survival was much better than predicted. The original Nottingham Prognostic Index was calculated on patients who did not receive adjuvant therapy. An updated version appeared in the abstract book for San Antonio but the authors failed to present their poster and the results are awaited.

EATIMS

The ear acupuncture for tamoxifen, anastrozole and letrozole-induced menopausal symptoms trial has a single-arm quasi-experimental design (whatever that means) where participants act as their own controls.

SUMMARY

Despite fears about the European legislation, the research community continues to actively investigate new treatments for patients with breast cancer. The majority of the trials listed above will report in the next 3–5 years. These will not necessarily provide definitive answers and are more likely to pose more questions that will require more trials. It is thus not surprising that a whole trials industry has sprung up. Organisation of trial groups is an important start. Funding for non-commercial trials remains a problem.

• **Key points**

- Trials are increasingly difficult to fund, manage and organise.
- Prevention trials have shown that tamoxifen reduces the risk of estrogen receptor-positive breast cancer by 40–50%.
- Third-generation aromatase inhibitors have shown superiority to tamoxifen in the adjuvant, switching and extended endocrine settings.
- Chemotherapy trials show incremental small benefits.
- Radiotherapy trials are focusing on partial breast radiotherapy and fractionation.
- Breast cancer mortality has fallen as a result of trial activity.

REFERENCES

1. Cuzick J, Forbes J, Edwards R et al. First results from the International Breast Cancer Intervention Study (IBIS-I): a randomised prevention trial. Lancet 2002; 360:817–24.

   This was a major randomised study demonstrating the benefits of tamoxifen in the prevention setting.

2. Cummings SR, Duong T, Kenyon E et al. Serum estradiol level and risk of breast cancer during treatment with raloxifene. Multiple Outcomes of Raloxifene Evaluation (MORE) Trial. JAMA 2002; 287:216–20.

3. Hartmann LC, Degnim A, Schaid DJ. Prophylactic mastectomy for BRCA1/2 carriers: progress and more questions. Clin Oncol 2004; 22:981–3.

4. Kaufmann M, Jonat W, Blamey R et al. Survival analyses from the ZEBRA study. Goserelin (Zoladex) versus CMF in premenopausal women with node-positive breast cancer. Zoladex Early Breast Cancer Research Association (ZEBRA) Trialists' Group. Eur J Cancer 2003; 39:1711–17.

5. Jakesz R, Hausmaninger H, Kubista E et al. Randomized adjuvant trial of tamoxifen and goserelin versus cyclophosphamide, methotrexate, and fluorouracil: evidence for the superiority of

282

Chapter Sixteen • What we can expect from trials in the next 5 years?

treatment with endocrine blockade in pre-menopausal patients with hormone-responsive breast cancer. Austrian Breast and Colorectal Cancer Study Group Trial 5. J Clin Oncol 2002; 20:4621–7.

6. Boccardo F, Rubagotti A, Amoroso D et al. Italian Breast Cancer Adjuvant Chemo-Hormone Therapy Cooperative Group Trials. GROCTA Trials: recent results. Cancer Res 1998; 152:453–70.

7. Davidson NE, O'Neill A, Vukov A et al. Effect of chemohormonal therapy in premenopausal, node-positive, receptor-positive breast cancer: an Eastern Cooperative Oncology Group Phase III Intergroup Trial (E5188, INT-0101) (abstract O69). Breast 1999; 8:232–3.

8. Baum M, Houghton J, Odling-Smee W et al. Adjuvant Zoladex in premenopausal patients with early breast cancer: results from the ZIPP trial (abstract P64). Breast 2001; 10(suppl. 1):S32–S33.

9. ATAC Trialists' Group. Anastrozole alone or in combination with tamoxifen versus tamoxifen alone for adjuvant treatment of postmenopausal women with early-stage breast cancer: results of the ATAC (Arimidex, Tamoxifen Alone or in Combination) trial efficacy and safety update analyses. Cancer 2003; 98:1802–10.

10. Coombes RC, Hall E, Gibson LJ et al. A randomized trial of exemestane after two to three years of tamoxifen therapy in postmenopausal women with primary breast cancer. Intergroup Exemestane Study. N Engl J Med 2004; 350: 1081–92.

11. Boccardo F, Rubagotti A, Puntoni M et al. The Italian Tamoxifen Anastrozole Trial. Breast Cancer Res Treat 2003; 82(suppl. 1):S6–S7.

These two studies (10 and 11) were large, powerful, randomised trials and provide important information about the role of aromatase inhibitors.

12. Jakesz R, Kaufmann M, Gnant et al. Benefits of switching postmenopausal women with a hormone-sensitive early breast cancer to anastrozole after two years adjuvant tamoxifen: combined results from 3123 women enrolled in the ABCSG trial and the ARNO 95 trial. Breast Cancer Res Treat 2004; 88(suppl. 1):abstract 2.

13. Powles T, Paterson S, Kanis JA et al. Randomized, placebo-controlled trial of clodronate in patients with primary operable breast cancer. J Clin Oncol 2002; 20:3219–24.

14. Albain KS, Green SJ, Peter M, Ravdin PM et al. Adjuvant chemohormonal therapy for primary breast cancer should be sequential instead of concurrent: initial results from intergroup trial 0100 (SWOG-8814). Proc Am Soc Clin Oncol 2002; 21:37a.

15. Pico C, Martin M, Jara C et al. Epirubicin-cyclo-phosphamide (EC) chemotherapy plus tamoxifen (T) administered concurrent (Con) versus sequential (Sec): randomized phase III trial in postmenopausal node-positive breast cancer (BC) patients. GEICAM 9401 study. Proc Am Soc Clin Oncol 2002; 21:37a.

16. Beral V and Million Women Study Collaborators. Breast cancer and hormone-replacement therapy in the Million Women Study. Lancet 2003; 362: 419–27.

17. Holmberg L, Anderson H for the HABITS steering and data monitoring committees. HABITS (hormonal replacement therapy after breast cancer: is it safe?), randomised comparison: trial stopped. Lancet 2004; 363:453–5.

18. Sainsbury R, Perren T, Croft SR et al. Does timing of breast cancer surgery in relation to the menstrual cycle phase affect prognosis? The Yorkshire Breast Cancer Group Intervention, Timing and Survival Study. Breast Cancer Res Treat 2004; 88(suppl. 1): S112.

19. Grant CS, Hartmann LC, Suman V et al. Menstrual cycle and surgical treatment of breast cancer. Breast Cancer Res Treat 2004; 88(suppl. 1):S213.

Seventeen

Litigation in breast disease

Tim Davidson and
Tom Bates

INTRODUCTION

Litigation in breast disease has accelerated at an alarming rate. In the USA, legal action over delay in the diagnosis of breast cancer has reached such an extent that the value of malpractice claims is second only to that for neurological damage to neonates.[1,2] Poor cosmetic outcome after cosmetic or reconstructive surgery is also a frequent cause for litigation and the saga of silicone breast implants has heightened public awareness and increased expectation of recompense for real or perceived injury.

Doctors have been made increasingly aware of the need to warn patients of the risks involved with any procedure, be it diagnostic or therapeutic, to involve patients in decision-making, and to seek informed consent after having discussed all alternative options, likely outcomes and potential complications. Patient information leaflets, involvement of breast care nurses and more detailed consent forms signed by the operating surgeon are now standard practice but have done little to stem the tide of litigation as patients' expectations continue to rise.

BASIC PRINCIPLES

The legal process differs between countries and although the present account is based on civil law in England and Wales, the general principles in use elsewhere are similar.[3] For a claimant (plaintiff) to succeed in law, she must satisfy the court (in the UK a judge, or in some countries a jury) that there was a failure or **breach of duty** of care (liability) and that as a foreseeable result she suffered an injury (causation). For the case to succeed, the court must find in favour of the claimant with regard to both liability and causation. Negligence cases are heard in civil court and the judge determines whether the defendant is liable (entirely different from a criminal court determining guilt or innocence). If the court finds in favour of the claimant, the court awards financial recompense to redress, as far as money is able, the injury that she has suffered.

The award of damages

The sole remedy available to the successful claimant in medical negligence litigation is an award of damages – a sum of money intended to restore the claimant to the position she would have been in but for the negligent act. Explanation and apology to the claimant or her family, desirable though they may be, are not within the power of civil law, nor are recommendations for retraining, suspension or deregistration of doctors who find themselves as defendants.

The award comprises two components, general and special damages. General damages are intended to compensate for pain, suffering and loss of amenity and are based upon judicial guidelines that are upgraded regularly to allow for inflation. Special damages are specific to the individual plaintiff and include past losses, which can be identified with some accuracy, and future losses, which can only be estimated. It is the future loss of earnings and the costs of providing care for the claimant and/or dependents that generate very high value claims. A young woman with dependent children earning a high income will attract a high value award if she (or her surviving spouse) can demonstrate that her premature death resulted from lack of care. The all-or-none principle adopted in English law means that the successful claimant will normally recover damages in full, although in one recent case where the claimant was held to have lost an 80% chance of cure, a deputy high court judge directed that damages should be calculated accordingly.[4]

In English law the magnitude or perceived culpability of the negligent act has no bearing whatsoever on the sum awarded and the principles of calculating the value of a claim are followed whether the matter is settled by direct negotiation or is heard in court, where damages, if not agreed, are determined by a judge. This contrasts with the position in the USA where cases that proceed to trial (the minority) rely on jury decisions which often incorporate an element of 'aggravated' or exemplary (punitive) damages, a sum the jury considers warranted by the wrongfulness of the defendant's act. The extent to which this affects the magnitude of the award can be seen by comparing the average value of claims concluded by settlement ($282 244) with the $869 766 secured by jury verdict in the 1995 Physician Insurers Association of America (PIAA) survey.[2]

Liability

DUTY OF CARE

Any doctor – radiologist, surgeon or pathologist – owes each individual patient a duty of care. This is rarely an issue. In the public sector the doctor acts as a servant of the hospital trust or community health authority and in this capacity he or she is covered by Crown Indemnity. When acting in a private capacity, the doctor is covered by a professional defence organisation of his or her choice.

BREACH OF DUTY

If a patient is referred to a breast clinic or is treated by a breast surgeon and the standard of care falls below that which the patient could reasonably have expected from a breast specialist, there has been a breach of the duty of care.

THE BOLAM TEST

A doctor is not negligent if he or she acts in accordance with a practice accepted at the time as proper by a responsible body of medical opinion. The Bolam test arises from the case of a patient who received electroconvulsive therapy and sustained fractures.[5] Negligence was alleged because the patient was not given muscle relaxants and was inadequately restrained. Some doctors would have used muscle relaxants and restraints, others not. The doctor was not found negligent because he acted in accordance with a practice accepted at the time, even though other doctors may have advocated a different practice.

The Bolam test requires a higher degree of skill from a specialist in his or her own field than from a general practitioner (GP). The Bolitho modification of Bolam adds the requirement that for the practice or opinion formed to be acceptable, it must be based on logical argument; an irrational practice cannot be claimed as acceptable in court simply because a body of medical opinion agrees with its use.[6]

GUIDELINES

National and local guidelines of good clinical practice are now in standard use throughout most disciplines in the NHS. Breast practice has been in the vanguard, with established and revised guidelines covering patient referral, diagnosis, treatment (both surgical and oncological) and organisational arrangements within breast units. Breaches of guidelines are in no way indicative of, or equivalent to, negligent clinical practice and guidelines are constantly being amended in the light of scientific knowledge, health-care resources, government targets, etc. However, medical practice that complies with guidelines is inevitably much easier to defend against allegations of negligence. A diagnostic excision biopsy exceeding 20 g, the current NHS Breast Screening Programme (BSP) guideline, is a common occurrence and does not equate to negligent practice; however, a patient claiming excessive deformity after such a procedure is unlikely to succeed in litigation if her biopsy specimen weighed under 20 g.

There is still considerable concern regarding the medicolegal implications of clinical practice guidelines for surgeons.[7] Carrick et al.[8] reported that whereas 41% of surgeons surveyed believed that guidelines would protect them against medicolegal claims, 37% believed that they would increase their exposure to claims. Of interest, significantly more breast surgeons compared with general surgeons believed that their exposure to claims would increase.

CONSENT

Great emphasis is now placed on warning patients of the risks of any proposed management but the principle of informed consent remains largely untested in English law. Consent obtained by a junior doctor who is not capable of undertaking the intended procedure is no longer considered acceptable. Standardised consent forms have recently been introduced throughout the UK. The degree of disclosure 'must primarily be a matter of clinical judgement' but catastrophic complications (such as total loss of a flap in breast reconstruction) must be included even if their occurrence is considered very rare.[9]

Causation

The second hurdle to be overcome by the claimant is to prove that the negligent act of the doctor, or more usually in the UK the NHS trust (which is vicariously liable for its employees), actually caused an injury which was forseeable. Causation may be obvious where there is a poor cosmetic outcome from breast reduction, but it may be difficult to prove cause and effect where there has been a delay in the diagnosis of breast cancer.

DID THE DELAY NECESSITATE MORE RADICAL TREATMENT?

Where the patient has had a mastectomy it is often plausible to suggest, on the balance of probabilities, that an earlier diagnosis would have made breast conservative surgery a real option. When the patient has received chemotherapy it is sometimes argued that this would not have been necessary if the diagnosis had been made sooner when, for example, the axillary lymph nodes would probably have been negative. However, this line of argument is open to counter-attack on the basis that failure to give chemotherapy would have omitted the only treatment likely to have made a real difference to prognosis.

DOES DELAY IN DIAGNOSIS REDUCE LIFESPAN?

This is a controversial area since there is public expectation, promoted over the years by health campaigners, that earlier diagnosis offers better chance of a cure and a longer lifespan. Where expert opinion is divided, the court often prefers the evidence in favour of delay having caused a reduced survival time.

DOES DELAY IN DIAGNOSIS REDUCE THE CHANCE OF A CURE?

Loss of a chance of cure is not a concept endorsed by the English courts,[10] but it is a cause for action in the USA. Cure is a difficult concept in breast cancer and this is discussed further below.

THE BURDEN (LEVEL) OF PROOF

In civil litigation the court determines the facts, which means that the judge makes a decision on the balance of probabilities, i.e. more likely than not (51% vs. 49%). This level of proof is quite different from that in criminal cases where proof of guilt is required beyond reasonable doubt. The 'all-or-none' nature of civil litigation in awarding damages is one of the areas most open to criticism. For example, if the court finds that as a result of negligence a woman has suffered a reduction in her chance of survival of 60%, she will be awarded the full amount to compensate her (or her family) as though the injury or loss had definitely occurred on the basis that *on balance* she is now more likely to die. If the court finds that her chance of survival is reduced by only 40%, it may award her nothing on the basis that *on balance* her chance of survival remains unchanged.

DELAY IN THE DIAGNOSIS OF BREAST CANCER

Delay in diagnosis may occur as a result of failure to refer the patient from primary care, false-negative mammography, failure to perform triple assessment, misinterpretation of fine-needle aspiration cytology (FNAC) or the misfiling of a positive test result. There are three phases that should be considered in breast cancer diagnosis, where the major responsibility often rests with the patient herself, with the referring GP or with the breast specialist in the clinic.[11]

Phase 1: patient delay

When a woman first becomes aware of a breast cancer, she may delay seeking advice for fear of the diagnosis or the treatment. She may be over-optimistic about the likely diagnosis or she may deny the possibility that she has cancer. The causes of patient delay are not relevant to the present discussion. Delay is longer on average in disadvantaged populations and at the extremes of age but the absence of a palpable lump may also be an important factor in falsely reassuring a woman that her symptoms are not serious.

Phase 2: delay in primary care

The GP who sees many cases of symptomatic breast disease each year but only one or two breast cancers is in an increasingly difficult position. The patient's perception is that she needs to see a specialist but the practitioner feels confident that the condition is benign especially in young women. Breast cancer is very uncommon in women under 35 years of age (3% of cancers) but when it does occur it is more difficult to diagnose.

It is usually inappropriate for a GP to needle the breast for cytology, unless there is a history of recurrent cysts. To rely on a negative mammogram without an expert clinical examination or FNAC to complete a triple assessment may increase the risk of false reassurance, although the evidence for this consensus opinion is not supported by the available data.[12] The GP is therefore faced with referring most women over 35 with breast symptoms for a specialist opinion without significant delay and GP referral guidelines have been in use in the UK since 1995.[13,14]

Administrative delay

Referral guidelines are now widely followed in order to avoid administrative delay between primary and secondary care, with urgent GP referrals ideally seeing a specialist within 2 weeks. Breast units throughout the UK submit audit data on compliance with 'target' (suspected cancer) referrals and these data are now in the public domain.[15] However, the prioritisation of referral letters is counter-productive if non-urgent cases have to wait longer, with several recent reports indicating that about 25% of breast cancers are found in patients who are non-urgent referrals.

Phase 3: after specialist referral

This occurs in the setting of specialist diagnosis between the first breast clinic visit and the definitive diagnosis and treatment of breast cancer. The role of triple assessment, and the circumstances and settings in which it fails, are critical to this phase and are dealt with in greater detail below. The specialist centre is also faced with the problem that women under 35 form the majority of the diagnostic workload (66%), the fewest number of breast cancers (3%)[12] and, paradoxically, the highest rate of medical malpractice claims.[2]

The North American experience

Two studies have been commissioned by the PIAA,[1,2] an association of 33 insurance companies representing over 90 000 physicians. Failure or delay in the diagnosis of breast cancer was the commonest cause of all medical litigation in the USA, and in terms of indemnity payout was second only to claims arising from neurologically impaired neonates.[2] One of the most striking features of both studies was the relatively young age of the claimants: women under 50 accounted for 69% of the claimants and received 84% of the indemnity paid. These figures are all the more surprising when one considers that only 25% of breast cancers occur in women under 50 years of age.[16]

The most common reasons cited for the delay were (in descending order): physical findings failed to impress, failure to adequately follow up the patient, negative mammogram report, misreading of the mammogram and failure to perform a biopsy.

False-negative and equivocal mammography results, whether used to diagnose a breast lump or as part of a screening programme, were cited in 80% of the cases and, not surprisingly, radiologists were the most frequent defendants. Radiologists are particularly at risk when the patient refers herself, since triple assessment may be incomplete because of lack of a clinical examination.

In 487 cases where liability was admitted by the defendant, the mean delay was 14 months. Mean damages of $227 000 were awarded for delays of less than 5 months. The mean payout for all delays was $301 000, with higher payouts being awarded for longer delays and to younger patients.[2] There are now statistical models for predicting the outcome and size of indemnity payout in malpractice lawsuits for breast cancer.[17]

That younger women, with the lowest incidence of breast cancer, have the highest incidence of malpractice claims is a paradox that may be explained by clinical lack of awareness or by unrealistic expectations of our ability to diagnose breast cancer in younger women. In any event, the diagnosis is more emotive and especially when the patient has young children the economic consequences of a reduced lifespan are more severe.

DIAGNOSIS OF BREAST CANCER

Approximately two-thirds of patients presenting at a symptomatic breast clinic are under 36 years of age and most will have benign disease, since only 3% of breast cancers occur in this age group.[18] Triple assessment, comprising expert clinical examination, imaging by mammography and/or ultrasound together with needle biopsy, is the foundation upon which clinicians diagnose breast lumps. However, it is not well appreciated the extent to which the accuracy of these tests is reduced in younger women (**Fig. 17.1**). It has been recently suggested that perfection of diagnosis will require removal of every solid mass,[19] but this would represent a retrograde step. The practice of defensive medicine, in place of conventional wisdom, will certainly be encouraged by a private health-care system, a litigious public and diagnostic tests whose sensitivity falls below 95%.

Physical examination

About 70% of all breast cancers are palpable, but in tumours measuring 0.6–1 cm diameter this figure

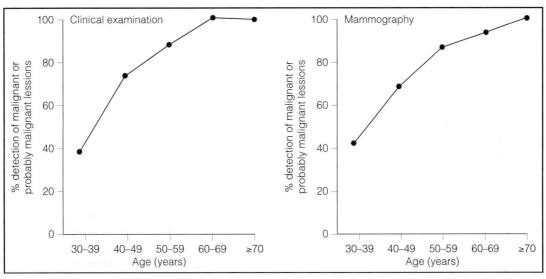

Figure 17.1 • Sensitivity of clinical and mammographic examination by age. With permission from Dixon JM, Mansel RE. Symptoms, assessment and guidelines for referral. In: Dixon JM (ed.) ABC of breast diseases, 2nd edn. London: BMJ Books, 2000, p. 6. Blackwell Publishing Ltd.

falls to 50%.[21] The larger the breast and the greater the density of breast tissue, the more difficult physical examination becomes. Cyclical changes in breast parenchyma may require repeated examination at different phases of the menstrual cycle, and it has been suggested that the optimal time to examine premenopausal women is a week after the onset of the menstrual period. Coexisting benign lumps, scars and distortion produced by previous surgery, the ridge of tissue above the inframammary fold and the underlying ribs all add to the uncertainty of clinical examination.

The small but real risk of breast cancer during pregnancy and lactation should also be appreciated. The changes in breast tissue increase the difficulties of clinical examination and may be a pitfall for the obstetrician who wishes to reassure an anxious patient at prenatal assessment. Other difficulties include inflammatory cancers masquerading as infection; the presence of silicone implants with an associated fibrous capsule in patients who have had breast augmentation; and the effect of hormone replacement therapy (HRT), which increases the density of breast parenchyma both clinically and radiologically.

The sensitivity of clinical examination for the detection of breast cancer, carried out by a senior and a junior member of the surgical team in women aged 30–39 years, can be as low as 25%.[22] A sensitivity of 90% can only be expected in older women, when the atrophic nature of the breast parenchyma and the low incidence of benign disease combine to make clinical diagnosis a relatively simple task.

The low sensitivity of clinical examination, coupled with the low incidence of breast cancer and the considerable numbers of young women attending breast clinics, must largely explain why failure of physical findings to impress the physician was one of the most common reasons for delay in diagnosis of breast cancer in the PIAA study.[2]

Mammography

False-negative mammography is one of the principal reasons for delay in diagnosis of breast cancer,[1,2,20,23–25] since a negative mammogram gives the clinician and patient a false sense of reassurance that the condition is benign. How much reliance can one place on a negative mammogram? Some authors suggest that the sensitivity of diagnostic mammography is greater than 90% but these findings are not universal.[26] The age of the patient is an important factor in false-negative reporting, since the high radiographic density of the breasts in young women (and with HRT) make detection of a similarly dense tumour more difficult.

Further analysis of data from the Health Insurance Plan Project estimated that the mean time by which the diagnosis of breast cancer can be advanced by screening (lead time) is 1.7 years;[27] other estimates vary from 0.4 to 3.0 years.[28,29] It is therefore probable that some cancers detected after the initial (prevalent) screening mammogram (interval cancers) were in fact present at the time of the prevalent mammogram but not detected. It has been shown that 25% of the cancers detected at the second screening mammogram (incident screen) 3 years after the prevalent screen in the NHS BSP represent a false-negative finding on the initial films.[30]

Screening issues are well discussed by Wright and Mueller.[31] Data from the Breast Cancer Detection Demonstration Project (BCDDP) revealed that both clinical examination and mammography were less sensitive in women under 50 years of age.[14] Interval cancers are more often node positive but this may be due to length bias, where those cancers detected in the interval between screens are more aggressive than prevalent cancers detected at the initial screen. The number of cancers not detected by the initial screen is inversely proportional to age; 36% of cancers in women aged 40 attending for screening were not detected by the prevalent screen compared with just 9% in those aged 75.[16]

Ultrasound

The use of ultrasound to augment mammography has expanded since the mid-1990s. The expertise of breast radiologists in the use of this technique has improved considerably, the result of not only specialisation in breast imaging but also rapid improvements in the performance of ultrasound equipment. It is now considered good practice to carry out an ultrasound examination in a patient of any age complaining of a lump, especially when this is not detectable on clinical or mammographic examination. There is a trend for ultrasound-guided core biopsy to replace FNAC although both techniques are currently acceptable.

Fine-needle aspiration cytology

For many years FNAC was the principal method for obtaining a tissue diagnosis of a palpable lump, since it is both cost-effective and obviates the need for open biopsy. How much reliance can one place in the result of FNAC? Dixon et al.[22] reported that the sensitivity of FNAC could be increased from 66 to 99% by restricting the biopsy to one aspirator. In comparison, the sensitivity of FNAC in women under 36 years was found to be reduced to 78%.[18,32] Dixon et al.[22] found that the accuracy of this investigation was not related to the age of the patient, with the sensitivity of FNAC in women under 36 years at 100% if inadequate samples were excluded from the calculations.

In a review of 112 reports of FNAC of breast masses by Layfield et al.,[33] the overall accuracy was over 95% but concern was raised over the range of false-negative and false-positive reporting (1–35% and up to 18% respectively) and of unsatisfactory specimens (1–68%). Core biopsy is now advisable after inadequate (C1) FNAC of a mass.

Despite the introduction of FNAC, delay in diagnosis of greater than 50 days still occurred, and 85% of such delays were in women under 55 years of age.[34] It is possible that FNAC in isolation may fail to detect breast cancer in up to 25% of women under 36 years of age attending a breast clinic. In small tumours, a sampling error (where the clinician fails to sample the actual tumour) is probably more common than failure to achieve an adequate sample or misinterpretation of the cytology. Where a lump is very small or indefinite, but is apparent on ultrasonography, current practice is moving towards ultrasound-guided core biopsy to reduce sampling error. Increasingly core biopsy is replacing FNAC because core biopsy can differentiate invasive from in situ cancer; FNAC cannot. There are few if any false positives and providing core biopsy is image guided and a sufficient number of cores of the lesion are obtained, sensitivity is at least as good as FNAC.

Efficacy of triple assessment

If it is assumed that breast cancer detection by clinical examination, mammography and FNAC or core biopsy are independent of each other, it is

Table 17.1 • False-negative rates of triple assessment for women under 35 years old compared with the generally quoted results.[12,16,34]

	False-negative rate	
	Women <35 years	Overall
Clinical examination	0.75	0.12
Mammography	0.75	0.12
Fine-needle cytology	0.22	0.05
All three false negative	12.3%	0.072

possible to calculate the theoretical rate at which all three tests will give a false-negative result. The false-negative rates of the three investigations[18,32] have been multiplied and expressed as a percentage (**Table 17.1**). It is probable that the sensitivities of these tests are not totally independent of each other, and therefore the predicted rate that all three tests will be false negative for an individual is a conservative estimate. The sensitivity of the three tests means that for a woman under 36 years with breast cancer, there may be a 12% chance that all three tests will give a false-negative result. If the generally accepted overall sensitivities are taken, the chance that all three tests will produce a false-negative result falls to approximately 1 in 1000 patients. However, the data from which these sensitivities are calculated will be skewed towards the older age groups and the overall rate of false-negative triple assessment in the clinic may be as high as 4%.[35]

CURABILITY OF BREAST CANCER

Is breast cancer a curable disease? The 5- and 10-year survival rates are useful in the comparison of different treatment regimens but are not synonymous with cure. Since survival measurements are made from the date of histological diagnosis, earlier detection of the tumour by mammographic screening will improve survival data without necessarily having any real impact on cure. This phenomenon is known as lead-time bias.

Crude cure rates seldom take account of the histological nature of breast cancer. In a study of 133 long-term survivors of breast cancer, on histological review 10% were considered to be benign disease.[36] Of the remaining 119 survivors with a definite diagnosis of breast cancer, more than two-thirds had a special type of invasive cancer (e.g. cribriform, tubular), tumours generally considered to be less aggressive than invasive ductal or lobular cancer.

Three concepts of cure

Haybittle[37] has discussed three concepts of cure: statistical cure, clinical cure and personal cure.

STATISTICAL CURE: DEATH FROM ALL CAUSES

Statistical cure can be applied to a group of patients rather than to individuals by comparing the survival of a group of patients treated for breast cancer with the survival of an age-matched normal population. If after a long period of follow-up a fraction of the original group of patients shows an annual death rate from all causes similar to the age-matched normal population, that fraction can then be said to be statistically cured.

By expressing the observed number of deaths in the treated group as a ratio of the expected number of deaths in the age-matched normal population (O/E ratio), statistical cure would be demonstrated by a ratio of unity. In four long-term studies of patients treated for breast cancer, statistical cure has not been convincingly demonstrated. In a French study from Villejuif, the 95% confidence intervals included unity between 15 and 25 years but over the next 5 years the ratio was significantly greater than 1.[38] In a Cambridge study which followed 704 patients for 31 years, the O/E ratio and 95% confidence intervals remained greater than 1. In the Edinburgh study, the O/E ratio reached 1.47 at 17–20 years (95% confidence limits 1.00–2.07), and in the Birmingham study the O/E ratio was 1.34 (95% confidence limits 0.95–1.84) at 35+ years. Even after 40 years, an excess mortality among young patients treated for breast cancer has been demonstrated by Rutqvist and Wallgren.[39] The evidence is against a statistically cured group of breast cancer patients. It seems that a population of patients who have had breast cancer will always have a higher death rate from all causes than a matched control population, even after 20 or 30 years.

CLINICAL CURE: FREE OF BREAST CANCER AT POST-MORTEM

Clinical cure is demonstrated if a group of patients treated for breast cancer is at no greater risk of dying from breast cancer than an age- and sex-matched normal population.[37] This definition of cure as applied to a disease considered fatal is used by actuaries for life insurance policies. To establish a clinical cure for breast cancer would be the most satisfactory outcome of any study but accurate reporting of the cause of death for all subjects in such a study is essential, which perhaps explains the paucity of data relating to clinical cure. Long-term studies have failed to demonstrate a clinical cure for breast cancer. The Edinburgh study showed that 15–20 years after initial treatment, patients were 20 times more likely to die from breast cancer than the normal population. In the Cambridge study,[37] deaths from breast cancer were 19-fold greater than the expected rate between 20 and 25 years of age and 15-fold greater between 25 and 35 years of age. An excess mortality in patients with breast cancer has also been reported after 18 years in Stockholm and Connecticut.[40]

PERSONAL CURE

Personal cure relates to the individual, so that a personal cure can be claimed if the patient has no further symptoms from breast cancer at the time of death and the patient dies from another cause. Accurate death certification is essential and in the Cambridge study, 26% of deaths were assessed as being from another cause without overt signs of breast cancer being present. Mueller et al.[41] investigated the cause of death in 3558 patients with breast cancer reported to the Upstate Medical Center Cancer Registry, Syracuse, New York. They found that 20 years after diagnosis, 80% of women diagnosed as having breast cancer were dead; 88% of these deaths were due to breast cancer. Cancer of the breast was the ultimate cause of death in 96.5% of patients aged 21–50 years at the time of diagnosis, in 90.0% of patients aged 51–70 years and in 77.5% of patients aged 71–100 years. It is only in the oldest group of patients that death from other causes competes significantly with breast cancer, so that a personal cure rate of 22.5% can be claimed. This finding is supported by a number of studies in the literature but these largely pre-date the use of adjuvant chemotherapy. If adjuvant therapy postpones death, rather than eliminating the disease completely, the lifespan of patients will be increased. Such an increase in lifespan would result in more deaths being due to other causes and so the number of personal cures of breast cancer would increase.

Cancer control window

The theory that early detection of a tumour will lead to cure depends on the concept that at the time of earlier detection and treatment the tumour has not metastasised. There is therefore a theoretical window of opportunity to cure patients with cancer by surgery. The period of time between the earliest possible detection of the cancer and the time at which the tumour metastasises has been described as the cancer control window.[42] If the tumour has already metastasised by the time it reaches the threshold size for detection, there is no window and only effective systemic therapy might cure the patient.

Tumour doubling time

Patients presenting to a symptomatic breast clinic typically have a tumour diameter of 3 cm. Assuming the cancer cell has a diameter of 10 μm and exhibits exponential growth, this equates to 10^{10} cells and 33 tumour doublings. The usual threshold diameter for detection of a breast cancer by physical examination is 1 cm; such a tumour consists of 10^9 cells and is the result of 30 doublings. It is possible for mammography to detect tumours as small as 2 mm diameter, which equates to a tumour of 10^7 cells and about 23 doublings.

Assuming a constant doubling time, early detection of breast cancer is a misnomer, since at least two-thirds of the biological life of the tumour will have been completed at the time of detection.[43] In medicolegal terms, if the alleged delay in diagnosis was 14 months for a cancer with a doubling time of 90 days, such a delay would equate to the number of cells increasing by one order of magnitude (i.e. from 10^9 to 10^{10} cells) (Fig. 17.2). This represents a major increase in tumour load but is a very short period in the lifespan of the tumour and it is difficult to be sure that this period of delay would have a significant effect. In civil law, however, the court wants to know whether such an effect is more

likely than not to alter the patient's prognosis or treatment.

Lymph node status is the most important prognostic indicator at the time of surgical excision. Rutqvist and Wallgren[39] found that 61% of women under 51 years of age had axillary disease at the time of surgery. Assuming the growth rate of the nodal metastasis approximates to that of the primary tumour, it is possible to estimate the theoretical time at which the tumour must have metastasised (Fig. 17.3). Not infrequently this would have occurred long before the threshold size for detection of the primary tumour.[43]

Tubiana and Koscielny[44] suggested that breast cancer represents a continuum from slow-growing tumours with late axillary involvement and distant dissemination to the most aggressive, rapidly growing and early metastasising subtype. In medicolegal terms the major variable at issue is the delay in starting treatment. It is generally assumed by the claimant and her legal advice that delay in diagnosis and treatment is the cause of the metastasis rather than the inherent biology of the tumour itself.

As with other cancers, it is generally accepted that breast cancer begins as a single cell or a small group of cells that exhibit an exponential growth pattern. The length of time taken for a tumour to double in volume is known as the doubling time, usually expressed in days. Actual doubling times for breast cancers have been estimated by measuring the size of mastectomy scar recurrences[45] and also by serial mammographic evaluation;[46] both estimations assume exponential growth of the tumour. There is great variation in doubling times between different breast cancers, ranging from less than 25 days to more than 1000 days, and tumour doubling times appear to exhibit a log-normal distribution.[45]

Pearlman[45] categorised patients as having fast (<25days), intermediate (26–75 days) and slow-growing (>76 days) tumours based on measurement of tumour doubling time; 5-year survival rates were 5, 62 and 100% respectively. However, if patient survival was plotted against the lifespan of a patient expressed as the number of tumour doublings that a patient survived (e.g. a patient who survived 6 years and had a tumour doubling time of 25 days would have survived 88 tumour doublings), the difference in survival between the fast-growing and the intermediate/slow-growing tumours disappeared.

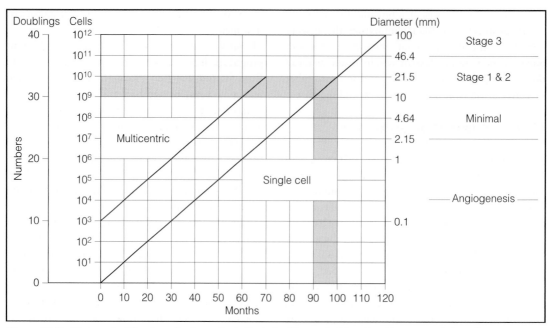

Figure 17.2 • Tumour doubling time: the theoretical effect of a 10-month delay. Graphic representation of tumour growth for a breast cancer with a doubling time of 90 days, assuming an exponential growth pattern. Growth rates (measured by the number of cells, number of tumour doublings and size of the tumour) of tumours that begin as a single cell and as a group of 1000 cells are plotted. By the time of diagnosis, typically two-thirds of the tumour's life will have passed. The theoretical effect that a 10-month delay in diagnosis would have on the size of the tumour is shown (shaded). With permission from Plotkin D, Blankenberg F. Breast cancer: biology and malpractice. Am J Clin Oncol 1991; 14:254–66.

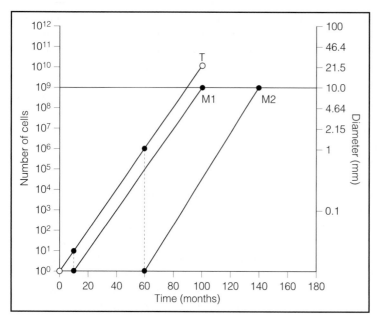

Figure 17.3 • Tumour doubling time: theoretical timing of metastatic growth. The time at which metastatic spread would have occurred is estimated. A 10-mm metastatic deposit is found at the time of surgery (M1) and 40 months following sugery (M2). Assuming that the growth rate of the metastatic deposit is similar to that of the primary tumour, dissemination of M1 occurred within 10 months of the development of the primary tumour (T), while that of M2 occurred within 5 years of development of the primary tumour. Both these events would have occurred long before detection of the primary tumour would have been possible. With permission from Plotkin D, Blankenberg F. Breast cancer: biology and malpractice. Am J Clin Oncol 1991; 14:254–66.

This implies that there was little therapeutic response for any of the patients, despite there being differences in the actual periods of survival, i.e. patients tended to survive a similar number of tumour doublings.

Although lymph node metastases are more commonly found in fast-growing tumours, it would be wrong to assume that the survival of patients was entirely a consequence of tumour doubling time. Galante et al.[46] emphasised the importance of the metastatic potential of the tumour, suggesting that within fast-, intermediate- and slow-growing tumours there may be subsets with high and low metastasising potential.

VIGNETTES ON LIABILITY

The following vignettes illustrate the areas of breach of duty that arise in medicolegal breast cases, most of which concern either a delay in diagnosis of breast cancer or a poor cosmetic outcome after cosmetic or reconstructive surgery. However, there are other issues of liability, including pneumothorax caused by FNAC and false-positive cytology leading to unnecessary surgery. The comments following each vignette should not be taken as a definitive opinion but do raise the issues which would be discussed in conference with counsel. Consideration must be given to the time at which the alleged breach of duty took place since the practice of breast surgery is changing rapidly. If any authority or guideline is to be relevant, it must have been in the public domain at the time.

Vignette 1: Radiological delay in diagnosis

A woman aged 54 years attended for the second round of breast screening (incident screen) and was found to have an opacity on mammography that proved malignant. Having been shown the films she asked to see the previous films taken 3 years earlier. When these were reluctantly produced it was evident to her experts that the cancer had been present 3 years previously.

COMMENTS

- One-quarter of screen-detected cancers are apparent with hindsight 3 years earlier on mammograms and, very occasionally, 6 years earlier. Most often the tumour is seen only as one of a number of similar opacities on the original mammogram.

- Such a 'missed diagnosis' may be obvious to a radiologist with knowledge of the outcome but if the mammograms are interspersed with normal films, as in the screening situation, more often than not they will be passed as normal. However, in perhaps one-third of such cases expert opinion will state that any competent breast radiologist working to an acceptable standard should have reported the abnormality and in this situation liability has to be admitted.

- It is important in any screening programme that the number of women who have benign mammographic abnormalities who are recalled for further tests, and even excision biopsy, is kept to a minimum. The radiological quality standard for recall rate is 7%.

- Breast radiologists in the NHS BSP who have a high detection rate (sensitivity) for breast cancer also have a high recall or false-positive rate (low specificity). Conversely, radiologists with a lower detection rate recall fewer patients unnecessarily.

- A recent Appeal Court judgement in a controversial cervical screening case ruled that relatively minor abnormalities which eventually proved malignant should have been referred for more expert opinion. If this level of sensitivity were to be required of breast screening, it might put the whole programme at risk.

- The net result of the increasing medicolegal threat to breast radiologists has been an increase in the recall rate and the core biopsy rate of doubtful lesions. The recruitment of radiologists into breast imaging is proving difficult.

- The increasing expertise with ultrasound examination of the breast, the use of guided core biopsy and the specification (and cost) of equipment have placed breast imaging outside the competency of the general radiologist. The breast surgeon using ultrasound in the clinic may be similarly compromised unless training in the technique can be verified.

- The practice of repeating mammography after an interval for an appearance that is very probably benign may be difficult to defend if it eventually proves malignant. This particularly applies to microcalcification, where core biopsy is the safest course, with specimen radiography to confirm that sampling of representative tissue contains calcification.

Vignette 2: False-positive cytology, lymphoedema and alteration of records

A 60-year-old patient was referred to a breast clinic with a clinically suspicious breast lump. Mammography was also suspicious of malignancy (R4) and FNAC was malignant (C5). The patient underwent wide local excision and axillary lymph node clearance for what subsequently proved to be a histologically benign condition. She complained of a poor cosmetic outcome and a painful swollen arm which she had not been warned about. The nursing records stated 'patient was warned of the risk of lymphoedema'.

COMMENTS

- A false-positive cytology result is a rare but potentially devastating event. From a medicolegal standpoint, an external expert review of the cytology should be the first step. If one or more experts are agreed that the cytologist acted reasonably in reporting the slides as unequivocally malignant, attention will then focus on the surgeon.
- The surgeon has to be aware that a false-positive cytology may very occasionally occur in the best hands and for this reason increasing numbers of surgeons will not carry out mastectomy without histological confirmation from a core biopsy. Histology is mandatory in the absence of a fully concordant malignant triple assessment including R5 imaging and should have been obtained in this case. A full axillary clearance for a benign condition is a potentially significant injury and it is unfortunate that this patient developed lymphoedema.
- The risk of lymphoedema is not well quantified since it may occur a long time after the treatment, vary considerably in extent and may occur after a variety of treatments.[47] Communicating the level of risk of lymphoedema before axillary surgery is a difficult task since any treatment option will carry some risk, but the patient must be made aware of this potential morbidity.
- The tense of the warning about lymphoedema suggested that this was a retrospective note made after the event. Judges place most credence on handwritten contemporaneous records, which are often brief and poorly legible. Any addition, alteration or amendment to the record must be clearly identified as such by signing and dating the record. Any temptation to alter the record after the event must be firmly resisted even if it is a computer-generated entry. Lawyers are constantly on the alert for alterations to the records, which are often quite obvious. Senior counsel: 'nurses are always doing it – doctors do it too but they are usually a little more subtle'.

Vignette 3: Cosmetic defect after benign biopsy and the benefit of preoperative diagnosis

A 50-year-old woman who was symptom-free was invited to attend the NHS BSP. Mammography showed a suspicious lesion in one breast and a diagnostic excision biopsy was carried out after stereotactic wire localisation. The pathology proved benign but the specimen weight was not recorded. The cosmetic outcome was unsatisfactory, with loss of volume and distortion of the nipple.

COMMENTS

- The current quality guidelines for the NHS BSP[48] indicate that 80% of benign excision biopsies should weigh less than 20 g. The target in the original guidelines was 90% but the subsequent UK national average indicated that over 50% of such biopsies weighed in excess of this target.[49] Failure to record the weight immediately places the surgeon in a difficult position but it is also important to document that an explanation of risk has been given to the patient. The surgeon who is experienced in the use of this technique is more likely to achieve an appropriate biopsy with the minimum of tissue loss.

- Surgeons are sometimes tempted to carry out a larger biopsy than absolutely necessary in the hope that the operation will be both diagnostic and therapeutic. This is a hazardous strategy since if the biopsy proves benign there may be an unnecessary cosmetic defect and if it is malignant an inadequate resection may compromise further surgery.
- Preoperative diagnosis by core biopsy is clearly preferable to excision biopsy and should have been attempted. The target for preoperative diagnosis of cancers in the NHS BSP of 90% is now being achieved in many centres.[49]

Vignette 4: Failure of preoperative assessment and postoperative management

A 65-year-old woman presented with a small but obvious carcinoma in the tail of the left breast. The surgeon performed FNAC, which showed malignant cells (C5), and he carried out wide local excision of the tumour without preliminary breast imaging and without performing an axillary node sample. The tumour was grade 2 but the resection margins and the presence of vascular invasion were not reported. The patient was started on tamoxifen but was not referred to an oncologist for consideration of radiotherapy.

COMMENTS

- The management of this patient falls short of an acceptable standard in a number of respects (breach of duty) but until such time as she develops evidence of recurrence, which may never occur, any harm (causation) remains potential.
- A preoperative mammogram might have shown widespread malignant microcalcification or multifocal tumour and in this situation conservative surgery would not have been appropriate and should not have been performed. There might also have been an undetected cancer in the contralateral breast.

- To manage a patient with conservative surgery without knowledge of the resection margins and without referring her for consideration of radiotherapy is unacceptable. A local recurrence of the order of 30% is to be expected.
- It is clear that this case was not discussed at a multidisciplinary meeting. The case history would certainly have alerted a member of the team to the inappropriate management.
- Knowledge of the axillary node status is considered to be important in patients with invasive carcinoma and has been recommended in UK guidelines since 1995.[50]

Vignette 5: Pneumothorax following FNAC

A dental nurse aged 32 years presented with a lump in the tail of the left breast. An ultrasound examination was negative and an experienced clinical assistant in the breast clinic carried out FNAC. Unfortunately, he pierced the pleura and caused a pneumothorax that required hospitalisation and pleural drainage. The patient was not warned of the risk and complained of persistent chest pain over a period of many months.

COMMENTS

- Did the clinician fail in his duty of care by advancing the needle too far or by failing to warn the patient? The literature suggests a risk of around 1 in 10 000.[51–53] It is not rare to strike a rib with the needle at FNAC. Piercing the pleura could be more common than is recognised because a trivial pneumothorax may go undetected, and possibly the pain of a pneumothorax may be perceived to be in the breast.
- In several cases the court has found pneumothorax to be a rare but recognised complication that can occur without breach of duty although a recent case ruled this injury to be negligent, which was an unexpected judgement.[53] It is an unfortunate fact of current medicolegal practice in the UK that if the claimant receives legal aid the defendant does not recover costs even when the case is successfully defended. There is therefore a

reluctance on the part of health authorities to defend low-value cases in court and an even greater reluctance to appeal a judgement that seems open to doubt.

- In resisting a claim of negligence, it is important to be able to show that the clinician was experienced in the technique.[53] Were this to be a trainee, it would be important to show that he or she had been properly supervised.
- It is important that clinicians are aware of the risk of pneumothorax. The highest risk appears to be with lesions in the tail of the breast of a thin patient where the pectoral muscle does not provide an additional layer on the chest wall.
- Pneumothorax has been reported following needle localisation by a radiologist and following aspiration of a postoperative seroma of the axilla.
- Performing FNAC and/or core biopsy using image guidance should reduce the risk because the lesion is approached parallel to the chest wall rather than through the skin directly over the lesion.

Vignette 6: False-negative FNAC, trainees in the diagnostic setting and lobular carcinoma

A 38-year-old patient was referred to a breast clinic with a breast lump. Preliminary mammography was negative and a specialist registrar (senior trainee) found an indefinite lump of which he was not suspicious. He carried out FNAC but failed to achieve an adequate specimen (C1). The result was not available on the day of the clinic visit. At follow-up appointment 6 weeks later, she was seen by another specialist registrar who repeated the FNAC. On this occasion cytology showed an adequate sample of benign ductal cells (C2). She was discharged from the clinic but re-presented 6 months later with an invasive lobular carcinoma at the same site.

COMMENTS

- Trainees must be adequately supervised and only permitted to see patients by themselves

when their trainer is satisfied that they are entirely competent and understand local management protocols. The 1995 guidelines (British Association of Surgical Oncology Breast Surgeons Group) required that a trainee should also have been attending the breast clinic for at least 2 months.[50] This latter requirement has been omitted from the current revision of the guidelines.[54] Trainees should not be brought in to fill an unforeseen hiatus in the breast clinic and strict adherence to local protocols is essential.

- There is a learning curve in achieving adequate samples with FNAC and it is likely that this will be achieved more quickly with immediate reporting of cytology, since the trainee has immediate feedback and is then faced with repeating the procedure immediately. The rate of inadequate FNAC samples (C1) should be monitored for each clinician. This should be less than 20%, although an adequate sample of benign ductal cells (C2) does not ensure a representative sample of the palpable lump.
- False-negative cytology may be due to cytological misinterpretation but is more commonly due to sampling error.
- Clinicians should be aware that lobular cancers are prone to false-negative mammography. There is also an increased rate of inadequate cytology (C1) and of difficulty with false-negative interpretation (C2).
- The diagnosis of breast cancer in young women is difficult and delay is more common. The cause of this delay is multifactorial but large numbers of women have benign breast nodularity whereas the number with breast cancer is small but significant. The sensitivity of triple assessment may be lower in young women, with consequent delay in diagnosis. Core biopsy is now being used increasingly with or without FNAC in an attempt to reduce the rate of missed diagnosis in these young women.
- In the situation where a patient complains of a lump but on clinical examination or mammography nothing is obvious, ultrasound is particularly useful. If a lesion is seen on ultrasound, a guided core biopsy is ideal.

IMPACT OF THE NHS BREAST SCREENING PROGRAMME

The introduction of screening has had a major influence on breast practice in the UK. The NHS BSP has for the first time enabled a public audit of radiologists, pathologists and surgeons. Radiologists will know their own detection and recall rates. Standard detection ratios, which allow for differences in case mix, are compared between screening units and are published. In most screening units the previous mammograms of all interval cancers that are notified are reviewed so that the radiologist will be aware of his or her false-negative cases. Radiologists in the BSP are expected to review 10 000 films annually in order to maintain their expertise, although it is unlikely that any radiologist doing purely symptomatic work would achieve this level of exposure.

It is axiomatic that patients with symptomatic and screen-detected cancers should receive the same quality of care and although this has not always been easy to achieve, there is recognition that symptomatic breast services have benefited. Some professionals have been shown to be outliers, which has led to medicolegal action in both radiology and surgery. Retraining and revalidation or opting out of the specialty may be a difficult choice.

The mastectomy rate for small screen-detected invasive breast cancers varies by surgeon but also by region. In 1997–98 the highest rate was in Trent (43%) and the lowest in South Thames West (17%);[49] this is not to suggest that some women in Trent underwent inappropriate mastectomy since it is also possible that some women in South Thames West received inadequate surgery. Variations in radiotherapy techniques have also been highlighted by the screening programme and suboptimal treatment schedules have led to changes.

There has been considerable pressure on the occasional operator to stop work in a given sub-specialty. In breast surgery it may take many years for any difference in outcome due to suboptimal surgery to become apparent. An increased local recurrence rate would be the first difference to emerge but is entirely dependent on the availability of good data. It is quite possible that a unit providing suboptimal management of in situ and invasive breast cancer also has poor data and if patients are lost to follow-up, local recurrence rates may appear lower than they really are.

Breast cancer carries a high profile and once a perceived problem with a screening unit or hospital enters the public domain, considerable anxiety is generated in the local population. Openness is the best policy and any attempt to withhold potentially embarrassing information is counter-productive.

DELAY IN DIAGNOSIS: CAUSATION ISSUES

In a case of delay in diagnosis, it is often relatively straightforward to establish whether there has been a breach of duty of care. The next hurdle to be overcome by the claimant is to satisfy the court, on the balance of probabilities, that this period of delay actually caused her predictable harm. The public and the judiciary have the expectation, encouraged by widely publicised rapid referral guidelines, that an early diagnosis carries a better outlook for the treatment of cancer and a better chance of cure. It is not surprising therefore that counter-arguments of lead-time bias and predeterminism of tumour biology tend to fall on deaf ears.

Having established liability for a delay in diagnosis, the issue of causation may include the allegation that less severe treatment would have been required with earlier diagnosis, e.g. a mastectomy would not have been necessary. It may also be argued that psychological damage has ensued. However, the main issue centres around the question as to whether the claimant has suffered a reduced expectation of life or if, as is often the case by the time the matter comes to court, she has already died whether she would have lived longer. Expert opinion is often divided and the court makes a judgement on the position that sounds most convincing on the day.

Richards et al.[55] carried out a systematic review of the literature on the effect of delay in diagnosis of breast cancer and, having apparently allowed for lead-time bias, found a reduction in 5-year survival of 7% with a delay of 3–6 months and 12% with a delay of more than 6 months. Dische et al.[56] extrapolated a 1.8% decrease in survival from Richards et al.'s data for each 1-month delay up to 6 months. In the same issue of the *Lancet*, Sainsbury et al.[57] reported no such effect but produced the apparently contradictory finding that patients with the shortest delay had the worst prognosis. This latter finding has been previously reported by Afzelius et al.[58] who found that the rapidly growing breast cancer with a poorer prognosis was more likely to be immediately apparent to the first clinician the patient consulted. The very slowly growing tumour with a good prognosis may be more difficult to diagnose.

The survival curves for patients with the best-prognosis tumours (small, special type, grade I, node negative) have a prognosis that is not very different from those of the normal population, and clearly a formula based on the findings in Richards et al.'s study that assessed reduction in survival for each month of delay would be inappropriate. However, if one accepts that this is a real effect overall, one would have to argue that some tumours with a worse prognosis would suffer a greater loss of survival.[56] It would nevertheless seem intuitive, bearing in mind the concept of the cancer control window, that the most aggressive tumours with rapid metastatic potential are likely to be incurable from so early on in their natural history that diagnostic delays are less likely to have a significant impact.

VIGNETTES ON CAUSATION

The following vignettes have been constructed to illustrate some of the issues that arise once liability has been accepted and the question of causation arises. Delay in diagnosis remains an area of considerable uncertainty and the comments reflect our opinions and experience of differing arguments presented to the court.

Vignette 7: 12-month delay in diagnosis of node-positive carcinoma

A 32-year-old woman was referred to a breast clinic with a lump in the breast. An ultrasound examination showed an indeterminate opacity 1.0 cm in diameter consistent with a fibroadenoma but no sample was taken by FNAC or core biopsy. She was discharged from the clinic but returned a year later with a clinical carcinoma at the same site. This measured 2.1 cm on both ultrasound and pathological examination and was grade 3; one of four nodes was positive. Liability for a delay in diagnosis and treatment was admitted for failure to carry out a biopsy at the first visit.

COMMENTS

- The Nottingham Prognostic Index (NPI)[59] is often used to determine the difference in outcome by calculating the change of value of the index over the period of delay. NPI is calculated as follows:

$$NPI = 0.2 \times \text{tumour size (cm)} + \text{node status} \ (1–3) + \text{grade} \ (1–3)$$

- The index has proved to be a robust indicator of prognosis but from a medicolegal standpoint it has the drawback that its application relies on unknown assumptions about the individual case.

Assumption 1: the tumour grade remains constant: this is usually agreed by both sides.

Assumption 2: the nodal status at the time of the breach of duty is usually unknown, but is often disputed by the experts for the claimant and the defendant. Axillary node status is invariably presumed to have been negative by the claimant, and this claim is supported by tables for tumour grade and tumour size which show the probability of positive nodes. Only in grade 2 and 3 tumours which are greater than 2.5 cm in diameter does the probability of positive nodes rise above 50%. Therefore on the balance of probabilities, which is the legal test, it is argued that the nodes would have been negative at the earlier time when the tumour was smaller and the diagnosis missed.

Assumption 3: in this particular case a record of tumour size at the first visit was available; however, if no clinical measurement was recorded and there was no imaging, an approximate tumour size (diameter) has to be derived from a putative tumour volume, itself derived by working back from the tumour volume at diagnosis using tumour doubling times. This type of calculation relies on the assumptions (i) that tumour growth is exponential, (ii) that in calculating tumour diameter the tumour approximates a sphere, and (iii) that the doubling time chosen from a wide range of values is appropriate for the tumour in question. The accuracy of this form of calculation can therefore only ever be approximate. The tumour size itself is a weak determinant of prognosis in the NPI but the derived earlier tumour size is further used to calculate the likely nodal status.

- The NPI at the first visit was 4.2 (size, 0.2; node, 1, presumed negative; grade, 3). The NPI a year later was 5.42 (size, 0.42; nodes, 2; grade, 3). The prognosis groups for NPI scores are shown in **Table 17.2**.[60] The patient has therefore moved from the moderate I prognosis group (73% survival at 10 years) to the poor prognosis group with a much poorer chance of long-term survival (26% at 10 years) (**Fig. 17.4**). However, if the tumour had only increased to 2.0 cm, the patient would have remained within the moderate II prognosis group.
- The NPI is often used by expert opinion but it has not been validated as a method for calculating differences in survival in this way. Whenever an estimation is given as to reduction in survival following a delay in diagnosis, allowance should be made for lead-time bias.

Table 17.2 • Nottingham Prognostic Index

Group	Index value	10-year survival (%)
Excellent (EPG)	2.0–2.4	96
Good (GPG)	2.41–3.4	93
Moderate I (MPGI)	3.41–4.4	82
Moderate II (MPGII)	4.41–5.4	75
Poor (PPG)	5.41–6.4	53
Very poor (VPG)	≥6.41	39

From the Nottingham Primary Breast Cancer Series. Data relate to patients with primary operable breast cancer, treated from 1990 to 1996.

Vignette 8: 2-year delay in diagnosis of node-negative grade 1 carcinoma

A 40-year-old woman presented with a lump in the breast and a triple assessment was carried out. The tumour measured 1.5 cm on ultrasound and mammography and FNAC was reported as benign (C2). She was discharged from the clinic but 2 years later returned with a carcinoma 3.0 cm in diameter on histology. The tumour was grade 1 and the four axillary nodes sampled were clear. Review of the

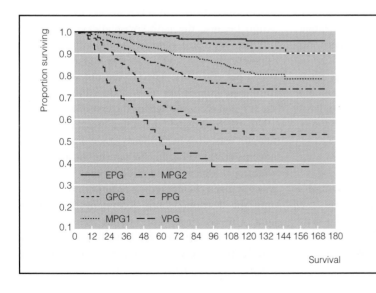

Figure 17.4 • Overall survival by Nottingham Prognostic Index group (1990–96 data). Data from Nottingham Tenovus Primary Breast Cancer Series.[60] EPG, excellent prognostic group; GPG, good prognostic group; MPG1, moderate 1 prognostic group, MPG2, moderate 2 prognostic group; VPG, very poor prognostic group.

original cytology indicated that this had been under-reported and an expert opinion graded the slides unequivocally malignant (C5). Liability was admitted. The patient was treated by breast conservation and postoperative radiotherapy.

COMMENTS

- The standard of care must be judged by the standard reasonably expected of a cytologist working at the same level. It is inappropriate to ask a world expert in the field to judge the opinion of a doctor from a district general hospital.
- The NPI only changed from 2.3 to 2.6 and although the tumour doubled in size over the 2-year period of delay, it remains within the good prognosis group. The treatment would have been the same with an earlier diagnosis and therefore there is no causation on this test.

Vignette 9: 3-year delay in diagnosis of a carcinoma missed on screening

A woman of 50 years old responded to an invitation for mammographic screening and was recalled for magnification views of a localised area of microcalcification in one breast. There was a soft tissue opacity and the appearance was judged benign on further views and ultrasound. She was returned to routine screening but 3 years later the screening films showed an obvious carcinoma at the same site. This was a 2.0-cm, grade 2, infiltrating carcinoma with an extensive in situ component; 4 of 10 nodes were positive. The NPI was 5.4. An opinion from a breast screening radiologist rated the original films as suspicious of ductal carcinoma in situ (R4) and stated that the focus of microcalcification should have been biopsied by any competent breast radiologist.

COMMENTS

- Practice has changed and a radiologist is more likely to advise biopsy of microcalcification now than several years ago. It is important that the radiologist is judged on what was considered reasonable at the time the original decision was made.

- Delay due to radiological misinterpretation tends to be a matter of years rather than months. Breast screening by mammography every 3 years does reduce the number of breast cancer deaths by about 25%, but it is more likely than not that a delay in diagnosis of 3 years will affect survival in a proportion of cases.
- The potential loss of survival in this particular case would be considerable since the original lesion would, on the balance of probabilities, have been an area of high-grade ductal carcinoma in situ without evidence of invasion. This lesion would carry a near-normal expectation of life if it had been adequately treated at age 50. At age 53 the patient now has a poor prognosis tumour and more likely than not will fail to reach retirement age.

Vignette 10: 14-month delay in the breast clinic and failure to recommend chemotherapy

A 30-year-old woman was referred with a lump in the breast to a general surgeon in January 1989 but was seen by a succession of three registrars (surgeons in training). An initial ultrasound examination showed a 1-cm opacity consistent with a fibroadenoma but the FNAC was reported as mildly atypical (C3) and the pathologist advised 'consider biopsy to confirm'. However, the registrar took no action because the pathologist always seemed to produce equivocal reports. A 6-month follow-up appointment was given and this was repeated by two other registrars. The GP did not wait for the third appointment but referred the patient again to the surgeon who saw her for the first time in March 1990 and immediately diagnosed breast cancer. The tumour was 4 cm in diameter, grade 3 and heavily node positive (NPI 6.8). The patient was treated by wide local excision and radiotherapy alone. She was not given chemotherapy or hormone treatment until she developed bone secondaries 16 months later. The ER status was not determined (1990). Liability was admitted for the delay in diagnosis and the failure to give chemotherapy at the time of diagnosis of the primary tumour.

COMMENTS

- Ignoring advice to consider a biopsy because 'he always says that' suggests a failure of communication between clinician and cytologist. It is clear that there was no multidisciplinary meeting.
- Arranging a 6-month follow-up for a breast lump that is presumed benign is illogical. A follow-up at 2–6 weeks with review by a senior surgeon would have been appropriate, at which time excision biopsy or repeat FNAC would have been advisable. An ultrasound-guided core biopsy, which is what would be advised now, was not standard practice in 1990.
- The place of a trainee giving an independent opinion in a breast clinic is discussed elsewhere. However, UK guidelines for the management of breast cancer patients were not published until 1995.[50]
- The judge took evidence from five expert witnesses. It was agreed that when first seen that the tumour would have been grade 3, 1 cm in diameter and node negative and that chemotherapy would not have been given in 1989. The tumour had increased in size to 4.0 cm in the 14 months of delay and opinion was divided as to whether this was ever potentially curable. The experts for the claimant were far more optimistic than those for the defence but in the event the judge preferred the latter. The trial proceedings make good reading.[61] The Woolf recommendation that there might be only one expert responsible to the court is controversial but the concept that experts should not be in the pocket of one party is widely welcomed.
- The effect of the delay of 15 months in giving chemotherapy was also a matter of considerable variation between the experts. The estimated reduction in life-years ranged between a few months and 5 years. 'Doing the best that I can on the basis of all the evidence, I consider that on the balance of probabilities, the negligent failure to provide Mrs X with adjuvant chemotherapy in 1990 caused her to die 18 months before, sadly she would have died anyway.' One can only have sympathy

with the judge in taking an average of the opinions on offer.
- There was considerable sympathy for the family of the deceased patient, who were awarded damages. Unfortunately, the damages amounted to less than the defence had already paid into court. The claimant could have taken the sum paid in but chose to contest the case in court for a larger sum on the advice of their experts. Civil litigation rules resulted in the family winning the case but receiving none of the settlement.

SILICONE IMPLANTS

The litigation in North America surrounding silicone gel-filled prostheses is instructive since in the absence of any scientific evidence, the major manufacturer of implants was made bankrupt.[62,63] Silicone prostheses were introduced in 1964 but by 1980 there were anecdotal reports of an association between implants and various forms of auto-immune disease, of which scleroderma was the most common. However, the reported symptoms were often non-specific[64] and similar to those experienced in the general population.

Undoubtedly the prostheses did develop fibrous capsules and some ruptured, which introduced the concept of silicone leaking into the tissues. This evidence of complications heightened alarm and led to a number of high-profile cases against the manufacturers of the implants in which enormous sums were awarded in damages for flu-like symptoms.[65] The litigation subsequently led to the Food and Drug Administration in the USA placing a moratorium on the use of silicone gel implants until they were proved safe, since although there was little evidence of harm, the actual testing had been suboptimal. By 1995 nearly half a million women had joined in a class action against Dow Corning, the principal manufacturer of silicone implants, who were unable to withstand the cost of the litigation process and filed for bankruptcy.

There is now a large body of evidence showing that there is no association between leaking silicone implants and connective tissue disease,[66,67] and it is fortunate that the medicolegal malfeasance seen in North America was not repeated in Europe.

POOR COSMETIC OUTCOME

Litigation arising from poor cosmetic outcome after surgery for breast cancer has been relatively uncommon in the past. Perhaps this relates to patients' greater concerns regarding the diagnosis of malignancy and their ultimate survival rather than cosmesis. However, this situation is changing with the increasing practice of breast conservation surgery rather than mastectomy. The patient who has undergone mastectomy may later claim that she suffered a much poorer cosmetic outcome than if she had undergone breast conservation surgery. Had there been reasonable indications to support its use and had the option been fully discussed?

When mastectomy is required, there is now increasing demand for reconstruction, which is reflected in the UK national guidelines. When mastectomy is advised, there should be evidence of discussion regarding either immediate or later breast reconstruction. Informed consent is paramount in this situation and it will undoubtedly be to the clinician's benefit to record appropriately that alternative treatment options and potential compliations of surgery have been discussed. The help of a trained breast care nurse to augment and further document the surgeon's advice is an additional protection that is now seen as an essential requirement in the practice of breast surgery. The patient who has only recently confronted the diagnosis of breast cancer, and the need for mastectomy, is unlikely to be in a position to absorb and respond to the various options for breast reconstruction and may require several lengthy sessions of counselling.

The breast surgeon must make available to the patient the appropriate range of reconstructive options, whether he or she will be able to perform them personally or whether it might require a joint undertaking with a plastic surgery colleague or referral to another centre. Currently, there is no certificate of competency in training in breast reconstruction within the UK and the need for guidelines is currently being addressed.

Should a patient undertake litigation against the breast surgeon on the basis of dissatisfaction with her cosmetic outcome following reconstruction, the Bolam principle would apply in determining liability, i.e. the practice would be compared with that held to be reasonable by a similar body of professionals, in this case breast surgeons trained to undertake breast reconstruction. Concerns have been raised that plastic surgeons might present in court expert opinions that demand a higher standard of reconstructive skill (such as free flap techniques), which might persuade the judge that the breast surgeon had not met his or her duty of care, but these fears remain as yet unfounded.

On the other hand, purely cosmetic breast surgery poses even greater expectations from the patient and potentially more risks for the surgeon. Evidence that appropriate discussions about potential risks and complications and poor cosmetic outcome in the realm of cosmetic surgery needs to be adequately recorded, with the use of appropriate information brochures, photographs and documented consultation notes or correspondence to explain adequately the proposed procedure. In addition, the surgeon should consider obtaining both standard evidence of consent as well as evidence that the literature has been received and understood.

Auditing of operative results may also be required in the future to demonstrate that a particular complication was simply bad luck and within the expected percentage risk of this occurrence. Audit evidence may well confirm that a particular surgeon's complication rate was at or below the accepted rate for that particular procedure. Alternatively, audit evidence that a particular surgeon had a complication rate far exceeding the accepted norm may well lead to litigation should that information become available to the patient. However, in a subspeciality of surgery where success or failure is not a matter of mortality but a value judgement and where complications will inevitably be underreported, any audit would lack the finality of the cardiac surgeon's results. The general principle of informed consent seems again to be at the forefront of defensive medical practice.

Vignette 11: Poor cosmetic outcome after reconstruction by a breast surgeon

A 52-year-old patient with multifocal cancer was advised to have a mastectomy by a breast surgeon, but after discussion with the breast care nurse she requested immediate reconstruction. He offered her a tissue expander, which was inserted at the time of mastectomy, but it was not subsequently possible to achieve symmetry with the large contralateral breast. Contralateral breast reduction was carried out, with a poor cosmetic outcome. She was subsequently referred to a plastic surgeon.

COMMENTS

- Patient expectation of a good cosmetic outcome is arguably less demanding for post-mastectomy reconstruction than for cosmetic surgery of the breast. Nevertheless, there is growing demand for a wider choice and more sophisticated reconstruction techniques and a better outcome.
- The first question that must be addressed is the adequacy of training in reconstructive surgery that the surgeon has undertaken. If that training was entirely appropriate, the second question is whether the standard of advice and operative skill met that which the patient could reasonably have expected. Very often a poor outcome is due to bad luck rather than poor judgement and provided the patient has been warned of the risk, she does not have a case against the surgeon. However, unless the answer to both questions is in the affirmative, the surgeon is liable and in the sphere of cosmetic and reconstructive surgery, the damage is self-evident, i.e. causation is less of an issue than liability. With delay in diagnosis the converse is the case.
- A more senior general surgeon who with the passage of time has become a breast surgeon will often have become competent in the use of implants and tissue expanders. Many breast surgeons in the UK have now attended training courses on the use of the latissimus dorsi flap and their experience with this robust and safe flap has on the whole proved satisfactory. Some breast surgeons have mastered the art of pedicled transverse rectus abdominis muscle reconstruction, but free tissue transfer is beyond the capability and theatre time constraints of most breast surgeons.
- The move towards immediate reconstruction at the time of mastectomy has made it more difficult to offer the patient what may be the most appropriate reconstruction for her and yet not breach time guidelines for commencement of her surgical treatment. This tension is now starting to present as a medicolegal issue and patients who have been offered a more basic form of reconstruction may, once the cancer has been dealt with, feel that the advice they have received fell below that which they could reasonably have expected.
- Reduction mammoplasty (as in this case) and surgery for gynaecomastia, both procedures on normal tissues undertaken mainly for cosmetic reasons, remain high-risk areas for patient dissatisfaction and should never be undertaken on an occasional basis.

THE WOOLF REPORT

In a review of the UK civil justice system, Lord Woolf singled out medical negligence cases as being worthy of special attention.[68] The difficulty of proving both causation and negligence, which arises more particularly in medical negligence than in other personal injury cases, accounts for much of the excessive cost. The root of the problem, however, lies less in the complexity of the law or procedure than in the climate of mutual suspicion and defensiveness. Patients feel let down when treatment goes wrong, sometimes because of unrealistic expectations as to what could be achieved. Doctors feel they are under attack from aggrieved patients and react defensively. The patients' disappointment is then heightened by what they perceive to be a refusal to acknowledge fault and an attempt to cover up.

Lord Woolf identified medical negligence as the area generating most expense, delay and confrontation and the highest proportion of claims which failed. In cases valued at less than £12 500, the median figure for the costs of litigation was 137% of the value of the claim. This financial background has a profound effect on the conduct of litigation. The general rule is that 'costs follow the event': the unsuccessful party is responsible for the costs of both sides. Privately financed claimants are therefore reluctant to pursue actions where the chances of success are equivocal. In the UK, if the claimant is supported by legal aid and loses the case, costs are not recoverable by the defendant. The health authority or defence society cannot recover their own costs, even if successful; if unsuccessful, they will be responsible not only for all their own but for all the claimant's costs as well. It is small wonder there is pressure to settle low-value claims, even if defensible. Perhaps more importantly there is a reluctance to appeal when an important point of principle has been left uncontested.

Over 90% of medical claims that reach litigation in the UK are legally aided because of the high costs of medical litigation. Most often the defendant is the health authority or hospital trust; hence expenses incurred by both the claimant and defendant are funded from the public purse.

It is anticipated that two recent changes in the UK will improve the position of the claimant and reduce the need for litigation. Firstly, the National Patient Safety Agency (NPSA, formerly the NHS Litigation Authority) administers a voluntary scheme that acts as a mutual insurer for those hospital trusts which participate. Secondly, the NHS Ombudsman's jurisdiction has been extended to include complaints against all NHS staff, once the internal complaints system has been exhausted. The latter is a free service that provides an inquisitorial investigation but has no jurisdiction over financial compensation.

The recommendations of the Woolf report are intended to improve the resolution of disputes between patients and doctors, reduce the delay and cost, while treating both parties fairly. These recommendations include the following.

1. Training of health professionals in the rudiments of medical negligence law.
2. The General Medical Council should consider whether a rule of professional conduct is needed to clarify the responsibility of health-care professionals to their patients when they discover an act or omission in which they may have been negligent.
3. The NHS should improve methods of tracing former hospital staff.
4. A pre-litigation protocol for medical negligence cases. Claimants should notify defendants with a written intention to sue 3 months before action. If liability is disputed, defendants should provide a reasoned answer.
5. Alternatives to litigation, such as the Health Service Ombudsman, should be proffered to patients by solicitors.
6. The special lists on the Queen's Bench should include a medical negligence list of judges familiar with medical negligence cases.
7. Training of trial judges in medical issues.
8. Standard tables to quantify medical negligence claims.
9. Courts should facilitate a pilot study of the various 'fast-track' options for dealing with claims under £10 000, so that these claims can be litigated on a modest budget.

The new Civil Procedure Rules 1998 have introduced a fundamental change to medical negligence litigation in England and Wales. There are now tight timetables in order to reduce delays to a minimum and medical experts will be required to address their report to the court and not to the party from whom the expert has received instructions (part 35).[69] 'The expert witness has a duty ... to provide objective unbiased opinion to the court on matters within his expertise, never assuming the role of an advocate.'

RISK MANAGEMENT

Failure of communication and poor physician–patient relationships often prompt patients into taking legal action. A woman who feels that her complaints have been taken seriously and investigated thoroughly is less likely to sue her clinician. In cases where the patient–doctor relationship breaks down, referral to another specialist may be the best course of action.

Extensive risk management strategies have been proposed for radiologists[70] and clinicians[2,71] in an attempt to improve the quality of patient care and to reduce the likelihood of defending costly legal cases. The recommendations of the PIAA study[2] cover the most common problems and are listed below. Many of these recommendations will best be realised by the establishment of a multidisciplinary approach to the care of breast patients, now considered central to good practice. Other recommendations, such as the physical examination by radiologists of all women attending screening mammography, would require considerable additional resources.

Risk management recommendations of the PIAA

Practitioners involved in the diagnosis of breast cancer should undertake the following actions. (Square brackets indicate our interpolations.)

ALL PRACTITIONERS

- Document all patient complaints relative to the breast, including a gynaecological history (menarche, age of first pregnancy, termination of pregnancy, breast-feeding, menopause/hysterectomy, oral contraceptive use, HRT) and previous mantle irradiation for lymphoma.
- Document any family history of breast cancer, including age of the first-degree relative at diagnosis, bilaterality and associated cancers (e.g. ovarian with *BRCA1* families).
- Document the results of previous mammographic studies.
- Document the recommendations for subsequent diagnostic studies and follow-up.
- Follow up with other consultants the results of investigations.
- Obtain a tissue or cytological diagnosis in those with a palpable mass with a negative mammogram.
- Use appropriate diagnostic tests even in the case of pregnancy.

PRIMARY CARE PHYSICIANS INCLUDING OBSTETRICIANS AND GYNAECOLOGISTS

- Do not abandon diagnostic pursuit because the clinical findings are unimpressive.
- Perform a thorough breast examination on every female patient as part of the physical examination regardless of age or complaint. [This recommendation must be contentious.]

- If a mass is detected, further studies must be undertaken to rule out malignancy.
- Ensure that the patient understands the need for further studies and document the fact.
- Perform regular follow-up examinations on patients who present with breast complaints. [This recommendation must be contentious.]

RADIOLOGISTS

- Repeat the study if a mammogram results in a film of poor technical quality.
- Recommend a repeat study, additional views, follow-up studies or other imaging modalities (e.g. ultrasound) as appropriate if the mammogram results are equivocal.
- Ensure an adequate physical examination was performed and documented. [This would cause difficulty for screened patients.]
- Compare the results of the present study with previous studies.
- Promptly report findings to the referring physician; if the patient was self-referred, the result should be sent directly to her. If there is any suspicion of an abnormality, the patient should be advised and told to consult her physician or surgeon promptly.
- If performing a screening mammogram on a self-referred patient, ensure a thorough breast examination is caried out or advise the patient of the importance of a physical examination to complement the mammographic study. In cases where the patient is self-referred, ensure that she receives proper follow-up visits. Double reading (two radiologists) increases the sensitivity of screening mammography.

SURGEONS

- Always perform an adequate examination and document findings, especially when the referring physician's findings were unimpressive.
- When performing a localisation biopsy, ensure the correct lesion was removed, in both open and needle procedures. Radiography of the biopsy specimen should always be done.
- Promptly report consultation and biopsy results to the referring physician.

REFERENCES

1. Physician Insurers Association of America. Breast cancer study. Rockville, MD: PIAA, 1990.

2. Physician Insurers Association of America. Breast cancer study. Rockville, MD: PIAA, 1995; pp. 1–27.

3. Branthwaite M. Law for doctors: principles and practicalities. London: Royal Society of Medicine Press, 2000.

4. Judge v. Huntington Health Authority (1995) 6 Med LR 223.

5. Bolam v. Friern Hospital Management Committee [1957] 2 All ER 118; [1957] 1 WLR 582.

6. Bolitho v. City & Hackney Health Authority [1997] 4 All ER 771; [1997] 3 WLR 1151.

7. Hurwitz B. Clinical guidelines and the law. Br Med J 1995; 311:1517–18.

8. Carrick SE, Bonevski B, Redman S et al. Surgeons' opinions about the NMRC clinical practice guidelines for the management of early breast cancer. Med J Aust 1998; 169:300–5.

9. Sidaway v. Bethlem R. Hospitals [1985] AC 871.

10. Brahams D. Loss of chance of survival. Lancet 1996; 348:1604.

11. Andrews BT, Bates T. Delay in the diagnosis of breast cancer: medico-legal implications. Breast 2000; 9:223–7.

12. Salih A, Webb MW, Bates T. Does open-access mammography and ultrasound delay the diagnosis of breast cancer? Breast 1999; 8:129–32.

13. Davidson T. Delay in diagnosing breast cancer: medicolegal implications. Trends Urol Gynaecol Sexual Health 1998; 3:11–12.

14. Austoker J, Mansel R, Baum M et al. Guidelines for referral of patients with breast problems. Sheffield: NHS Breast Screening Programme, 1995.

15. Dr Foster Guide to Hospitals and Consultants. Available at http://hospital.drfoster.co.uk

16. Lannin DR, Harris RP, Swanson FH et al. Difficulties in diagnosis of carcinoma of the breast in patients less than fifty years of age. Surg Gynecol Obstet 1993; 177:457–62.

17. Zylstra S, Bors-Koefoed R, Mondor M et al. A statistical model for predicting the outcome in breast cancer malpractice lawsuits. Obstet Gynecol 1994; 84:392–8.

18. Yelland A, Graham MD, Trott PA et al. Diagnosing breast carcinoma in young women. Br Med J 1991; 302:618–20.

19. Donegan WL. Evaluation of a palpable breast mass. N Engl J Med 1992; 327:937–42.

20. Woodman CBJ, Threlfall AG, Boggis CRM, Prior P. Is the three year breast screening interval too long? Occurrence of interval cancers in NHS Breast Screening Programme's north western region. Br Med J 1995; 310:224–6.

21. Wolfe JN. Analysis of 462 breast carcinomas. Am J Radiol 1974; 121:846–53.

22. Dixon JM, Anderson TJ, Lamb J et al. Fine needle aspiration cytology, in relationship to clinical examination and mammography in the diagnosis of a solid breast mass. Br J Surg 1984; 71:593–96.

23. Mitnick JS, Vazquez MF, Plesser KP et al. Breast cancer malpractice litigation in New York State. Radiology 1993; 189:673–6.

24. Joensuu H, Asola R, Holli K et al. Delayed diagnosis and large size of breast cancer after a false negative mammogram. Eur J Cancer 1994; 30A:1299–302.

25. Tennvall J, Moller T, Attwell R. Delaying factors in primary treatment of breast cancer. Acta Chir Scand 1990; 156:591–6.

26. Walker QJ, Langlands AO. The misuse of mammography in the management of breast cancer. Med J Aust 1986; 145:185–7.

27. Walter SD, Day NE. Estimation of the duration of a pre-clinical disease state using screening data. Am J Epidemiol 1983; 118:865–6.

28. Dubin N. Benefits of screening for breast cancer: application of a probabilistic model to a breast cancer detection project. J Chron Dis 1979; 32:145–51.

29. Fox H, Moskowitz M, Saenger L et al Benefit/risk analysis of aggressive mammographic screening. Radiology 1978; 128:359–65.

30. Daly CA, Apthorp L, Field S. Second round cancers: how many were visible on the first round of the UK National Breast Screening Programme, three years earlier? Clin Radiol 1998; 53:25–8.

31. Wright CJ, Mueller CB. Screening mammography and public health policy: the need for perspective. Lancet 1995; 346:29–32.

32. Ashley S, Royle GT, Corder A et al. Clinical, radiological and cytological diagnosis of breast cancer in young women. Br J Surg 1989; 76:835–7.

33. Layfield LJ, Glasgow BJ, Cramer H. Fine needle aspiration in the management of breast masses. Pathol Annu 1989; 24:23–62.

34. Bates AT, Bates T, Hastrich DJ et al. Delay in the diagnosis of breast cancer: the effect of the introduction of fine needle aspiration cytology to a breast clinic. Eur J Surg Oncol 1992; 18:433–7.

35. Jenner DC, Middleton A, Webb WM et al. In-hospital delay in the diagnosis of breast cancer. Br J Surg 2000; 87:914–19.

36. Dixon JM, Page DL, Anderson TJ et al. Long-term survivors after breast cancer. Br J Surg 1985; 72:445–8.

37. Haybittle JL. Is breast cancer ever cured ? Rev Endocr Relat Cancer 1983; 13:13–18.

38. Le MG, Hill C, Rezvani A et al. Long-term survival of women with breast cancer. Lancet 1984; ii:922.

39. Rutqvist LR, Wallgren A. Long-term survival of 458 young breast cancer patients. Cancer 1985; 55:658–65.

40. Ederer F, Cutler SJ, Goldenberg IS et al. Causes of death among long-term survivors from breast cancer in Connecticut. J Natl Cancer Inst 1963; 30:933–47.

41. Mueller CB, Ames F, Anderson GD. Breast cancer in 3,558 women: age as a significant determinant in the rate of dying and causes of death. Surgery 1978; 83:123–32.

42. Spratt JS, Spratt SW. Medical and legal implications of screening and follow-up procedures for breast cancer. Cancer 1990; 66:1351–62.

43. Plotkin D, Blankenberg F. Breast cancer: biology and malpractice. Am J Clin Oncol 1991; 14:254–66.

44. Tubiana M, Koscielny S. Cell kinetics, growth rate and the natural history of breast cancer. The Heuson Memorial Lecture. Eur J Clin Oncol 1988; 24:9–14.

45. Pearlman AW. Breast cancer: influence of growth rate on prognosis and treatment evaluation. A study based on mastectomy scar recurrences. Cancer 1976; 38:1826–33.

46. Galante E, Gallus G, Guzzon A et al. Growth rate of primary breast cancer and prognosis: observations on a 3- to 7-year follow up in 180 breast cancers. Br J Cancer 1986; 54:833–6.

47. Forrest APM, Everington D, McDonald CC et al. The Edinburgh randomised trial of axillary sampling or clearance after mastectomy. Br J Surg 1995; 82:1504–8.

48. National Coordination Group for Surgeons Working in Breast Cancer Screening. Quality assurance guidelines for surgeons in breast cancer screening. Sheffield: NHS Breast Screening Programme publication no. 20, 1996.

49. NHS Breast Screening Programme and British Association of Surgical Oncology. An audit of screen detected breast cancers for the year of screening April 1997 to March 1998. Sheffield: NHS Breast Screening Programme, 1999.

50. Breast Surgeons Group of the British Association of Surgical Oncology. Guidelines for surgeons in the management of symptomatic breast disease in the United Kingdom. Eur J Surg Oncol 1995; 21(suppl. A):1–13.

51. Christie R, Bates T. The risk of pneumothorax as a complication of diagnostic fine needle aspiration or therapeutic needling of the breast: should the patient be warned? Breast 1999; 8:98–9.

52. Gately CA, Maddox PR, Mansel RE. Pneumothorax: a complication of fine needle aspiration of the breast. Br Med J 1991; 303:627–8.

53. Bates T, Davidson T, Mansel R. Litigation for pneumothorax as a complication of fine-needle aspiration of the breast. Br J Surg 2002; 89:134–7.

54. Breast Surgeons Group of the British Association of Surgical Oncology. Guidelines for surgeons in the management of symptomatic breast disease in the United Kingdom (1998 revision). Eur J Surg Oncol 1998; 24:464–76.

55. Richards MA, Westcombe AM, Love SB et al. Influence of delay on survival in patients with breast cancer: a systematic review. Lancet 1999; 353:1119–26.

56. Dische S, Bentzen G, Bond S. The influence of delay in diagnosis of breast cancer upon outlook. Clin Risk 2000; 6:4–6.

57. Sainsbury R, Johnston C, Haward B. Effect on survival of delays in referral of patients with breast-cancer symptoms: a retrospective analysis. Lancet 1999; 353:1132–5.

58. Afzelius P, Zedeler K, Sommer H et al. Patients' and doctors' delay in primary breast cancer. Acta Oncol 1994; 33:345–51.

59. Galea MH, Blamey RW, Elston CW et al. The Nottingham Prognostic Index in primary breast cancer. Br Cancer Res Treat 1992; 22:207–19.

60. Thompson AM, Pinder SE. Prognostic factors. In: Dixon JM (ed.) The ABC of breast diseases, 3rd edn. Oxford: Blackwell Publishing, 2006; pp. 77–80.

61. Taylor v. West Kent Health Authority (1997) 8 Med LR 251–7.

62. Price JM, Rosenberg ES. The silicone gel breast implant controversy: the rise of expert panels and the fall of junk science. J R Soc Med 2000; 93:31–4.

63. Renwick SB. Silicon breast implants: implications for society and surgeons. Med J Aust 1996; 165:338–41.

64. Duffy MJ, Woods JE. Health risks of failed silicone gel breast implants: a 30 year clinical experience. Plast Reconstr Surg 1994; 94:295–9.

65. Angell M. Science on trial: the clash of medical evidence and the law in the breast implant case. New York: WW Norton, 1996.

66. Medical Devices Agency. Silicone implants and connective tissue disease. London: Department of Health, 1995.

67. Silicone gel implants: the report of the Independent Review Group. London: Independent Review Group, 1998.

68. Woolf HK. Medical negligence. In: Access to justice: final report to the Lord Chancellor on the

civil justice system in England and Wales. London: HMSO, 1996; pp. 169–96.

69. Civil Procedure Rules. 1998.

70. Brenner RJ. Medico-legal aspects of breast imaging: variable standards of care relating to different types of practice. Am J Roentgenol 1991; 156:719–23.

71. Osuch JR, Bonham VL. The timely diagnosis of breast cancer: principles of risk management for primary care providers and surgeons. Cancer 1994; 74:271–8.

Index